Contents

Introduction

Welcome to the study of human disease. Your textbook, *An Introduction to Human Disease*, was based on courses given to undergraduate and graduate students like you who have mastered the essential concepts of human disease. Many have gone on to careers in biology, medicine, nursing, and other health fields. Each chapter in your book begins with learning manifestations, and principles of treatment of the important diseases considered in each chapter. Each chapter then finishes with an annotated bibliography that points you toward important articles in the medical literature related to the subjects considered in the chapter.

This workbook will help you navigate through the course. It includes diagrams, Power-Point presentations, and various types of exercises to test and reinforce your comprehension of the essential features of the diseases you will be studying. To get you started on your journey of discovery, the workbook begins with a listing of the important points considered in the first five chapters of your book. You will build on these concepts as you continue into other chapters dealing with specific organ system derangements.

I believe that you will be pleasantly surprised to find that the basic concepts relating to human disease are quite straightforward, easy to understand, and extremely interesting. You have undoubtedly completed a course in anatomy and physiology, and you already know that every organ system has key structural features and physiologic functions. All is well when the systems function properly. When you know normal structure and function, it is not hard to understand what happens when systems don't function properly, producing disease. Moreover, when you understand the anatomic and physiologic changes associated with a disease, you can usually deduce the clinical manifestations of the disease and can understand how treatment favorably influences its course and outcome.

The benefit you derive from the course will depend to a large extent on your own efforts. The course follows the class schedule closely. To get the most from the class, read over the material to be covered before you attend the lecture or classroom exercise so that you are familiar with what is to be covered. Then you will be in a better position to get more out of the lectures and other classroom activities dealing with the subjects considered in the assigned chapters. After the class, reread the materials covered in class while the material is still fresh in your mind, and use the workbook material to help you. This approach will help you "nail down" your comprehension of the material. Such a systematic approach to learning the material will pay big dividends, and you will derive tremendous satisfaction from watching your knowledge base relating to human disease grow by "leaps and bounds" as you proceed through the course.

Enjoy your adventure. Have a pleasant journey.

Leonard Crowley

EIGHTH EDITION

An Introduction to
HUMAN DISEASE

PATHOLOGY AND PATHOPHYSIOLOGY CORRELATIONS

STUDENT WORKBOOK

LEONARD V. CROWLEY
Biology Department
Century College
University of Minnesota Medical Center, Fairview
Minneapolis, Minnesota

JONES AND BARTLETT PUBLISHERS

Sudbury, Massachusetts

BOSTON   TORONTO   LONDON   SINGAPORE

World Headquarters
Jones and Bartlett Publishers
40 Tall Pine Drive
Sudbury, MA 01776
978-443-5000
info@jbpub.com
www.jbpub.com

Jones and Bartlett Publishers
 Canada
6339 Ormindale Way
Mississauga, Ontario L5V 1J2
Canada

Jones and Bartlett Publishers
 International
Barb House, Barb Mews
London W6 7PA
United Kingdom

Jones and Bartlett's books and products are available through most bookstores and online booksellers. To contact Jones and Bartlett Publishers directly, call 800-832-0034, fax 978-443-8000, or visit our website, www.jbpub.com.

Substantial discounts on bulk quantities of Jones and Bartlett's publications are available to corporations, professional associations, and other qualified organizations. For details and specific discount information, contact the special sales department at Jones and Bartlett via the above contact information or send an email to specialsales@jbpub.com.

The author, editor, and publisher have made every effort to provide accurate information. However, they are not responsible for errors, omissions, or for any outcomes related to the use of the contents of this book and take no responsibility for the use of the products and procedures described. Treatments and side effects described in this book may not be applicable to all people; likewise, some people may require a dose or experience a side effect that is not described herein. Drugs and medical devices are discussed that may have limited availability controlled by the Food and Drug Administration (FDA) for use only in a research study or clinical trial. Research, clinical practice, and government regulations often change the accepted standard in this field. When consideration is being given to use of any drug in the clinical setting, the health care provider or reader is responsible for determining FDA status of the drug, reading the package insert, and reviewing prescribing information for the most up-to-date recommendations on dose, precautions, and contraindications, and determining the appropriate usage for the product. This is especially important in the case of drugs that are new or seldom used.

Production Credits
Publisher: Cathleen Sether
Acquisitions Editor: Shoshanna Goldberg
Senior Associate Editor: Amy L. Bloom
Production Director: Amy Rose
Senior Production Editor: Renée Sekerak
Associate Marketing Manager: Jody Sullivan
V.P., Manufacturing and Inventory Control: Therese Connell
Cover Design: Kristin E. Parker
Cover and Title Page Image: Courtesy of Leonard V. Crowley
Composition: Auburn Associates, Inc.
Printing and Binding: Courier Stoughton
Cover Printing: Courier Stoughton

ISBN: 978-0-7637-7467-7
6048

Printed in the United States of America
13 12 11 10   10 9 8 7 6 5 4 3 2

How This Book Can Help You Learn

All of us have different learning styles. Some of us are visual learners, some more auditory, some learn better by doing an activity. Some students prefer to learn new material using visual aids. Some learn material better when they hear it in a lecture; others learn it better by reading it. Cognitive research has shown that no matter what your learning style, you will learn more if you are actively engaged in the learning process.

This Student Workbook will help you learn by providing a structure to your notes and letting you utilize all of the learning styles mentioned above. Students don't need to copy down every word their professor says or recopy their entire textbook. Do the assigned reading, listen in lecture, follow the key points your instructor is making, and write down meaningful notes. After reading and lectures, review your notes and pull out the most important points.

This Student Workbook is your partner and guide in note-taking. Your Workbook provides you with a visual guide that follows the chapter topics presented in your textbook. If your instructor is using the PowerPoint slides that accompany the text, this guide will save you from having to write down everything that is on the slides. There is space provided for you to jot down the terms and concepts that you feel are most important to each lecture. By working with your Workbook, you are seeing, hearing, writing, and later, reading and reviewing. The more often you are exposed to the material, the better you will learn and understand it. Using different methods of exposure significantly increases your comprehension.

Your Workbook is the perfect place to write down questions that you want to ask your professor later, interesting ideas that you want to discuss with your study group, or reminders to yourself to go back and study a certain concept again to make sure that you really got it.

Having organized notes is essential at exam time and when doing homework assignments. Your ability to easily locate the important concepts of a recent lecture will help you move along more rapidly, as you don't have to spend time rereading an entire chapter just to reinforce one point that you may not have quite understood.

Your Student Workbook is a valuable resource. You've found a wonderful study partner!

Note-Taking Tips

1. It is easier to take notes if you are not hearing the information for the first time. Read the chapter or the material that is about to be discussed before class. This will help you to anticipate what will be said in class, and have an idea of what to write down. It will also help to read over your notes from the last class. This way you can avoid having to spend the first few minutes of class trying to remember where you left off last time.

2. Don't waste your time trying to write down everything that your professor says. Instead, listen closely and only write down the important points. Review these important points after class to help remind you of related points that were made during the lecture.

3. If the class discussion takes a spontaneous turn, pay attention and participate in the discussion. Only take notes on the conclusions that are relevant to the lecture.

4. Emphasize main points in your notes. You may want to use a highlighter, special notation (asterisks, exclamation points), format (circle, underline), or placement on the page (indented, bulleted). You will find that when you try to recall these points, you will be able to actually picture them on the page.

5. Be sure to copy down word-for-word specific formulas, laws, and theories.

6. Hearing something repeated, stressed, or summed up can be a signal that it is an important concept to understand.

7. Organize handouts, study guides, and exams in your notebook along with your lecture notes. It may be helpful to use a three-ring binder, so that you can insert pages wherever you need to.

8. When taking notes, you might find it helpful to leave a wide margin on all four sides of the page. Doing this allows you to note names, dates, definitions, etc., for easy access and studying later. It may also be helpful to make notes of questions you want to ask your professor about or research later, ideas or relationships that you want to explore more on your own, or concepts that you don't fully understand.

9. It is best to maintain a separate notebook for each class. Labeling and dating your notes can be helpful when you need to look up information from previous lectures.

10. Make your notes legible, and take notes directly in your notebook. Chances are you won't recopy them no matter how noble your intentions. Spend the time you would have spent recopying the notes studying them instead, drawing conclusions and making connections that you didn't have time for in class.

11. Look over your notes after class while the lecture is still fresh in your mind. Fix illegible items and clarify anything you don't understand. Do this again right before the next class.

Chapter Outline

The chapter outline provides you with an organizational guide to the topics and ideas presented in this chapter of the text.

Introductory Concepts in Chapter 1

The following material is provided as a guide to some of the fundamental concepts in the first five chapters. It may help you organize the material as you get started in this course. You will build on these concepts as you begin to study diseases involving various organ systems.

1. Disease is a disturbance of the structure or function of the body.
2. Disease produces various manifestations: signs, symptoms, and abnormal laboratory test results.
3. The clinician's task is to determine the nature of the disease (make a diagnosis), estimate the probable outcome of the disease (prognosis), and then treat the patient (symptomatic and specific treatment).
4. Look over the various diagnostic procedures available to the physician, but learning the details of them is not necessary now.
5. We talk about screening for disease in a population. Screening requires three things: a "screenable population" (significant frequency of disease); a reliable, cost-effective test to identify the disease that can be performed without risk to the patient; and evidence that early detection of the disease will favorably influence outcome.

Study Questions

The following questions are provided as a test for comprehension and as a study guide for use with the text chapters. Additional study material is located at http://health.jbpub.com/humandisease/8e, which contains useful tools such as an A&P review, animated flashcards, an interactive online glossary, crossword puzzles, and web links.

Key Terms

Define the following terms:

1. Etiology _____

2. Symptom of disease _____

3. Sign of disease _____

4. Diagnosis _____

5. Prognosis _____

6. Specific treatment _____

7. Symptomatic treatment _____

8. Pathogen _____

9. Pathogenesis _____

Fill-in-the-Blank

1. A test based on echoes produced in tissues by high-frequency sound waves is _____.

2. A young woman has a skin rash caused by an allergic reaction to an antibiotic. This patient's condition would be classified as _____.

3. The opinion of a physician concerning the eventual outcome of a disease in a patient is called _____.

4. A disease in which the principal manifestation is an abnormal growth of cells leading to formation of tumors is called _____.

Identify

1. Identify the five major categories of diseases, and indicate the characteristic features of each type.

   a. _____

   b. _____

   c. _____

   d. _____

   e. _____

2. Identify the nine major categories of diagnostic tests and procedures available to help the physician or other health practitioner diagnose and treat a patient properly.

   a. _____

   b. _____

   c. _____

   d. _____

e. _____

f. _____

g. _____

h. _____

i. _____

3. Identify three tests that measure the electrical impulses associated with various body functions and activities.

a. _____

b. _____

c. _____

4. Identify the tests or procedures that would be useful to assist the physician in evaluating the following conditions in a patient.

a. Urinary tract infection _____

b. Fractured wrist _____

c. Possible "heart attack" _____

d. A lump in the breast _____

e. Amenorrhea in a young woman _____

f. The maturity of a fetus and the location of the placenta within the mother's uterus _____

_____

Discussion Questions

1. Describe the differences between a diagnosis and a prognosis. _____

_____

_____

_____

2. Describe the steps a physician or other health practitioner uses to make a diagnosis of a specific disease or condition in a patient. _____

_____

_____

_____

3. What is the difference between symptomatic treatment and specific treatment? _____

_____

_____

_____

4. You wish to develop a program to screen for a specific disease, such as diabetes. Describe the requirements for a successful screening program. _____

_____

_____

_____

5. A middle-aged man consults his physician because of cough, fever, chest pain, and purulent sputum. What diagnostic measures will assist the physician in determining the cause of the patient's illness? _____

_____

_____

_____

6. A governmental agency proposes a pilot program to screen a population for a disease by means of a blood test. The characteristics of the disease and the screening test are listed here. Which of these characteristics indicate that the proposed screen is likely to be worthwhile, and which indicate that it is likely not to be worthwhile? Explain your answers.

   a. The disease occurs with some frequency (1 per 1000 persons screened).

   _____

   b. The disease progresses slowly in affected persons.

   _____

   c. No specific method of treatment is available at the present time.

   _____

   d. The test can detect the disease in its early stage and is relatively inexpensive (about $42.50).

   _____

   e. The test is quite specific, producing few false-positive or false-negative results.

   _____

Notes

_____
_____
_____
_____
_____
_____
_____
_____
_____
_____
_____
_____
_____
_____
_____
_____
_____
_____
_____
_____
_____
_____
_____
_____
_____
_____
_____
_____
_____
_____
_____
_____
_____
_____
_____
_____
_____
_____

Chapter 1

General Concepts of Disease:
Principles of Diagnosis

Learning Objectives

- Define:
  - Disease
  - Lesions
  - Organic and functional disease
  - Symptomatic and asymptomatic disease
  - Etiology
  - Pathogenesis
- Categories of human disease
- Types of diagnostic tests and procedures

Characteristics of Disease (1 of 3)

- **Disease:** disturbance of body structure or function
- **Lesions:** well-defined, characteristic structural changes in organs and tissues as a result of disease
- Organic disease
  - Associated with <u>structural</u> changes
  - Gross examination
  - Histologic examination
- Functional disease
  - No morphological abnormalities yet body functions are profoundly disturbed

Characteristics of Disease (2 of 3)

- **Pathology**: study of disease
  - Pathologist: physician who specializes in diagnosing and classifying diseases by studying the morphology of cells and tissues
  - Clinician: physician/health care professional that cares for patients
- **Symptoms:** subjective manifestations such as pain or weakness
- **Signs**: physical findings or objective manifestations such as swelling or redness

Characteristics of Disease (3 of 3)

- Symptomatic disease: with symptoms and/or signs
- Asymptomatic disease: no signs or symptoms
  - Distinction between asymptomatic and symptomatic depends on extent
  - Early stages of disease, usually asymptomatic
  - If not treated, progresses to symptomatic
- Etiology: cause of disease
- Etiologic agent: agent responsible for causing disease
- Pathogenesis: process of development of disease
- Pathogen: any microorganism that causes disease

Classifications of Disease (1 of 3)

- Congenital and hereditary diseases
  - Developmental disturbances
  - Causes: genetic abnormalities; abnormalities in chromosome number or distribution; intrauterine injury; interaction of genetic and environmental factors
  - Hemophilia (hereditary), German measles (congenital)

Classifications of Disease (2 of 3)

- Inflammatory diseases: Body reacts to injury through an inflammatory process
  - Bacteria or microbiologic agents: sore throat
  - Allergic reaction: hay fever
  - Autoimmune diseases: SLE, diabetes type 1
  - Unknown etiology
- Degenerative diseases
  - Tissue or organ degeneration as a result of aging or breakdown
  - Arthritis, atherosclerosis

Classifications of Disease (3 of 3)

- Metabolic diseases: Disturbance in metabolic process in body
  - Diabetes, hyper- or hypothyroidism, fluid and electrolyte imbalance
- Neoplastic diseases: Uncontrolled cell growth
  - Benign: lipoma
  - Malignant: Lung cancer
- Basis of classification
  - 1. Similarity of lesions
  - 2. Similarity of pathogenesis
- Diseases with similarities may not necessarily be closely related

Health and Disease

- Good health: more than the absence of disease
- Condition in which body and mind function efficiently and harmoniously as an integrated unit
- Traditional medicine: goal is to cure or ameliorate disease.
- Modern medicine: advances relieve suffering and advance human welfare but do not guarantee good health.

Continuum of Health and Disease

Good Health   Serious Illness

←——————————→

• Everyone is somewhere <u>between the midpoint and good health</u>
• Good health requires active participation, assuming responsibility for one's health
  – Eat properly, exercise, avoid harmful excesses such as overeating, smoking, heavy drinking, or using drugs
  – Use one's mind constructively, express emotions appropriately, nurture a positive mental attitude

Principles of Diagnosis

• Diagnosis: determination of nature and cause of illness
  – Clinical history
  – Physical examination
  – Differential diagnosis
• Prognosis: eventual outcome of disease
• Treatment
  – Specific treatment – directed at underlying cause
  – Symptomatic treatment – alleviates symptoms but does not influence course of disease

Clinical History (1 of 2)

• 1. History of current illness
  – Severity, time of onset, and character of patient's symptoms
• 2. Medical history
  – Details of general health and previous illnesses that may shed light on current problems
• 3. Family history
  – Health of patient's parents and family members; diseases that run in families

Clinical History (2 of 2)

- 4. Social history
  - Patient's occupation, habits, alcohol and tobacco consumption, general health, current problems
- 5. Review of symptoms
  - Symptoms other than disclosed in history of present illness, suggesting other parts of the body affected by disease

Physical Examination

- Physical examination
  - Systematic examination of patient, with emphasis on parts of body affected by illness
  - Abnormalities noted correlated with clinical history
- Differential diagnosis
  - Consideration of various diseases or conditions that may also explain patient's symptoms and signs
  - Diagnostic possibilities narrowed by selected laboratory tests or other diagnostic procedures
  - Opinion of medical consultant may be sought

Screening Tests

- Screening tests for detection of disease
  - Detect early asymptomatic diseases amenable to treatment to prevent or minimize late-stage organ damage
- Screening for some genetic diseases
  - To screen for carriers of some genetic diseases transmitted from parent to child as either dominant or recessive trait
  - Identifying carriers allows affected persons to make decisions on future childbearing or management of current pregnancy
  - Example: recessive gene for sickle cell anemia in 8% of Black population

Requirements for Effective Screening

- A significant number of persons must be at risk for the disease in the group being screened.
- A relatively inexpensive noninvasive test must be available to screen for the disease that does not yield a high number of false-positive or false-negative results
- Early identification and treatment of the disease will favorably influence course of disease.

Diagnostic Tests and Procedures (1 of 13)

- Clinical laboratory tests
  - Purpose: To determine concentration of substances in blood or urine frequently altered by disease
  - Uses:
    - Determine concentration or activity of enzymes in the blood
    - Evaluate function of organs
    - Monitor response of certain cancers to treatment
    - Detect disease-producing organisms in urine, blood, feces
    - Determine response to antibiotics

Diagnostic Tests and Procedures (2 of 13)

- Tests of electrical activity: to measure electrical impulses associated with bodily functions and activities
  - ECG: measures serial changes in electrical activity of the heart in various phases of the cardiac cycle
    - Identify disturbances in heart rate, rhythm, abnormal impulses
    - Recognize heart muscle injury from ECG abnormalities
  - EEG: measures electrical activity of brain; brain waves
  - EMG: measures electrical activity of skeletal muscle during contraction and at rest

Diagnostic Tests and Procedures
(3 of 13)

- Radioisotope (radionuclide) studies: evaluate organ function by determining rate of uptake and excretion of substances labeled with a radioisotope
- Uses:
  - Anemia: radioisotope-labeled vitamin B12
  - Hyperthyroidism: radioactive iodine
  - Pulmonary blood flow: albumin; to detect presence of blood clots
  - Cancer spread: phosphorus; to determine presence of tumor deposits in bone or spine
  - Heart muscle damage: evaluate blood flow

Diagnostic Tests and Procedures
(4 of 13)

- Endoscopy
  - To examine interior of body using rigid or flexible tubular instruments equipped with lens and light source
  - To perform surgery formerly done through large abdominal incisions
    - Bronchoscope: trachea and major bronchi
    - Cystoscope: bladder
    - Laparoscope: abdomen
- Ultrasound
  - Mapping echoes produced by high-frequency sound waves transmitted into body; echoes reflect change in tissue density, producing images

Diagnostic Tests and Procedures
(5 of 13)

- X-ray
  - Principle: use of high-energy radiation waves at lower doses to produce images to help diagnose disease
  - Can penetrate through tissues at varying degrees depending on tissue density
  - Act on a photographic film or plate (roentgenogram) as the rays leave the body
- Radiopaque: appears white on film; high-density tissues such as bone absorb most of the rays
- Radiolucent: appears dark on film; low-density tissues allow rays to pass through

Notes

Notes

_____

_____

_____

_____

_____

_____

_____

_____

_____

_____

_____

_____

_____

_____

_____

_____

_____

_____

_____

_____

_____

_____

_____

_____

_____

_____

_____

_____

_____

_____

_____

_____

_____

Diagnostic Tests and Procedures (6 of 13)

- X-ray can include use of contrast media to outline structures not otherwise visualized on standard films
  - Barium sulfate: intestinal tract
  - Radiopaque oil: bronchogram
  - Intravenous dye: intravenous pyelogram; urinary tract
  - Radiopaque tablets: visualize gallstones
  - Arteriogram: visualize blood flow, identfy narrowing or obstruction
  - Cardiac catherization: blood flow through heart, detect abnormal communications between chambers

Diagnostic Tests and Procedures (7 of 13)

- Computed tomographic (CT) scans
  - Principle: radiation detectors record amount of X-rays or ionizing radiation absorbed by body and feed data into a computer that reconstructs the data into an image
  - Radiopaque and radiolucent tissues appear white and dark as in a conventional x-ray
  - Individual organs sharply demarcated by planes of fat that appear dark because of its low density
  - Delivers higher dose of ionizing radiation than x-ray

Diagnostic Tests and Procedures (8 of 13)

- Uses of computed tomographic (CT) scans
  - Cancer screening asymptomatic individuals
  - Detect abnormalities in internal organs that cannot otherwise be identified by standard x-ray

Diagnostic Tests and Procedures
(9 of 13)

- Magnetic resonance imaging (MRI)
  - Principle: computer-constructed images of body based on response of hydrogen protons in water molecules when placed in a strong magnetic field
    - Protons align in the direction of the magnetic field
    - Protons are temporarily dislodged and wobble when radiofrequency waves are directed at them
    - Protons emit a measurable signal (resonance) that can be used to construct images
    - Intensity of resonance depends on water content of tissues, strength and duration of radiofrequency pulse

Diagnostic Tests and Procedures
(10 of 13)

- MRI: advantages over CT scan
  - Does not use ionizing radiation
  - Can detect abnormalities in tissues surrounded by bone, such as spinal cord, orbit, skull
  - Bone interferes with scanning because of its density but does not produce an image in MRI because of its low water content
- Uses
  - Multiple sclerosis
  - Superior to mammography in detecting breast cancer

Diagnostic Tests and Procedures
(11 of 13)

- Positron emission tomography (PET)
  - Principle: Measures metabolism of biochemical compounds that are labeled with positron-emitting isotopes to measure organ function, example glucose
  - Disadvantages
    - Very expensive and not widely available
    - Requires facilities for incorporating the isotopes into the biochemical compound

Notes

Diagnostic Tests and Procedures (12 of 13)

- Uses of PET
  - Assess biochemical functions in brain
  - Determine metabolic activities of organ or tissue; specific site in an organ where compound is metabolized
  - Evaluate changes in blood flow in heart muscle following a heart attack
  - Distinguish benign from a malignant tumor (increased glucose uptake in malignant versus benign tumors)

Diagnostic Tests and Procedures (13 of 13)

- Cytologic and histologic examinations
  - Papanicolau (Pap) smear: identifies abnormal cells in fluids or secretions; for recognizing early changes that may be associated with cervical and other cancers
  - Biopsy: tissue samples obtained for histologic examination to determine abnormal structural and cellular patterns accompanying disease
    - Liver, kidney, bone marrow

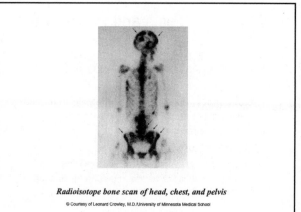

Radioisotope bone scan of head, chest, and pelvis

© Courtesy of Leonard Crowley, M.D./University of Minnesota Medical School

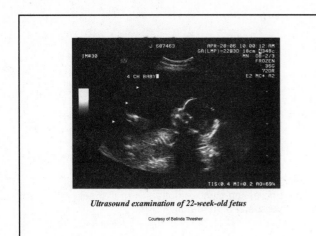

Ultrasound examination of 22-week-old fetus

Courtesy of Belinda Thresher

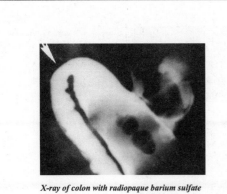

X-ray of colon with radiopaque barium sulfate

© Courtesy of Leonard Crowley, M.D./University of Minnesota Medical School

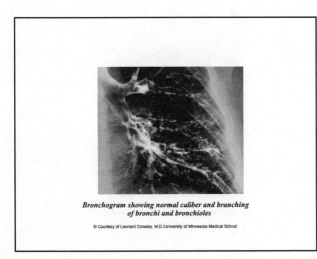

Bronchogram showing normal caliber and branching of bronchi and bronchioles

© Courtesy of Leonard Crowley, M.D./University of Minnesota Medical School

Notes

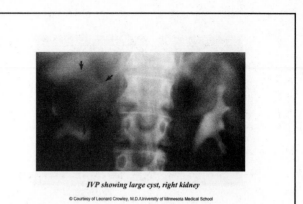

IVP showing large cyst, right kidney

© Courtesy of Leonard Crowley, M.D./University of Minnesota Medical School

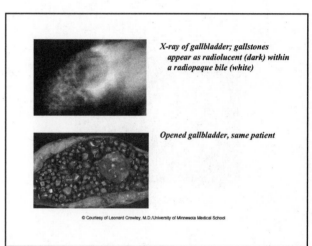

X-ray of gallbladder; gallstones appear as radiolucent (dark) within a radiopaque bile (white)

Opened gallbladder, same patient

© Courtesy of Leonard Crowley, M.D./University of Minnesota Medical School

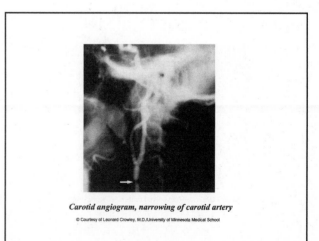

Carotid angiogram, narrowing of carotid artery

© Courtesy of Leonard Crowley, M.D./University of Minnesota Medical School

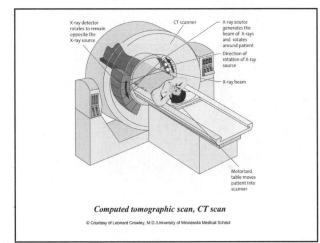

X-ray detector
rotates to remain
opposite the
X-ray source

CT scanner

X-ray source
generates the
beam of X-rays
and rotates
around patient

Direction of
rotation of X-ray
source

X-ray beam

Motorized
table moves
patient into
scanner

Computed tomographic scan, CT scan

© Courtesy of Leonard Crowley, M.D./University of Minnesota Medical School

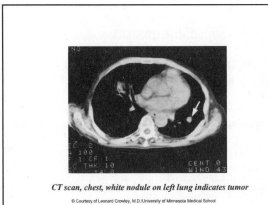

CT scan, chest, white nodule on left lung indicates tumor

© Courtesy of Leonard Crowley, M.D./University of Minnesota Medical School

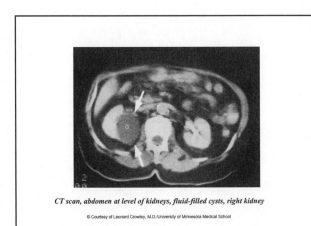

CT scan, abdomen at level of kidneys, fluid-filled cysts, right kidney

© Courtesy of Leonard Crowley, M.D./University of Minnesota Medical School

Notes

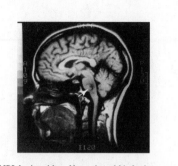

MRI, brain, with malformation within brain stem

© Courtesy of Leonard Crowley, M.D./University of Minnesota Medical School

Discussion

- What are the underlying principles for these diagnostic procedures: x-ray, CT scan, MRI, PET?
- Explain the requirements for an effective screening.
- Differentiate:
  - Symptomatic versus specific treatment
  - Sign versus symptom
  - Symptomatic versus asymptomatic disease
  - Diagnosis versus prognosis

Chapter 2   Cells and Tissues: Their Structure and Function in Health and Disease

Chapter Outline

The chapter outline provides you with an organizational guide to the topics and ideas presented in this chapter of the text.

Introductory Concepts in Chapter 2

The following material is provided as a guide to some of the fundamental concepts in the first five chapters. It may help you organize the material as you get started in this course. You will build on these concepts as you begin to study diseases involving various organ systems.

1. The cell is the basic structural and functional unit of the body. All cells have similar features (nucleus, cytoplasm, organelles), but many cells are specialized to perform specific functions.
2. The nucleus contains the genetic material (23 pairs of chromosomes = the genome) that directs the functions of the cell (via messenger RNA). The cytoplasm contains the various organelles (e.g., mitochondria, ribosomes, endoplasmic reticulum, lysosomes) that carry out the functions specified by DNA (see Fig. 2-8).
3. Groups of similar cells form tissues. Tissues are organized to form organs, and groups of organs form organ systems.

4. Epithelium covers the exterior of the body, lines the interior of organs such as the respiratory and GI tracts, lines body cavities, forms glands, and forms the functional cells of organs that have excretory or secretory functions (such as the liver and kidneys). Epithelium is classified on the basis of its structure (simple or stratified; squamous, transitional, or columnar). Connective tissue connects and supports. Muscle contracts, and nerve tissue conducts.

5. Materials move in and out of cells across cell membranes by active transport, phagocytosis, and pinocytosis (active processes that require the cell to expend energy) and by diffusion and osmosis (passive, non–energy-requiring processes).

6. Cells adapt to changing conditions (atrophy, hypertrophy, hyperplasia, metaplasia, dysplasia, increased enzyme synthesis).

7. Injured cells exhibit structural and functional abnormalities—swelling, fatty change, and necrosis, for example.

8. Normal cells don't last forever. They have a predetermined life span, and they wear out. (As we see later, some tumor cells can proliferate indefinitely. They are "immortal.")

Study Questions

The following questions are provided as a test for comprehension and as a study guide for use with the text chapter. Additional study material is located at http://health.jbpub.com/humandisease/8e, which contains useful tools such as an A&P review, animated flashcards, an interactive online glossary, crossword puzzles, and web links.

Key Terms

Define the following terms:

1. Genetic code _____

2. Organelle _____

3. Hyperplasia _____

4. Dysplasia _____

5. Osmosis _____

6. Diffusion _____

7. Metaplasia _____

True/False

Tell whether each statement is true or false. If false, explain why the statement is incorrect.

1. The nucleus directs the metabolic functions of the cell. _____

_____

2. Organelles are small chromosome fragments present in the nucleus. _____

_____

3. Lysosomes digest material brought into the cell by phagocytosis. _____

_____

4. All cells survive the same length of time within the body. _____

_____

5. Migration of water molecules from a more dilute solution to a more concentrated solution across the semipermeable membrane is called diffusion. _____

_____

Identify

1. Identify eight components within a typical cell, and indicate the function of each.

    a. _____

    b. _____

    c. _____

    d. _____

e. _____

f. _____

g. _____

h. _____

2. Identify the four major types of tissues, and briefly describe the functions of each type.

   a. _____

   b. _____

   c. _____

   d. _____

3. Identify the three germ layers that develop from the fertilized ovum, and indicate what structures develop from each layer. (*Hint:* see Fig. 2-5.)

   a. _____

   b. _____

   c. _____

4. Identify the five ways in which cells adapt to changing conditions.

   a. _____

   b. _____

   c. _____

   d. _____

   e. _____

Discussion Questions

1. Diagram the structure of a typical cell. Indicate the functions of the major organelles.

2. What is the difference between cell hyperplasia and dysplasia? _____

_____

_____

_____

3. How does the cell respond to injury? _____

_____

_____

_____

4. What are the major difference between epithelium and connective tissue? _____

_____

_____

_____

5. Briefly describe the structures and main functions of the various types of epithelium. _____

_____

_____

_____

6. List and describe the various ways that materials move in and out of cells across the cell membrane. _____

_____

_____

_____

7. Describe how osmosis differs from diffusion. _____

_____

_____

_____

8. Describe the difference between cell metaplasia and cell dysplasia. _____

_____

_____

_____

9. Describe some of the important changes that occur in an aging cell, and describe ways by which we can retard aging changes in cells. _____

_____

_____

_____

Chapter 2   Cells and Tissues: Their Structure and Function in Health and Disease

Notes

_____

_____

_____

_____

_____

_____

_____

_____

_____

_____

_____

_____

_____

_____

_____

_____

_____

_____

_____

_____

_____

_____

_____

_____

_____

_____

_____

_____

_____

_____

_____

_____

_____

_____

_____

_____

_____

_____

_____

Chapter 2

Cells and Tissues: Their Structure and Function in Health and Disease

---

Learning Objectives

- Explain
  - Organization of cells
  - Types of tissues
  - Organ systems
  - Germ layers and derivatives
- Describe
  - Cell function and genetic code
  - DNA and enzyme synthesis
- Movement of materials in and out of cells
- Cell adaptation to changing conditions
- Cell injury, cell death, cell necrosis

Organization of Cells

- Cells
- Tissues
- Organs
- Organ systems
- Functioning organism
- An abnormality at any level of organization can cause disease

---

Notes

Basic Structure and Organization of Cells

- Nucleus: contains genetic information; directs metabolic function of cells
- Cytoplasm: surrounds nucleus; structures carry out directions of the nucleus
- Cell: basic structural and functional unit of the body
- Tissues: group of similar cells performing the same functions
- Organs: groups of tissues
- Organ Systems: groups of organs functioning together
- Functioning Organisms: integrated organ systems

The Cell

- Nucleus
- Cytoplasm
  - Mitochondria
  - Endoplasmic reticulum
  - Golgi apparatus
  - Lysosomes
  - Centrioles
  - Cytoskeleton
- Membranes of lipid and protein molecules

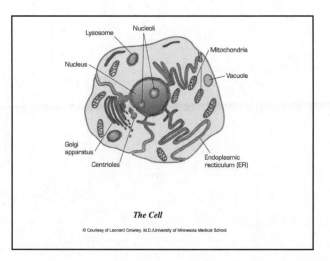

The Cell

© Courtesy of Leonard Crowley, M.D./University of Minnesota Medical School

Nucleus and Cytoplasm

- Nucleus
  - Two types of nucleic acid combined with protein
  - Nuclear membrane: double-layered; with pores; separates nucleus from cytoplasm
    - Deoxyribonucleic acid (DNA): in chromosomes in the nucleus, contains genetic information
    - Ribonucleic acid (RNA): in nucleoli; component of messenger, transfer, ribosomal RNA
- Cytoplasm
  - Mass of protoplasm surrounded by a selectively permeable cell membrane
  - Contains organelles

Organelles (1 of 4)

- Mitochondria
  - Rod-shaped structures capable of converting food material into energy to manufacture ATP (adenosine triphosphate) that fuels chemical reactions in the cell
- Endoplasmic reticulum
  - Interconnected network of tubular channels enclosed by membranes; communicates with nuclear and cellular membranes
  - Rough endoplasmic reticulum (RER): with ribosomes
  - Smooth endoplasmic reticulum (SER): with lipids

Organelles (2 of 4)

- Golgi apparatus
  - Flattened membrane-like sacs near the nucleus
  - For synthesis of large carbohydrate molecules
  - Connected with the tubules of the RER
  - Proteins from ribosomes → RER tubules → Golgi apparatus → combine with carbohydrate molecules→ form secretory granules
- Lysosomes: "digestive system" of cell
  - Cytoplasmic vacuoles with digestive enzymes
  - Digestion occurs within phagocytic vacuole to prevent leakage of enzymes
  - Peroxisome: with enzymes that decompose hydrogen peroxide, H_2O_2

Notes

Notes

Organelles (3 of 4)

- Centrioles
  - Short cylindrical structures adjacent to nucleus
  - Move to opposite poles of the cell during cell division to form the mitotic spindle
- Cytoskeleton
  - Form cell's structural framework, shape, and cell movements (e.g. phagocytosis)
  - Consists of 3 types of protein tubules
    - Microtubules: largest
    - Intermediate filaments
    - Microfilaments: smallest

Organelles (4 of 4)

- Cytoskeleton: intermediate filaments
  - Small, tough protein filaments
  - Reinforce cell's interior and keep its shape by holding the organelles in proper position
  - Identification and characterization of intermediate filaments provide diagnostic and prognostic information
    - Alzheimer disease
    - Cancer diagnosis: helps determine the cell of origin

Tissues

- Group of cells that perform a similar function
- Four types:
  - 1. Epithelium
  - 2. Connective and supporting
    - Fibrous   Cartilage
    - Elastic   Bone
    - Reticular   Hematopoietic
    - Adipose   Lymphatic
  - 3. Muscle
  - 4. Nerve

Epithelium (1 of 2)

- Covers exterior of the body
- Lines interior of body surfaces communicating with the outside: GIT, urinary tract, and vagina
- Forms glands and parenchymal (functional) cells of excretory or secretory organs (liver and kidneys)
- Contains no blood vessels but nourished by diffusion
- Functions
  - All types of epithelium protect
  - Absorb
  - Secrete: mucus, sweat, oil, enzymes, hormones

Epithelium (2 of 2)

- Exocrine glands: discharge secretions through a duct
  - Pancreas: both an exocrine and endocrine gland
- Endocrine glands: discharge secretions directly into the bloodstream
  - Example: thyroid and adrenals
- Endothelium: layer of simple squamous epithelium
- Mesothelium: layer of simple squamous epithelium lining pleural, pericardial, and peritoneal cavities

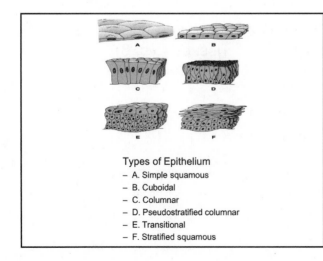

Types of Epithelium
- A. Simple squamous
- B. Cuboidal
- C. Columnar
- D. Pseudostratified columnar
- E. Transitional
- F. Stratified squamous

Notes

Connective and Supportive Tissues (1 of 3)

- Types of connective tissue fibers
  - Collagen fibers
    - Connects and supports tissues
    - Contains collagen; long and flexible, strong but does not stretch
  - Elastic fibers
    - Responsible for distensibility of arteries
    - Contains elastin, not as strong but stretches
  - Reticulin fibers
    - Form supporting framework of organs
    - Similar to collagen but thin and delicate

Connective and Supportive Tissues (2 of 3)

- Examples
  - Hematopoietic (blood-forming)
  - Lymphatic (lymphocyte-forming)
  - Loose and dense fibrous tissues
  - Elastic tissue
  - Reticular tissue
  - Adipose tissue
  - Cartilage: hyaline, elastic, fibrocartilage
  - Bone
  - Subcutaneous tissue

Connective and Supportive Tissues (3 of 3)

- Ligaments
- Tendons
- Blood vessel wall membranes
- Bronchi walls
- Trachea
- Supporting framework of organs
  - Liver, spleen and lymph nodes

Muscle

- Smooth muscle
  - Located in walls of hollow internal organs
    - Gastrointestinal, biliary, and reproductive tracts
    - Blood vessels
  - Functions automatically, not under conscious control
- Striated muscle
  - Moves skeleton
  - Under conscious control
- Cardiac muscle
  - Found only in the heart
  - Resembles striated but with features common to both smooth and striated muscle

Nerve

- Neurons: nerve cells, transmit nerve impulses
- Neuroglia: supporting cells
  - More numerous than neurons
  - Astrocytes: long, star-shaped cells, numerous highly branched process
  - Oligodendroglia: small cells, scanty cytoplasm, surround nerve cells
  - Microglia: phagocytic cells

Organ

- Groups of different tissues integrated to perform a specific function
  - One tissue performs primary function
  - Other tissues perform supporting function
- Parenchymal cells: primary functional cells of an organ
- Parenchyma: functional cells of an organ
- Stroma: tissue that forms the supporting framework of an organ

Notes

Notes

Germ Layers (1 of 2)

- Highly complex structure of entire body evolves from a single cell, fertilized ovum → multiplies, differentiates, and is organized to form organs and organ systems
- Fertilized ovum differentiates into:
  – Trophoblast: peripheral group of cells; form placenta and other structures to support and nourish embryo
- Inner cell mass: inner group of cells; will give rise to the embryo; arranged in three distinct germ layers
  – Ectoderm
  – Mesoderm
  – Entoderm

Germ Layers (2 of 2)

- Ectoderm: outer layer (external covering of body, nervous system, ears, eyes)
- Mesoderm: middle layer (connective tissue, muscle, bone, cartilage, heart, blood, blood vessels, and major portions of urogenital system)
- Entoderm: inner layer (epithelium of pharynx, respiratory tract, liver, biliary tract, pancreas, some parts of urogenital tract)

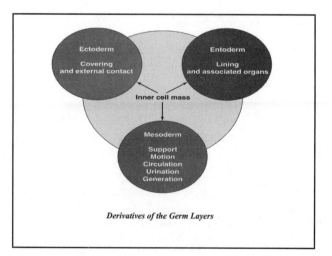

Derivatives of the Germ Layers

Cell Function, DNA, Genetic Code (1 of 3)

- Chromosomes: DNA combined with proteins
- DNA
  - Contains genetic code, transmitted to each newly formed cell in cell division
  - Nucleotide: basic structural unit of DNA; consists of
    - phosphate group
    - linked to a deoxyribose
    - joined to a nitrogen-containing base
  - Replication of DNA: original chain serves as model for synthesis of new chain; forms two double strands, each containing original strand and newly formed strand
  - Genetic code: regulates various functions of cells

Cell Function, DNA, Genetic Code (2 of 3)

- DNA bases
  - Purine base: adenine and guanine
  - Pyrimidine base: thymine and cytosine
- Base pairing
  - Only adenine can pair with thymine
  - Only guanine can pair with cytosine
- DNA molecule consists of two strands of DNA held together by weak chemical attractions between the bases of adjacent chains

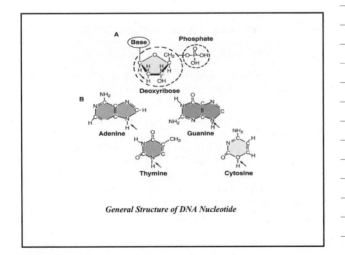

General Structure of DNA Nucleotide

Notes

Cell Function, DNA, Genetic Code (3 of 3)

- Genetic coding
  - DNA in nucleus "tells the cell what to do"
  - Directs synthesis of enzymes and other proteins by the ribosomes in the cytoplasm
  - Messenger RNA (mRNA) carries out the "instructions" encoded in the DNA to the ribosomes in the cytoplasm

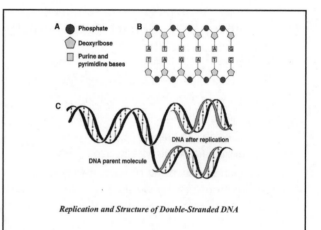

Replication and Structure of Double-Stranded DNA

Movement of Materials In and Out of Cells (1 of 2)

- Oxygen and nutrients must enter the cell and waste products must be eliminated by crossing through a selectively permeable membrane
- Diffusion: solutes move from concentrated → dilute solution
- Osmosis: water molecules move from dilute → concentrated solution
- Active transport: movement from ↓ concentration → ↑ concentration; requires cell to expend energy due to concentration gradient
- Phagocytosis; pinocytosis

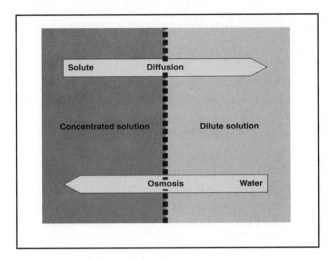

Movement of Materials In and Out of Cells (2 of 2)

- Phagocytosis: ingestion of particles too large to pass across cell membrane
  - Cytoplasm flows around the particle and cytoplasmic processes fuse to engulf particle within a vacuole into the cytoplasm
- Pinocytosis: ingestion of fluid rather than solid material

Adaptation of Cells to Changing Conditions (1 of 3)

- Atrophy: reduction in cell size in response to
  - Diminished function
  - Inadequate hormonal stimulation
  - Reduced blood supply
- Examples
  - Reduction of skeletal muscle size when extremity is immobilized in a cast for a prolonged period
  - Shrinkage of breasts and genitals following menopause due to diminished estrogen secretion

Notes

Adaptation of Cells to Changing Conditions (2 of 3)

- Hypertrophy: increase in cell size without increase in cell number
  - Muscles of a weight lifter
  - Heart of a person with high blood pressure
- Hyperplasia: increase in both cell size and number in response to increased demand
  - Glandular tissue of breasts during pregnancy in preparation for lactation
  - Enlargement of thyroid gland to increase output of hormones

Adaptation of Cells to Changing Conditions (3 of 3)

- Metaplasia: change from one type of cell to another
  - Example: lining of a chronically inflamed bladder
- Dysplasia: cell development and maturation are disturbed and abnormal
  - Individual cells vary in size and shape
  - Example: chronic inflammation of epithelial cells of uterine cervix may progress to cervical epithelial dysplasia and neoplasia
- Increased enzyme synthesis
  - Adaptive response as in inactivating/detoxifying drugs or chemicals through SER enzymes

Cell Injury, Cell Death, Cell Necrosis (1 of 2)

- Normal conditions: potassium actively transported into cell, sodium is moved out
- Changes resulting from cell injury
  - Cell swelling: sodium diffuses into cell together with water molecules
  - Fatty change: accumulation of fat droplets within the cytoplasm due to impairment of enzyme systems that metabolize fat
- Cell necrosis: cell damage + cell death
  - All necrotic cells are dead, but not all dead cells are necrotic.

Cell Injury, Cell Death, Cell Necrosis (2 of 2)

- Apoptosis: programmed cell death
  - All normal cells have a predetermined life span.
  - Number of functional cells determined by the balance between cell growth and cell death
- Cell aging
  - Genetic and environmental factors play a role in cell longevity.
  - Aging of cells may be caused by damage to cellular DNA, RNA, and cytoplasmic organelles.
  - The more efficient the cell's repair process, the greater the likelihood of survival.
  - As cell ages, its enzyme systems gradually decline, and cell is less able to protect self from injury.

Discussion (1 of 2)

- The cervix is normally lined by non-keratinizing squamous epithelium. In cases of chronic irritation, inflammation, or injury, the cells undergo abnormal development and maturation with larger and darker nuclei in a disorderly manner.
  - A. Atrophy
  - B. Hypertrophy
  - C. Hyperplasia
  - D. Metaplasia
  - E. Dysplasia

Discussion (2 of 2)

- All cell death occurs as a result of cell injury.
  - A. TRUE
  - B. FALSE

Chapter 3   Chromosomes, Genes, and Cell Division

Chapter Outline

The chapter outline provides you with an organizational guide to the topics and ideas presented in this chapter of the text.

Introductory Concepts in Chapter 3

The following material is provided as a guide to some of the fundamental concepts in the first five chapters. It may help you organize the material as you get started in this course. You will build on these concepts as you begin to study diseases involving various organ systems.

1. Chromosomes occur in pairs: 22 matched pairs of homologous chromosomes called autosomes (non-sex chromosomes) and one pair of sex chromosomes (XX = females; XY = male). One member of each chromosome pair comes from each parent.
2. Genes occupy specific sites on chromosomes called *gene loci*. There are paired gene loci on the paired chromosomes. At any gene locus, any one of several related genes can occupy the locus. These alternative forms of genes are called *alleles* or *allelic genes*. A person is homozygous for a gene if both gene loci possess the same allelic gene; a person is heterozygous if the alleles are different. See the text for descriptions of dominant, recessive, codominant, and sex-linked genes and their effects.
3. There are two types of cell division: *mitosis,* characteristic of somatic cells, and *meiosis,* which occurs in germ cells. Each cell has already duplicated its DNA before it ever starts to divide.
4. Mitosis is simply a separation of already duplicated chromosomes. Each precursor (parent) cell produces two daughter cells, each one identical to the parent cell.
5. Meiosis is a two-phase process. In the *first division,* some intermixing of genetic material between homologous chromosomes occurs, and then the chromosomes separate without dividing. Each parent cell produces two daughter cells, each having only one member of each homologous pair of chromosomes (these homologous chromosomes are slightly different than those in the parents because of the intermixing of genetic material between homologous chromosomes). The *second division* is just like mitosis, but only 23 chromosomes separate. Each of the daughter cells from the first division, in turn, gives rise to two more daughter cells. The final result is that each precursor cell eventually gives rise to daughter cells in two divisions.

6. See the text for a description of the differences between spermatogenesis and oogenesis. These differences will be important when we consider chromosomal abnormalities such as Down syndrome.
7. The HLA (MHC) system is a system of interconnected (linked) genes located at gene loci on one pair of homologous chromosomes that determine specific proteins (self-antigens) called HLA or MHC proteins on the surface of cells. The HLA genes are transmitted in sets called *haplotypes,* with one set being provided by each parent (see Fig. 3-9). There are multiple possible alleles at each gene locus, and there are so many possible gene combinations that each individual has a unique set of HLA antigens (except identical twins, who possess identical genes). Certain HLA types appear to be associated with increased susceptibility to certain diseases.

Study Questions

The following questions are provided as a test for comprehension and as a study guide for use with the text chapters. Additional study material is located at http://health.jbpub.com/humandisease/8e, which contains useful tools such as an A&P review, animated flashcards, an interactive online glossary, crossword puzzles, and web links.

Key Terms

Define the following terms:

1. Allele _____

2. Dominant gene _____

3. Recessive gene _____

4. Homozygous _____

5. Heterozygous _____

6. Hemizygous _____

7. Human leukocyte antigen (HLA) _____

8. Haplotype _____

9. Gene therapy _____

True/False

Tell whether each statement is true or false. If false, explain why the statement is incorrect.

1. The human genome consists of about 3 billion pairs of DNA bases, and most of the DNA on chromosomes consists of genes that regulate cell structure and functions. _____
   _____

2. The Human Genome Project has identified all of the genes on the human chromosomes and has determined the function of each of these genes. _____
   _____

3. Minor variations in the sequence of the nucleotides within the same genes of different individuals (gene polymorphism) may lead to differences in the way the genes are expressed. _____
   _____

4. A gene inherited from a female parent does not always have the same effect as the identical gene inherited from the male parent. _____
   _____

5. Chromosomes normally exist in pairs called homologous chromosomes. _____
   _____

6. Certain HLA types appear to predispose a person to specific diseases. _____
   _____

7. Genes exist in pairs, and the members of each pair are located at corresponding sites (gene loci) on homologous chromosomes. _____

8. An individual is heterozygous for a gene if the genes at the corresponding loci on homologous chromosomes are the same and homozygous for the gene if the genes are different. _____

9. A dominant gene expresses itself in either the homozygous or heterozygous state. _____

10. An X-linked gene is one that occurs in *only* the female. _____

11. A defective X-linked gene may not cause clinical manifestations in the female, but may be associated with major clinical manifestations in the male. _____

12. Tell whether each of the following statements regarding identification of inherited disease in newborn infants by screening tests is true or false. If false, explain why the statement is incorrect.

    a. Screening is unlikely to be useful because most inherited diseases do not respond to treatment. _____

    b. Long-term harmful effects of inherited diseases can often be prevented by early treatment. _____

    c. Identification of a hereditary disease in a newborn may allow parents to make an informed decision regarding future pregnancies, based on the nature of the inherited disease and its prognosis. _____

Discussion Questions

1. Describe the major differences between mitosis and meiosis. _____

2. Describe how spermatogenesis differs from oogenesis. _____

3. What is the Human Genome Project? _____

_____

_____

_____

4. Describe the Lyon hypothesis relating to X chromosome inactivation. _____

_____

_____

_____

5. What is a karyotype? How is it determined? _____

_____

_____

_____

6. Describe what goals must be achieved for gene therapy to be successful. _____

_____

_____

_____

Notes

Chapter 3

Chromosomes, Genes, and Cell Division

Learning Objectives

- Chromosomes analysis and karyotype
- Mitosis versus meiosis
- Spermatogenesis versus oogenesis: implications of abnormal chromosome separations in older women
- Inheritance pattern of genes: dominant, recessive, codominant, sex-linked
- HLA system: application to organ transplantation, disease susceptibility
- Gene therapy: applications and limitations

Genes

- Segments of DNA chains that determine cell properties (structure and functions)
- Basic units of inheritance
- Exist in pairs or alleles one in each chromosome; occupy a specific site on a chromosome (locus)
- Paired in same way as chromosomes except in sperm and ova
- Homozygous: both alleles are the same
- Heterozygous: alleles are different

Genes and Inheritance

- Expression of genes
  - 1. Dominant gene: expressed in either homozygous or heterozygous state
  - 2. Recessive gene: expressed only in homozygous state
  - 3. Codominant gene: both alleles of a pair are expressed
  - 4. Sex-linked gene: genes carried on sex chromosomes producing sex-linked traits
- Female carrier of recessive X-linked trait is normal, effect of defective allele offset by normal allele on other X chromosome
- Male carrier of recessive X-linked trait, defective X chromosome functions like a dominant gene

Genome (1 of 2)

- Sum total of all genes in a cell's chromosomes
- Human Genome Project: international collaboration of scientists that mapped nucleotide sequence of the entire human genome by determining the specific locations of individual genes
- Genomics: study of gene structure to correlate gene structure with gene expression in individual

Genome (2 of 2)

- Gene product: enzyme or protein coded by a gene
- Exons: parts of chromosomal DNA chain that code for a specific protein or enzyme
- Introns: noncoding parts of chromosomal DNA in between exons

Single Nucleotide Polymorphisms, SNPS

- Structural variations in single gene nucleotides of different individuals
- Affect gene functions resulting in individual differences in body functions:
  - How rapidly cell inactivates drug or environmental toxin or repairs DNA damage
  - Variations in responses to food, antibiotics, or drugs
  - Ability to detoxify potential carcinogens or susceptibility to cancers
- Gene profile: determination of genetic susceptibility to chronic diseases and cancer

Chromosomes (1 of 2)

- Double coils of DNA combined with protein
- Present in the nucleus and control cell activities
- Exist in pairs, one derived from the male parent and one from the female parent
- Autosomes: 22 pairs in humans; similar in size, shape, appearance

Chromosomes (2 of 2)

- Sex chromosomes: one pair in humans
  - Determine genetic sex by composition of X and Y chromosomes
  - Normal female: XX; one X inactivated and appears attached to nuclear membrane
  - Normal male: XY chromosomes; Y chromosome appears as bright fluorescent spot in intact cell

Chromosome Analysis (1 of 2)

- Study composition and abnormalities in chromosomes in terms of number and structure
- Methods
  - Use human blood as source of cells and then cultured
  - Lymphocytes induced to undergo mitotic division

Chromosome Analysis (2 of 2)

- Division of cells stopped in metaphase and cells caused to swell. Cell has 46 chromosomes. Each chromosome consists of 2 chromatids joined at centromere
- Prepare stained smears of chromosomes
- Chromosomes arranged in standard pattern (karyotype)

X Chromosome Inactivation: Lyon Hypothesis

- X-inactivation or lyonization: only one of the two X chromosomes in females is genetically active; one is inactivated around 16th day of embryonic development; theorized by Mary Frances Lyon
- Barr body or sex chromatin body: inactive X chromosome
- X-inactivation occurs so female with two X chromosomes does not have twice as many X chromosome gene products as the male
- Choice of which X chromosome will be inactivated is random; once inactivated, remains inactive throughout the lifetime of the cell

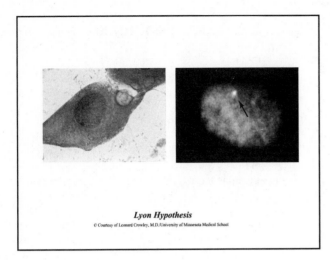

Lyon Hypothesis
© Courtesy of Leonard Crowley, M.D./University of Minnesota Medical School

Mitosis (1 of 2)

- Characteristic of somatic cells
- Each somatic cell contains 46 chromosomes
  - Not all mature cells able to divide (cardiac, skeletal muscle, nerve cells)
  - Connective tissue and liver cells divide as much as needed
  - Cells lining testicular tubules that produce sperm cells divide continually
  - Blood-forming cells in bone marrow divide continually to replace circulating cells in bloodstream

Mitosis (2 of 2)

- No reduction in chromosomes
- Each of two new daughter cells receives same number of chromosomes as in the parent cell
  - Each chromosome and its newly duplicated counterpart lie side by side; called chromatids
  - Each chromosome duplicates itself before beginning cell division

Notes

_____

_____

_____

_____

_____

_____

_____

_____

_____

_____

_____

_____

_____

_____

_____

_____

_____

_____

_____

_____

_____

_____

_____

_____

_____

_____

_____

_____

_____

_____

Mitosis: Sequence

- Sequence of mitosis
  - Prophase
  - Metaphase
  - Anaphase
  - Telophase

Mitosis: Prophase

- Each chromosome shortens and thickens
- Centrioles move to opposite poles of the cell and form mitotic spindle consisting of small fibers radiating in all directions
- Some fibers attach to the chromatids
- Nuclear membrane breaks down

Mitosis: Metaphase and Anaphase

- Metaphase
  - Chromosomes line up at center of the cell
  - Chromatids partially separated but remained joined at centromere, a constricted area where the spindle fibers are attached
- Anaphase
  - Chromatids separate to form individual chromosomes, which are pulled to opposite poles of the cell by spindle fibers

Mitosis: Telophase

- Nuclear membranes of two daughter cells reform
- Cytoplasm divides
- Two daughter cells are formed, each an exact duplicate of the parent cell

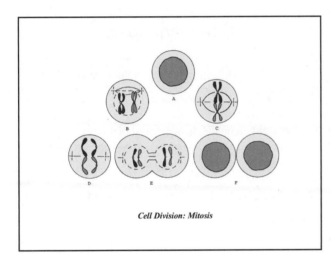

Cell Division: Mitosis

Meiosis

- Characteristic of germ cells
- Intermixing of genetic material between homologous chromosomes; chromosomes reduced by half
- Entails two separate divisions
  - First meiotic division: reduces number of chromosomes by half
    - Daughter cells receive only half of number of chromosomes by the parent cell
    - Chromosomes are not exact duplicates of those in parent cell
  - Second meiotic division: similar to mitosis, but each cell contains only 23 chromosomes

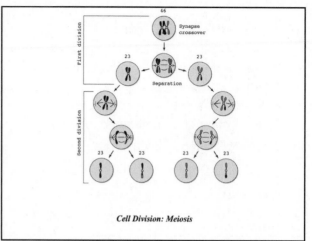

Cell Division: Meiosis

Gametogenesis

- Process of forming gametes (mature germ cells)
  - Gonads (testes and ovaries): contain precursor cells called germ cells capable of developing into mature sperm or ova
- Spermatogenesis: development of sperm
  - Spermatogonia: precursor cells in the testicular tubes
- Oogenesis: development of ova
  - Oogonia: precursor cells
- Both processes have similarities and differences

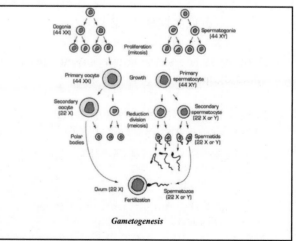

Gametogenesis

Spermatogenesis

- Spermatogonia form primary spermatocytes by mitosis (46 chromosomes)
  - ↓
- Primary spermatocytes form secondary spermatocytes by meiosis (23 chromosomes)
  - ↓
- Secondary spermatocytes form spermatids (23 chromosomes)
  - ↓
- Spermatids
  - ↓
- Sperm

Oogenesis (1 of 2)

- Oogonia form primary oocytes by mitosis in fetal ovaries (46 chromosomes)

  ↓

- Primary oocyte forms primary follicle and begins prophase of meiosis

  ↓

- Primary follicle matures under influence of FSH-LH; one mature follicle is ovulated each month

  ↓

Oogenesis (2 of 2)

- Primary oocyte forms secondary oocyte by first meiotic division

  ↓

- Secondary oocyte begins second meiotic division to form mature ovum
- Meiotic division completed when mature ovum is fertilized

Notes

_____
_____
_____
_____
_____
_____
_____
_____
_____
_____
_____
_____
_____
_____
_____
_____
_____
_____
_____
_____
_____
_____
_____
_____
_____
_____
_____
_____
_____
_____
_____
_____
_____
_____
_____
_____

Spermatogenesis and Oogenesis (1 of 2)

- Spermatogenesis
  - 1. Four spermatozoa formed from each precursor cell
  - 2. Spermatogenesis occurs continually, carried to completion in two months, seminal fluid always containing "fresh" sperm
- Oogenesis
  - 1. One ovum formed from each precursor cell, other three cells discarded as polar bodies
  - 2. Oocytes not produced continually
  - 3. Oocytes in ovary formed before birth and remained in prolonged prophase of first meiotic division in fetal life until ovulated

Spermatogenesis and Oogenesis (2 of 2)

- Congenital abnormalities from abnormal separation of chromosomes more frequent in older women
- Ova released late in woman's reproductive life have been held in prophase for a long time before assuming meiosis at time of ovulation (about 45 years)
- Ova have been exposed for years to potentially harmful radiation, chemicals, and injurious agents
- Predisposes to abnormal chromosome separation when cell division resumes at ovulation = excess or deficient number of chromosomes

Gene Imprinting (1 of 2)

- Genes occur in pairs on homologous chromosomes
- Each parent contributes one gene to the pair
- Modification process by adding methyl groups to DNA molecules of gene
- Does not change gene structure; only its expression in offspring
- Genes modified during gametogenesis
- Identical genes contributed by male and female parent may have different effects

Gene Imprinting (2 of 2)

- Gene from female parent may be imprinted differently from same gene in male parent; modifies expression of gene in offspring
- Manifestations of some hereditary diseases depend on which parent contributed the defective gene

Mitochondrial Genes and Inheritance (1 of 2)

- Chromosomes not the only site where genes are located in the cell
- Small amounts of DNA are present in mitochondria
- Mitochondrial DNA contains genes that code for ATP-generating enzymes
- Human ova contain several mitochondria; sperm contain very few mitochondria
- Inherited differently than genes on chromosomes; are not transmitted from parent to child like chromosomes

Mitochondrial Genes and Inheritance (2 of 2)

- Hereditary diseases resulting from mitochondrial DNA mutations are inherited differently from genetic mutations carried on chromosomes
- Mutations of mitochondrial DNA may affect ATP generation
- Transmission of abnormal mitochondrial DNA from parent to child is almost invariably from the mother
- Paternal transmission is extremely rare

Notes

Notes

_____
_____
_____
_____
_____
_____
_____
_____
_____
_____
_____
_____
_____
_____
_____
_____
_____
_____
_____
_____
_____
_____
_____
_____
_____
_____
_____
_____
_____
_____
_____
_____
_____
_____
_____
_____

Histocompatibility Complex Genes (1 of 3)

- Antigens present in organ donor cells must closely resemble those of the recipient for successful organ transplantation
- Human leukocyte antigens (HLA antigens)
  - Genetically determined antigens on cell surface that make individuals distinct from one another
  - Determined by a group of genes or major histocompatibility complex, MHC, on chromosome 6
  - Also referred to as HLA complex, MHC complex, and MHC antigens

Histocompatibility Complex Genes (2 of 3)

- Involved in generating immune responses to foreign antigens
- Antigenicity depends on whether they are
  - Self antigens or HLA proteins on person's own cells and recognized as self by the immune system or
  - Proteins from another (non-self antigens) that are recognized as foreign, triggering an immune response
- HLA complex consists of 4 separate, closely-linked gene loci: HLA – A; HLA – B; HLA – C; HLA – D (with additional subdivisions)

Histocompatibility Complex Genes (3 of 3)

- Designated by specific letter (for locus) and number (for allele) such as HLA-B27
- Haplotype: set of HLA genes on one chromosome that is transmitted as a set
- Surface proteins within the HLA system
  - MHC Class I proteins: determined by HLA-A, HLA-B, HLA-C genes; found in all nucleated cells and platelets; not in mature red blood cells as they are unnucleated
  - MHC Class II proteins: determined by HLA-D genes; found only on a few cells such as macrophages

Recombinant DNA Technology (1 of 2)

- Recombinant DNA: bacteria-foreign gene combination that can produce the desired biologic product
- Areas of practical application
  - Increase understanding of the molecular basis of genetic disease by studying normal gene structure and function
  - Prenatal diagnosis of genetic disease
    - Identifying abnormal genes and gene products in fetal cells
    - Identifying mutations of the gene in the fetal cell from the amniotic fluid cells

Recombinant DNA Technology (2 of 2)

- Process requires insertion of a gene that directs the synthesis of a biologic product, such as insulin, into bacterium (through a plasmid) or yeast
- Methods
  - 1. Recombinant DNA technology: genes from two different sources recombined in a single organism
  - 2. Genetic engineering: manipulations of genes
  - 3. Gene splicing: a piece of genetic material is cut open and another piece of genetic material is introduced

Gene Therapy (1 of 2)

- Extension of the principles of recombinant DNA technology
- Normal gene inserted into a defective cell lacking an enzyme or structural protein to compensate for the missing or dysfunctional gene
  - 1. Cells are removed from patient, treated, and reinfused
  - 2. Virus carrying the gene is introduced into the patient to treat defective cells

Notes

Notes

_____

_____

_____

_____

_____

_____

_____

_____

_____

_____

_____

_____

_____

_____

_____

_____

_____

_____

_____

_____

_____

_____

_____

_____

_____

_____

_____

_____

_____

_____

_____

_____

_____

Gene Therapy (2 of 2)

- Goals for successful application
  - 1. Identify and select correct gene to insert into the cell
  - 2. Choose the proper cell to receive the gene
  - 3. Select an efficient means of getting the gene into the cell
  - 4. Ensure that the newly inserted gene can function effectively long enough within the cell to make the therapy worthwhile

Chapter Outline

The chapter outline provides you with an organizational guide to the topics and ideas presented in this chapter of the text.

The Inflammatory Reaction
    Chemical Mediators of Inflammation
    The Role of Lysosomal Enzymes in the Inflammatory Process
    Inflammation Caused by Antigen–Antibody Interaction
    Harmful Effects of Inflammation
Infection
    Terminology of Infection
    Factors Influencing the Outcome of an Infection

Introductory Concepts in Chapter 4

The following material is provided as a guide to some of the fundamental concepts in the first five chapters. It may help you organize the material as you get started in this course. You will build on these concepts as you begin to study diseases involving various organ systems.

1. The inflammatory reaction is a nonspecific stereotyped response to cell injury. The response is always the same because any tissue injury triggers the release of the same type of mediators of inflammation (see Fig. 4-1). Mediators come from *mast cells* (mostly histamine), *platelets* (serotonin), and *other injured cells* (prostaglandins, leukotrienes); they also come from blood plasma (bradykinins) and from activation of blood proteins called *complement*.
2. Lysosomes (packs of digestive enzymes in the cytoplasm of white cells) release their digestive enzymes when white cells degenerate at the site of inflammation. The released lysosomal enzymes then cause further tissue injury.
3. Sometimes the tissue injury caused by the inflammation is so marked that it is necessary to suppress the inflammatory process by means of corticosteroids (such as cortisone) or nonsteroidal anti-inflammatory drugs (such as aspirin or ibuprofen).
4. Inflammation is a general term. If the inflammation is caused by a pathogenic microorganism, we use the term *infection*. Various terms are used to describe an infection: *cellulitis* (localized infection in the tissues), *lymphangitis* (infection spreading into lymphatic channels draining the site of infection, with red streaks running up the arm), *lymphadenitis* (regional lymph nodes involved), *abscess* (necrosis of tissue with a pocket of pus), and *septicemia* (bloodstream infection).
5. The outcome of an infection depends on whether the pathogen or body defenses win or whether they are evenly matched and a chronic infection results (see Fig. 4-14).

Study Questions

The following questions are provided as a test for comprehension and as a study guide for use with the text chapters. Additional study material is located at http://health.jbpub.com/humandisease/8e, which contains useful tools such as an A&P review, animated flashcards, an interactive online glossary, crossword puzzles, and web links.

Key Terms

Define the following terms:

1. Exudate _____

2. Infection _____

3. Inflammation _____

4. Leukocytes _____

5. Pathogenic _____

6. Plasma _____

7. Lymphadenitis _____

8. Septicemia _____

9. Antibodies _____

10. Mediators of inflammation _____

11. Phagocytosis _____

12. Fibrinogen _____

13. Lysosome _____

Fill-in-the-Blank

1. _____ is a specialized connective-tissue cell containing granules filled with histamine and other chemical mediators.

2. A platelet is a component of the blood—a roughly circular or oval disk concerned with _____.

3. Serotonin is a _____ mediator of inflammation released from platelets.

4. _____ is a prostaglandin-like mediator of inflammation.

5. Bradykinin is a chemical mediator of inflammation derived from components in the _____.

6. _____ is an acute spreading inflammation affecting the skin or deeper tissues.

7. Lymphangitis is an inflammation of _____ draining a site of infection.

8. _____ is an infection in which large numbers of pathogenic bacteria are present in the bloodstream.

True/False

Tell whether each statement is true or false. If false, explain why the statement is incorrect.

1. Mediators of inflammation are produced primarily by neutrophils. _____

_____

2. The inflammatory reaction is a nonspecific response to any agent that injures cells. _____

_____

3. The inflammatory reaction concentrates leukocytes and antibodies at the site of inflammation. _____

_____

4. The plasma cell is the most important cell in acute inflammatory reaction. _____

_____

5. Lymphocytes phagocytize debris produced by the inflammatory process. _____

_____

6. A serous exudate resulting from an inflammation is yellow because it consists primarily of inflammatory cells.

_____

7. A fibrinous exudate is rich in fibrinogen, which coagulates to form fibrin and create a sticky film on the surface of the inflamed tissue. _____

_____

8. Extensive destruction of tissue secondary to inflammation is often followed by scarring. _____

_____

Discussion Questions

1. What is the inflammatory reaction? Describe its clinical manifestations. (*Hint:* see Fig. 4-1.) _____

_____

_____

_____

2. What are mediators of inflammation? _____

_____

_____

_____

3. What is the source of the mediators of inflammation? _____

_____

_____

_____

4. Describe what part lysosomal enzymes play in perpetuating and intensifying the inflammatory reaction. _____

_____

_____

_____

5. What is the difference between the terms "infection" and "inflammation"? _____
_____
_____

6. What factors influence the outcome of an infection? (*Hint:* see Fig. 4-14.) _____
_____
_____

7. List the possible outcomes of an inflammation produced by a pathogenic bacteria. _____
_____
_____

8. What is the difference between serous and fibrinous exudates? _____
_____
_____

Notes

_____
_____
_____
_____
_____
_____
_____
_____
_____
_____
_____
_____
_____
_____
_____
_____
_____
_____
_____
_____
_____
_____
_____
_____
_____
_____
_____
_____
_____
_____
_____
_____
_____
_____
_____
_____

Chapter 4
Inflammation and Repair

Learning Objectives

- List characteristics and clinical manifestations
  - Acute inflammation
  - Types of exudates: serous, purulent, fibrinous, hemorrhagic
- Describe possible outcomes of an inflammatory reaction and its harmful effects
- Explain chemical mediators of inflammation and role in intensifying the inflammatory process
- Compare inflammation and infection

Inflammatory Reactions

- A nonspecific response to any agent that causes cell injury
- <u>Agents</u> may be
  - Physical (heat or cold)
  - Chemical (concentrated acid)
  - Microbiologic (bacterium or virus)

Local and Systemic Effects of Inflammation

- Local effects
  - Capillary dilatation
    - Increased blood flow, increased warmth and redness
  - Increased capillary permeability, leading to extravasation of fluid, leading to swelling
  - Attraction of leukocytes
    - Migrate to site of injury
    - Adhere to endothelium of small blood vessels
- Systemic effects: fever, leukocytes

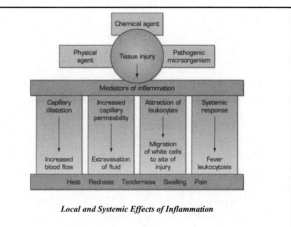

Local and Systemic Effects of Inflammation

Characteristic Signs of Inflammation

- Heat and redness
  - Dilated blood vessels and slowing of blood through vessels
- Swelling
  - Accumulation of fluid and exudate due to extravasation of plasma
- Tenderness and pain
  - Irritation of nerve endings

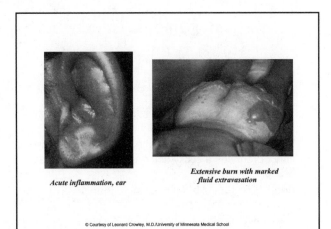

Acute inflammation, ear

Extensive burn with marked fluid extravasation

© Courtesy of Leonard Crowley, M.D./University of Minnesota Medical School

Inflammatory Process

- Acute inflammatory process
  - Polymorphonuclear leukocyte cell
    - Most important cell in acute inflammatory response; actively phagocytic cell
    - Mononuclear cells (monocytes, macrophages) follow later to clean up tissue debris
- Severe inflammatory process
  - Systemic effects become evident (feeling ill, fever)
  - Bone marrow accelerates production of leukocytes resulting in ↑ levels in bloodstream
  - Liver produces acute phase proteins such as C-reactive protein
- Mild inflammatory process
  - Self-limiting, subsides with tissue resolution

Outcome of Inflammation

- Depends on amount of tissue damage
  - Severe inflammatory process
    - Tissue damage → replacement of damage cells → heal with scarring
  - Mild inflammatory process
    - Self-limiting, subsides with tissue resolution
- Outcomes
  - Resolution
  - Repair
  - Areas of destruction replaced by scar tissue
  - Mediators intensify inflammatory process
  - Mediators generate more mediators

Exudate

- Fluid mixture of protein, leukocytes, and tissue debris
- Proportion of protein and inflammatory cells vary
- Serous: primarily fluid, little protein
- Purulent: largely inflammatory cells (pus)
- Fibrinous: rich in fibrinogen; coagulates and forms fibrin; produces a sticky film on surface of inflamed tissue
- Adhesions: bands of fibrous tissue that bind adjacent tissue together
- Hemorrhagic: increased red blood cells

Chemical Mediators of Inflammation

- Chemical agents that intensify the inflammatory process
- Cell-derived mediators
  - Mast cells: specialized connective tissue cells with granules filled with histamine, a vasodilator
  - Histamine and serotonin: also in blood platelets
  - Prostaglandins
  - Leukotrienes: synthesized from arachidonic acid
- Mediators from blood plasma
  - Bradykinin
  - Complement
    - Activated by antigen-antibody reaction
    - Series of proteins that interact in a regular sequence

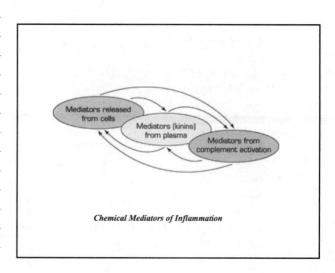

Chemical Mediators of Inflammation

Lysosomal Enzymes and Antigen-Antibody Reaction

- Lysosomal enzymes
  - From cytoplasm of phagocytic cells neutrophils and monocytes that can digest protein material
- Antigen-antibody reaction
  - Activates complements generating mediators
- Harmful effects of inflammation
  - Tissue injury results in part from the injurious agent and the inflammatory reaction itself
  - Adrenal corticosteroids: used to suppress a persistent inflammatory

Infection

- Inflammatory process caused by disease-producing organisms
- "itis": suffix indicates an infection or inflammatory process such as appendicitis, hepatitis, colitis
- Cellulitis: acute spreading infection at any site
- Abscess: infection associated with breakdown of tissues, formation of pus
- Septicemia: overwhelming infection where pathogenic bacteria gain access to bloodstream
- Pathogenic: capable of producing disease
- Virulence: a measure of severity of disease
- Host: affected individual or animal

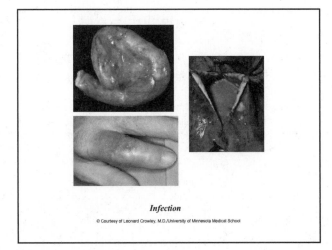

Infection

© Courtesy of Leonard Crowley, M.D./University of Minnesota Medical School

Infection

- Involves the relationship between invading organism and defenses of the body

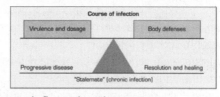

- •Factors influencing the outcome
  - –Virulence of organism
  - –Numbers of invading organisms
  - –Host resistance

Chronic Infection

- State in which the pathogenic organism and the host are evenly matched
- Relatively quiet, smoldering inflammation, associated with repeated attempts of the body at healing
- Predominant cells: lymphocytes, plasma cells, and monocytes

Discussion

- 1. How do the mediators of inflammation function?
- 2. What are the possible outcomes of an inflammation?
- 3. An exudate high in fibrinogen can coagulate producing fibrin that causes a sticky film on tissues that causes normally separate tissues to adhere together. This results from the production of:
  - – A.   Serous exudate
  - – B.   Purulent exudate
  - – C.   Fibrinous exudate
  - – D.   Hemorrhagic exudate
  - – E.   None of the above

Chapter 5   Immunity, Hypersensitivity, Allergy, and Autoimmune Diseases

Chapter Outline

The chapter outline provides you with an organizational guide to the topics and ideas presented in this chapter of the text.

The Body's Defense Mechanisms
Immunity
    The Role of Lymphocytes in Acquired Immunity
    Development of the Lymphatic System
    Response of Lymphocytes to Foreign Antigens
    The Role of Complement in Immune Responses
Antibodies (Immunoglobulins)
Hypersensitivity Reactions: Immune System–Related Tissue Injury
    Type I. Immediate Hypersensitivity Reactions: Allergy and Anaphylaxis
    Type II. Cytotoxic Hypersensitivity Reactions
    Type III. Tissue Injury Caused by Immune Complexes ("Immune Complex Disease")
    Type IV. Delayed (Cell-Mediated) Hypersensitivity Reactions
Suppression of the Immune Response
    Reasons for Suppression
    Methods of Suppression
    Tissue Grafts and Immunity
Autoimmune Diseases
    Autoimmune Disease Manifestations and Mechanisms of Tissue Injury
    Connective-Tissue (Collagen) Diseases
    Lupus Erythematosus

Introductory Concepts in Chapter 5

The following material is provided as a guide to some of the fundamental concepts in the first five chapters. It may help you organize the material as you get started in this course. You will build on these concepts as you begin to study diseases involving various organ systems.

1. Inflammation caused by a pathogenic microorganism (infection) differs from other types of inflammation caused by trauma or other types of tissue injury because the pathogen that causes the tissue injury is a *foreign substance* (non–self-antigen) that is introduced into the body. The body responds to its presence by generating an *immune response* to eliminate the foreign material in addition to giving rise to an inflammation.

2. The immune response may be *cell mediated* or *humoral*. Cell-mediated immunity is a property of T lymphocytes, which proliferate and accumulate around the foreign material, where they secrete destructive proteins called lymphokines. This is the main defense against viruses, fungi, parasites, and some bacteria such as the tubercle bacillus. Humoral immunity is a property of B lymphocytes. When stimulated by foreign material, they proliferate and "gear up" to produce large amounts of antibodies, which then combine with the foreign material. As B lymphocytes proliferate, they become transformed into cells with more cytoplasm that contains lots of ribosomes and rough endoplasmic reticulum. These cells are now called *plasma cells* and are very efficient "antibody-producing factories." This is our primary defense against most bacteria and bacterial toxins.

3. Several classes and types of antibodies (immunoglobulins) exist. See the fork analogy in the text (see Fig. 5-4). IgM, a large molecule, is the first antibody formed. IgG (gamma globulin) is formed soon thereafter and is the major immunglobulin. IgA is secreted by B lymphocytes in the mucosa of the GI and respiratory tracts and combines with inhaled or swallowed antigens so that they are not absorbed into the body. IgE is the allergy antibody. IgD is attached to the cell membranes of B lymphocytes; it has some special functions that need not be considered now.

4. Hypersensitivity reactions are important, and you should be familiar with them (see Table 5-3).
5. The IgE-mediated response triggers localized manifestations (allergy) or more serious systemic reactions to bee stings or penicillin reactions (anaphylaxis).
6. IgG-mediated hypersensitivity responses injure cells in two ways: by binding to cells and activating complement, which causes inflammation and tissue injury, or by forming antigen–antibody aggregates in tissues or in the circulation, which activates complement and induces inflammation.
7. A delayed hypersensitivity response (tuberculin-type hypersensitivity reaction) is a cell-mediated reaction and is not antibody related. Sensitized T lymphocytes accumulate at the site of contact with the foreign material and release lymphokines that attract macrophages and cytotoxic T lymphocytes. These attracted cells secrete cytokines (lymphokines and monokines) that cause the tissue injury and inflammation. A positive Mantoux test is an example of this type of reaction. Much of the tissue necrosis in tuberculosis is the result of a delayed hypersensitivity reaction to products of the tubercle bacillus.
8. Autoimmune disease occurs when the body develops an immune response to its own antigens (self-antigens), which damages the body's own cells and tissues. The nature of the autoimmune disease is determined by which organ or tissue is being attacked by the autoantibody.
9. Various mechanisms have been postulated to explain autoimmune disease (see Fig. 5-6). Defective regulation of the immune system by helper and suppressor lymphocytes is another mechanism of injury and one of the more important causes of autoimmune disease.
10. Table 5-4 provides examples of various autoimmune diseases, but the details of those diseases are not important now. Some examples will be illustrated in class.

Study Questions

The following questions are provided as a test for comprehension and as a study guide for use with the text chapters. Additional study material is located at http://health.jbpub.com/humandisease/8e, which contains useful tools such as an A&P review, animated flashcards, an interactive online glossary, crossword puzzles, and web links.

Key Terms

Define the following terms:

1. Acquired immunity _____

2. Cell-mediated immunity _____

3. Humoral immunity _____

4. Hypersensitivity _____

5. Active immunity _____

6. Passive immunity _____

7. Autoantibody _____

True/False

Tell whether the following statements are true or false as they apply to viral infections. If false, explain why the statement is incorrect.

1. Many viral infections cause acute cell necrosis and degeneration. _____

_____

2. Some viruses cause warts. _____

_____

3. Some viruses may persist indefinitely in the tissues of the host and become reactivated periodically, causing disease.

_____

4. Some viruses cause slowly progressive cell injury. _____

_____

5. Viruses are inhibited by adrenal corticosteroids. _____

_____

6. Some viruses respond to antiviral chemotherapeutic agents. _____

_____

Identify

1. Identify and describe the four major types of hypersensitivity reactions that cause tissue injury. (*Hint:* see Table 5-3.)

   a. _____

   b. _____

   c. _____

   d. _____

2. Identify and describe the four major categories of immunosuppressive agents used by physicians to treat autoimmune diseases or to perform organ transplants.

a. _____

b. _____

c. _____

d. _____

3. Identify and briefly describe three mechanisms postulated to explain the pathogenesis of autoimmune diseases.

a. _____

b. _____

c. _____

Discussion Questions

1. Describe the role of the lymphocyte in acquired immunity. (*Hint:* see Fig. 5-2.) _____
_____
_____
_____

2. Describe the role of the macrophage in acquired immunity. _____
_____
_____
_____

3. Describe the role of complement in immune responses. _____
_____
_____
_____

4. Draw and label a simple diagram of an immunoglobulin molecule. (*Hint:* see Fig. 5-4.)

5. List the major types of immunoglobulin molecules, and describe the function of each type.

_____
_____
_____

6. What is the difference between immunity and hypersensitivity? _____

_____

_____

7. What is the effect of autoantibody directed against the patient's own blood cells? _____

_____

_____

8. Describe what happens in a cell-mediated immune response secondary to a pathogenic microorganism. _____

_____

_____

9. Explain what happens when autoimmune diseases occur. How are they treated? _____

_____

_____

10. Describe what happens when a pathogenic organism enters the body. _____

_____

_____

11. Explain what happens when a person has a fungal infection. Are they treatable? _____

_____

_____

Matching

Match the cell in the left column with its function or activity in the right column.

1. _____ Macrophage

2. _____ Antigenic determinant (epitope)

3. _____ MHC complex

4. _____ Cytotoxic T cell

5. _____ Helper T lymphocyte

A. Regulates immune response

B. A small fragment of an antigen to which the immune system responds

C. Destroys abnormal or infected body cells

D. A group of unique self-antigens on body cells

E. Antigen processing cell

Chapter 5 Immunity, Hypersensitivity, Allergy, and Autoimmune Diseases

Notes

_____
_____
_____
_____
_____
_____
_____
_____
_____
_____
_____
_____
_____
_____
_____
_____
_____
_____
_____
_____
_____
_____
_____
_____
_____
_____
_____
_____
_____
_____
_____
_____
_____
_____

Chapter 5

Immunity, Hypersensitivity, Allergy, and Autoimmune Diseases

Learning Objectives

- Differentiate cell-mediated versus humoral immunity
- Compare immunity and hypersensitivity
- List and differentiate five classes of antibodies
- Hypersensitivity reaction
  - Describe pathogenesis
  - Role of IgA in allergy
  - Methods of treatment
- Autoimmune diseases
  - Summarize theories of pathogenesis
  - Clinical manifestations
  - Methods of treatment

The Body's Defense Mechanisms (1 of 2)

- Two separate mechanisms function together to protect us from disease
  - Inflammatory reaction: nonspecific response, phagocytosis of material by neutrophils and macrophages
  - Acquired immunity: develops after contact with pathogenic microorganism; depends on immune system; associated with stage of altered reactivity to foreign material (hypersensitivity)

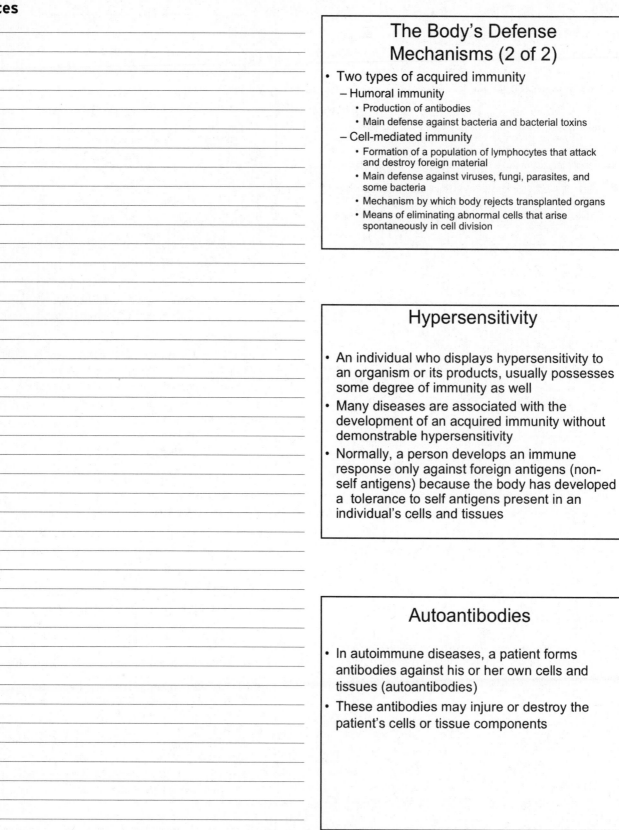

The Body's Defense Mechanisms (2 of 2)

- Two types of acquired immunity
  - Humoral immunity
    - Production of antibodies
    - Main defense against bacteria and bacterial toxins
  - Cell-mediated immunity
    - Formation of a population of lymphocytes that attack and destroy foreign material
    - Main defense against viruses, fungi, parasites, and some bacteria
    - Mechanism by which body rejects transplanted organs
    - Means of eliminating abnormal cells that arise spontaneously in cell division

Hypersensitivity

- An individual who displays hypersensitivity to an organism or its products, usually possesses some degree of immunity as well
- Many diseases are associated with the development of an acquired immunity without demonstrable hypersensitivity
- Normally, a person develops an immune response only against foreign antigens (non-self antigens) because the body has developed a tolerance to self antigens present in an individual's cells and tissues

Autoantibodies

- In autoimmune diseases, a patient forms antibodies against his or her own cells and tissues (autoantibodies)
- These antibodies may injure or destroy the patient's cells or tissue components

Acquired Immunity: Role of Lymphocytes

- Respond to foreign antigens
  - Cytokines: general term for chemical messengers involved in the immune process
  - Lymphokines: soluble proteins secreted by lymphokines that act as chemical messengers to exert their effects and to communicate with various cells of the immune system
  - Monokines: secreted by monocytes
  - Interferon: interferes with the multiplication of viruses within the cell
  - Interleukin: sends regulatory signals between cells of the immune system
  - Tumor necrosis factor: destroys foreign or abnormal cells and tumor cells

Lymphatic System (1 of 3)

- Precursor cells are formed initially from stem cells in the bone marrow, eventually developing into either of two groups:
  - T lymphocyte, thymus-dependent: Precursor cells that migrated from the marrow to the thymus
  - B lymphocyte, bone marrow: Precursor cells that remained within the bone marrow
- T and B cells need time to be activated and function effectively
- Natural killer cells: can destroy target cells as soon as they are encountered

Lymphatic System (2 of 3)

- Before birth, precursor cells of T and B lymphocytes migrate into spleen, lymph nodes, and other sites to proliferate and form masses of mature lymphocytes that will populate the various lymphoid organs
- Lymphocytes vary in lifespan
- Lymphocytes do not remain localized within lymphoid organs but circulate between bloodstream and lymphoid tissues
  - T lymphocytes = 2/3 of circulating lymphocytes
  - B lymphocytes = rest of circulating lymphocytes
  - Natural killer cells = 10%–15%; have neither T or B lymphocyte receptors; major targets are virus-infected cells and cancer cells

Lymphatic System (3 of 3)

- Each programmed lymphocyte develops antigen receptors on its cell membranes, allowing it to "recognize" and respond to a specific antigen
- Programming process allows T and B cells to be programmed to recognize and respond to a different antigen

Response of Lymphocytes to Foreign Antigens

- Entry of a foreign antigen into the body triggers a chain of events
  - Recognition of foreign antigen
  - Proliferation of lymphocytes that are programmed to respond to the antigen form a large group (clone) of cells
  - Destruction of foreign antigen by the responding lymphocytes

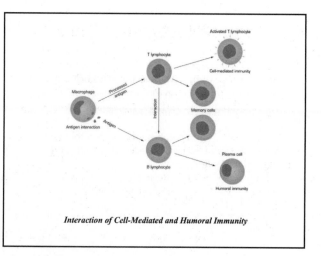

Interaction of Cell-Mediated and Humoral Immunity

Interaction of Cell-Mediated and Humoral Immunity (1 of 2)

- Antigen must first be "processed" and displayed on the cell membrane of the antigen processing cell before the immune response can be set in motion
- Lymphocytes interact with the antigen they are programmed to recognize
- When appropriately stimulated:
  - B lymphocytes proliferate and mature into antibody-forming plasma cells
  - T lymphocytes proliferate to form a diverse population of cells that regulate the immune response and generate a cell-mediated immune reaction to eliminate antigen

Interaction of Cell-Mediated and Humoral Immunity (2 of 2)

- Initial contact with a foreign antigen is followed by a lag phase of a ≥ week before an immune response is demonstrated
- Once body's immune mechanisms have reacted to a foreign antigen, some lymphoid cells retain a "memory" of the antigen that induced sensitization
- Memory is passed on to succeeding generations of lymphocytes
- Later contact with same antigen provokes a stronger and faster proliferation of sensitized lymphocytes or antibody-forming plasma cells

Types of Responding T Cells

- Regulator T cells: helper T cells that regulate immune system by establishing a balance between promoting and inhibiting the immune response
- Effector T cells: involved in delayed hypersensitivity reactions
- In AIDS, the virus attacks and destroys helper T lymphocytes

Notes

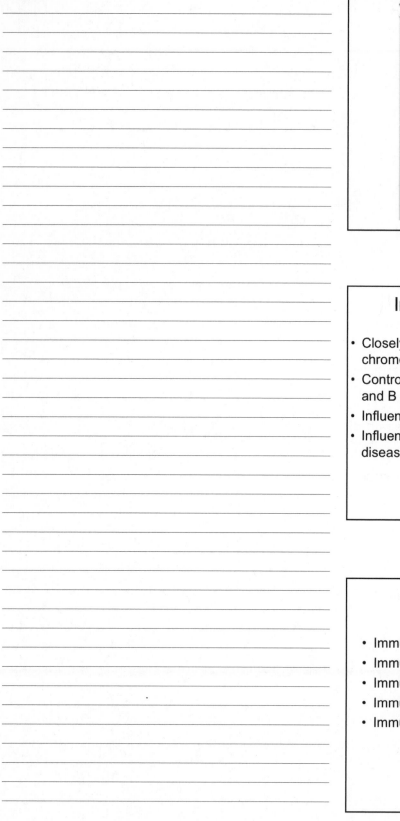

TABLE 5-1

Classification and functions of immune system cells

CELL FUNCTION	CELL TYPE	ACTION OF CELL
Antigen processing	Macrophages, B lymphocytes, dendritic cells	Process antigen and present to lymphocytes
Regulate immune response	Helper T cells (CD4+)	Cytokines regulate immune system activity
Promote cytotoxic immune response	Cytotoxic T cells (CD8+)	Produce cytokines that destroy foreign or abnormal cells displaying antigen fragments combined with MHC Class I antigens
Promote delayed hypersensitivity response	Delayed hypersensitivity T cells (CD4+)	Respond to antigen processing cells presenting foreign antigen fragments combined with MHC Class II antigens; produce cytokines that activate and stimulate macrophages, cytotoxic T cells, and NK cells
Destroy virus-infected cells and cancer cells	NK cells	Cytokine-mediated cell destruction; no previous contact with antigen required
Produce antibodies	Plasma cells	Antigen processed by B lymphocytes and presented to responding T cells stimulates B lymphocytes to mature into plasma cells and make antibodies

Immune Response Genes

- Closely related to the HLA complex on chromosome 6
- Control the immune response by regulating T and B cell proliferation
- Influence resistance to infection and tumors
- Influence likelihood of acquiring an autoimmune disease

Antibody Types

- Immunoglobulin G (IgG)
- Immunoglobulin A (IgA)
- Immunoglobulin M (IgM)
- Immunoglobulin E (IgE)
- Immunoglobulin D (IgD)

Antibodies (1 of 3)

- Globulins produced by plasma cells
- Can react only with the specific antigen that induced its formation

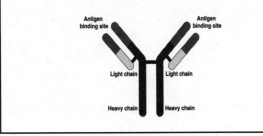

Antibodies (2 of 3)

- IgG
  - Smaller antibody
  - Principal antibody molecule in response to majority of infectious agents
- IgM
  - Large antibody, a macroglobulin
  - Very efficient combining with fungi
- IgE
  - Found in minute quantities in blood; concentration is increased in allergic individuals

Antibodies (3 of 3)

- IgA
  - Produced by antibody-forming cells located in the respiratory and gastrointestinal mucosa
  - Combines with harmful ingested or inhaled antigens, forming antigen-antibody complexes that cannot be absorbed, preventing antigens from inducing sensitization
- IgD
  - Found on cell membrane of B lymphocytes
  - Present in minute quantities in blood

Notes

Hypersensitivity Reactions (1 of 4)

- Antibody-mediated hypersensitivity
  - Type I: anaphylactic (immediate)
  - Type II: cytotoxic
  - Type III: immune complex

Hypersensitivity Reactions (2 of 4)

- Type I: anaphylactic (immediate)
  - Sensitizing antigen circulates throughout the body, triggers widespread mediator release from Ig-coated mast cells and basophils
  - May lead to anaphylaxis: severe generalized IgE-mediated reaction (fall in blood pressure, severe respiratory distress)
  - Prompt treatment required with epinephrine, other appropriate agents
  - Antihistamine drugs often relieve many of the allergic symptoms; histamine is one of the mediators released from IgE-coated cells
  - Later contact with same antigen triggers release of mediators (histamine) and related clinical manifestations
    - Ex: Localized response: hay fever, food allergy (peanuts)
    - Systemic response: bee sting, penicillin allergy
  - Atopic person: allergy-prone individual
  - Allergen: sensitizing antigen

Hypersensitivity Reactions (3 of 4)

- Type II: cytotoxic
  - Antibody combines to cell or tissue antigen resulting in complement-mediated lysis of cells or other membrane damage
  - Ex: Autoimmune hemolytic anemia, blood transfusion reactions,   RH hemolytic disease, some types of glomerulonephritis
- Type III: immune complex
  - Ag-Ab immune complexes deposited in tissues activate complements; PMNs attracted to site, causing tissue damage
  - Ex: rheumatoid arthritis, systemic lupus erythematosus (SLE), some types of glomerulonephritis

Hypersensitivity Reactions (4 of 4)

- Type IV: delayed hypersensitivity or cell-mediated hypersensitivity
  - T lymphocytes are sensitized and activated on second contact with same antigen.
  - Lymphokines induceinflammation and activate macrophages
  - Ex: Tuberculosis, fungal and parasitic infections, contact dermatitis

Suppression of Immune Response

- Reasons for suppression
  - Prevent undesirable effects
  - May be directed against individual's own cells or tissue components leading to autoimmune diseases
  - Responsible for rejection of transplanted organs
  - May lead to Rh hemolytic disease in newborn infants

Methods of Immune Suppression

- Main immunosuppressive agents
  - Radiation
  - Immunosuppressive drugs that impede cell division or cell function
  - Adrenal corticosteroid hormones
    - Suppress inflammatory reaction
    - Impair phagocytosis
    - Inhibit protein synthesis
  - Gamma globulin preparations contain potent antibodies preventing body from responding to corresponding antigen

Autoimmune Diseases (1 of 2)

- Pathogenesis
  - Alteration of patient's own (self) antigens causing them to become antigenic, provoking an immune reaction
  - Formation of cross-reacting antibodies against foreign antigens that also attack patient's own antigens
  - Defective regulation of the immune response by regulator T lymphocyte
- Treatment: corticosteroids, cytotoxic drugs

Autoimmune Diseases (2 of 2)

- Examples
  - Systemic lupus erythematosus
    - Systemic manifestations in various organs
  - Rheumatic fever
    - Inflammation in heart and joints
  - Glomerulonephritis
    - Inflammation in renal glomeruli
- Autoimmune blood diseases: anemia, leukopenia, thrombocytopenia
- Thyroiditis (hypothyroidism)
- Diffuse toxic goiter (hyperthyroidism)

TABLE 5-3

Etiology and clinical manifestations of common autoimmune diseases

	PROBABLE PATHOGENESIS	MAJOR CLINICAL MANIFESTATIONS
Rheumatic fever	Antistreptococcal antibodies cross-react with antigens in heart muscle, heart valves, and other tissues.	Inflammation of heart and joints
Glomerulonephritis	Some cases caused by antibodies formed against glomerular basement membrane; other cases caused by antigen-antibody complexes trapped in glomeruli.	Inflammation of renal glomeruli
Rheumatoid arthritis	Antibodies formed against serum gamma globulin.	Systemic disease with inflammation and degeneration of joints
Autoimmune blood diseases	Autoantibodies formed against platelets, white cells, or red cells; in some cases, antibody apparently is formed against altered cell antigens, and antibody reacts with both altered and normal cells.	Anemia, leukopenia, or thrombocytopenia, depending on nature of antibody
Lupus erythematosus and related collagen diseases	Various antinuclear antibodies cause widespread injury to several organs.	Systemic disease with manifestations in several organs
Thyroiditis	Antithyroid antibody causes injury and inflammatory cell infiltration of thyroid gland.	Hypothyroidism
Diffuse toxic goiter	Autoantibody mimicking thyroid-stimulating hormone (TSH) causes increased output of thyroid hormone.	Hyperthyroidism

Discussion (1 of 2)

- Which of the following does NOT characterize an active acquired immunity?
    - A. Requires repeated contact or exposure to the same antigen
    - B. Host produces own antibodies
    - C. Slow onset of action
    - D. Short-lived immunity
    - E. None of the above

Discussion (2 of 2)

- The first antibody formed in response to an antigenic stimulation
    - A. IgM
    - B. IgG
    - C. IgE
    - D. IgA
    - E. IgD

Chapter Outline

The chapter outline provides you with an organizational guide to the topics and ideas presented in this chapter of the text.

Types of Harmful Microorganisms
Bacteria
    Classification of Bacteria
    Identification of Bacteria
    Major Classes of Pathogenic Bacteria
    Antibiotic Treatment of Bacterial Infections
    Antibiotic Sensitivity Tests
    Adverse Effects of Antibiotics
Chlamydiae
Rickettsiae and Ehrlichiae
Mycoplasmas
Viruses
    Classification of Viruses
    Mode of Action
    Bodily Defenses Against Viral Infections
    Treatment with Antiviral Agents
Fungi
    Superficial Fungal Infections
    Highly Pathogenic Fungi
    Other Fungi of Medical Importance
    Treatment of Systemic Fungal Infections

Study Questions

The following questions are provided as a test for comprehension and as a study guide for use with the text chapters. Additional study material is located at http://health.jbpub.com/humandisease/8e, which contains useful tools such as an A&P review, animated flashcards, an interactive online glossary, crossword puzzles, and web links.

Key Terms

Define the following terms:

1. Virus _____

2. Human papillomavirus _____

3. *Histoplasma capsulatum* _____

4. *Neisseria* _____

5. Latent virus infection _____

6. Hemolysis _____

7. Antigens _____

8. Pathogenic _____

True/False

1. Tell whether each statement is true or false as it applies to streptococci. If false, explain why the statement is incorrect.

   a. The organisms are classified based on the carbohydrate antigens present in their cell walls and on the type of hemolysis produced by the organism growing on a blood agar plate. _____

   _____

   b. Most alpha hemolytic streptococci are very pathogenic. _____

   _____

   c. Group A beta streptococci may cause serious respiratory tract infections such as streptococcal pharyngitis, and such infections may be followed by rheumatic fever. _____

   _____

   d. Group B beta streptococci may colonize the genital tract of pregnant women and may lead to an infection in the infant caused by the streptococcus acquired by the infant during delivery. _____

   _____

2. Tell whether each statement is true or false as it applies to the organism causing anthrax (*Bacillus anthracis*). If false, explain why the statement is incorrect.

   a. The organism is a gram-positive, spore-forming aerobic bacillus. _____

   _____

   b. The organism can be used as a bioterrorism–germ warfare agent. _____

   _____

c. Inhalation of anthrax spores may cause a severe pulmonary infection. _____

_____

d. Pulmonary anthrax caused by inhalation of anthrax spores can be prevented by a short (1- to 2-week) course of antibiotics because the organism is sensitive to antibiotics. _____

_____

Identify

1. Identify and briefly describe the four potentially harmful side effects of antibiotics.

   a. _____

   b. _____

   c. _____

   d. _____

2. Identify the important diseases caused by

   a. Pneumococci _____

   b. Gonococci _____

   c. Acid-fast bacteria _____

3. Identify two highly pathogenic fungi and the type of diseases they produce.

   a. _____

   b. _____

4. Identify five possible effects of a virus invasion of a susceptible cell. (*Hint:* see Fig. 6-4.)

   a. _____

   b. _____

   c. _____

   d. _____

   e. _____

5. List the four major factors used to classify bacteria.

   a. _____

   b. _____

   c. _____

   d. _____

Matching 1

Match the diseases in the right column with the responsible organisms in the left column.

1. _____ Group A beta streptococcus
2. _____ Group B beta streptococcus
3. _____ Hemolytic staphylococcus
4. _____ Human papillomavirus
5. _____ *Histoplasma capsulatum*
6. _____ Herpes virus
7. _____ Varicella zoster virus
8. _____ Mumps virus
9. _____ *Bacillus anthracis*
10. _____ Meningococcus (*Neisseria meningitidis*)

A. Severe throat infection
B. Warts
C. Infection of newborn infant
D. "Fever blisters"
E. Pulmonary infection
F. Germ warfare agent
G. Wound infection
H. Skin rash
I. Parotid gland infection
J. Meningitis

Matching 2

Match the organism in the left column with the disease or condition in the right column.

1. _____ *Brucella*
2. _____ *Borrelia*
3. _____ *Ehrlichia*
4. _____ *Babesia*
5. _____ *Yersinia*

A. A malaria-like parasite transmitted by ticks
B. A febrile illness transmitted to people from unpasteurized milk or tissues of infected animals
C. Causes a febrile illness with a skin rash
D. Causes bubonic plague
E. A tick transmitted rickettsia-like agent that infects white blood cells

Discussion Questions

1. How is the Gram stain used to classify bacteria?_____

_____

_____

_____

2. How do antibiotics inhibit the growth of bacteria? (*Hint*: see Fig. 6-2.)_____

_____

_____

_____

3. How does penicillin kill bacteria? _____

_____

_____

_____

4. How do bacteria become resistant to an antibiotic? _____

_____

_____

_____

5. What factors render a patient susceptible to an infection by a fungus of low pathogenicity? _____

_____

_____

_____

Notes

_____

_____

_____

_____

_____

_____

_____

_____

_____

_____

_____

_____

_____

_____

_____

_____

_____

_____

_____

_____

_____

_____

_____

_____

_____

_____

_____

_____

_____

_____

_____

_____

_____

_____

_____

_____

Chapter 6

Pathogenic Microorganisms

Learning Objectives

- Explain
  - Characteristics of bacteria
  - Major groups of pathogenic bacteria
- Describe
  - Inhibition of microbial growth by antibiotics
  - Adverse effects of antibiotics
  - Antibiotic sensitivity testing and interpretation of results
- Explain
  - Mode of action of viruses
  - Body's response to viral infections
- Discuss infections caused by chlamydiae, mycoplasma, rickettsiae, and fungi

Pathogenic Microorganisms

- Bacteria
- *Chlamydiae*
- *Rickettsiae* and *Ehrlichiae*
- *Mycoplasma*
- Viruses
- Fungi

Classification of Bacteria

- Classified according to four major characteristics:
  - Shape and arrangement: coccus, bacillus, spiral
  - Gram stain reaction: gram-positive and gram-negative
  - Biochemical and growth characteristics
    - Aerobic and anaerobic
    - Spore formation
    - Biochemical profile
  - Antigenic structure: antigens in cell body, capsule, flagella

Shape and Arrangement

- Coccus (spherical)
  - Clusters: *staphylococci*
  - Chains: *streptococci*
  - Pairs: *diplococci*
  - Kidney bean-shaped, in pairs: *Neisseriae*
- Bacillus (rod-shaped)
  - Square ends: *bacillus anthracis*
  - Rounded ends: *mycobacterium tuberculosis*
  - Club-shaped: *corynebacteria*
  - Fusiform: *fusobacteria*
  - Comma-shaped: *vibrio*
- Spirochete (spiral)
  - Tightly-coiled: *treponema pallidum*
  - Relaxed coil: *borrelia*

Gram Staining

- Bacteria are classified as either gram-positive or gram-negative based on ability to resist or retain certain dyes
- Based on the chemical and physical properties of their cell walls
- Dried fixed suspension of bacteria prepared on a microscopic slide
  - Step 1: Crystal violet (purple dye)
  - Step 2: Gram's iodine (acts a mordant)
  - Step 3: Alcohol or acetone (rapid decolorization)
  - Step 4: Safranin (red dye)
- Gram-positive: resists decolorization and retains purple stain
- Gram-negative: can be decolorized and stains red

Readily Gram-Stained Organisms (1 of 2)

- **Gram-positive cocci**: *Staphylococcus, Streptococcus, Enterococcus*
- **Gram-negative cocci**: *Neisseria* (meningitis, gonorrhea)
- **Gram-positive rods**: *Bacillus, Corynebacterium, Clostridium, Listeria, Actinomyces, Nocardia*

Readily Gram-Stained Organisms (2 of 2)

- **Gram-negative rods**
- **Pathogenic inside and outside intestinal tract:** *Escherichia Salmonella*
- **Pathogenic inside intestinal tract**: *Shigella, Vibrio, Campylobacter, Helicobacter*
- **Pathogenic outside intestinal tract**: *Klebsiella, Enterobacter, Serratia, Pseudomonas, Proteus, Providencia, Morganella, Bacteroides*
- **Respiratory tract organisms**: *Hemophilus, Legionella, Bordetella*
- **Organisms from animal sources**: *Brucella, Francisella, Pasteurella, Yersinia*

Not Readily Gram-Stained Organisms

- Not Obligate Intracellular Parasites
  - *Mycobacterium*
  - *Mycoplasma*
  - *Treponema*
  - Leptospira
- Obligate Intracellular Parasites
  - *Chlamydia*
  - *Rickettsia*

Pathogenic Microorganisms

Notes

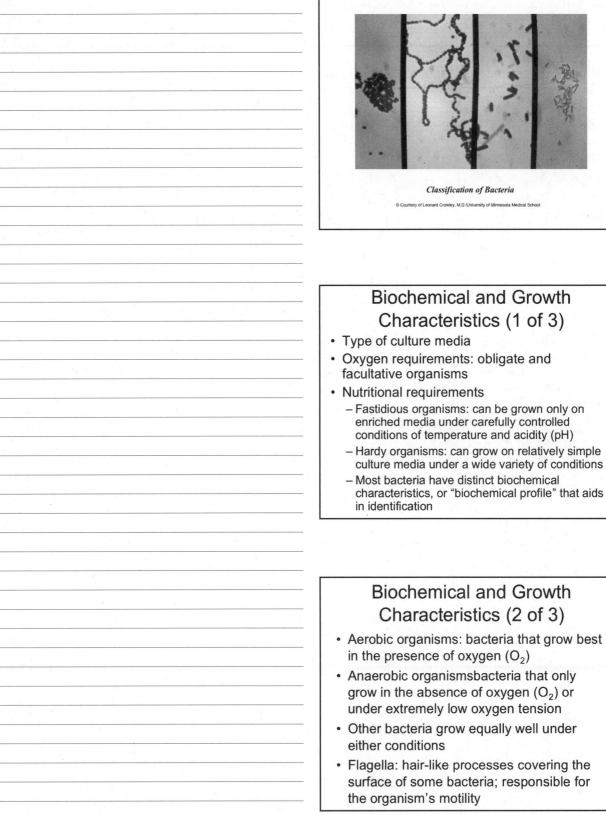

Classification of Bacteria

© Courtesy of Leonard Crowley, M.D./University of Minnesota Medical School

Biochemical and Growth Characteristics (1 of 3)

- Type of culture media
- Oxygen requirements: obligate and facultative organisms
- Nutritional requirements
  - Fastidious organisms: can be grown only on enriched media under carefully controlled conditions of temperature and acidity (pH)
  - Hardy organisms: can grow on relatively simple culture media under a wide variety of conditions
  - Most bacteria have distinct biochemical characteristics, or "biochemical profile" that aids in identification

Biochemical and Growth Characteristics (2 of 3)

- Aerobic organisms: bacteria that grow best in the presence of oxygen (O_2)
- Anaerobic organismsbacteria that only grow in the absence of oxygen (O_2) or under extremely low oxygen tension
- Other bacteria grow equally well under either conditions
- Flagella: hair-like processes covering the surface of some bacteria; responsible for the organism's motility

Biochemical and Growth Characteristics (3 of 3)

- Spores: dormant, extremely resistant bacterial modification formed under adverse conditions
- Spores can germinate and give rise to actively growing bacteria under favorable conditions

Antigen Structure

- Contained in:
  - Cell body
  - Capsule
  - Flagella
- The antigenic structure can be determined by special methods, defining a system of antigens unique for each group of bacteria

TABLE 6-1

Important pathogenic bacteria

| TYPE | GRAM-STAIN REACTION | |
	GRAM-POSITIVE	GRAM-NEGATIVE
Cocci	Staphylococci Streptococci Pneumococci	Gonococci Meningococci
Bacilli	Corynebacteria Listeria Bacilli Clostridia	Hemophilus Gardnerella Francisella Yersinia Brucella Legionella Salmonella Shigella Campylobacter Cholera bacillus Colon bacillus (Escherichia coli) and related organisms
Spiral organisms	Treponema pallidum Borrelia burgdorferi	
Acid-fast organisms	Tubercle bacillus Leprosy bacillus	

Notes

Staphylococci

- Gram-positive cocci arranged in grapelike clusters
- Normal inhabitants of
  - Skin (Staphylococcus epidermidis)
  - Nasal cavity (Staphylococcus aureus)
- Commonly found on skin and in nose of patients and hospital staff
- Normally not pathogenic
- Opportunistic organisms
- Cause disease by producing toxins
  - Vomiting and diarrhea; toxic shock
  - Tissue necrosis
  - Hemolysis)
- Cause disease by causing inflammation

Staphylococci Infections

- Skin infections: impetigo; boils (furuncles, carbuncles); nail infection (paronychia); cellulitis; surgical wound infection; eye infection; postpartum breast infections (mastitis)
- Sepsis: wounds and IV drug use
- Endocarditis: infection of lining of heart and valves
  - Normal and prosthetic valves, IV drug use
- Osteomyelitis and arthritis
- Pneumonia
- Abscess
- Some strains are highly resistant to antibiotics (MRSA or Methicillin-resistant *Staphylococcus aureus*

Streptococci Classification

- Based on type of hemolysis and differences in carbohydrate antigens in the cell walls or C carbohydrate (Lancefield Classification Groups A to U)
- Beta hemolysis: complete lysis of red cells
  - Group A (*Streptococcus pyogenes*): causes pharyngitis
  - Group B (*Streptococcus agalactiae*): genital tract of women, neonatal meningitis, sepsis
  - Group D (*Enterococcus faecalis, Streptococcus bovis*) urinary, biliary, cardiovascular infections
- Non-beta hemolysis
  - Alpha hemolysis: incomplete lysis of red cells (*Streptococcus pneumoniae*)
  - Gamma hemolysis: non-hemolytic, no lysis

Streptococci

- Gram-positive cocci arranged in chains or pairs
  - Normal inhabitants of skin, mouth, pharynx (Viridans strep), gut, female genital tract (Peptostreptococci)
  - Opportunistic organisms
- Diseases:
  - Pyogenic: pharyngitis, cellulitis, endocarditis, UTI
  - Toxigenic: scarlet fever, toxic shock syndrome
  - Immunologic: rheumatic fever, glomerulonephritis

Antibiotics

- One of the great discoveries and advances in medicine
- Antibiotic resistance
  - 1. Over-prescribing
  - 2. Inappropriate prescribing
  - 3. Overuse as feed supplement for livestock
  - 4. Improper use
  - 5. Spread of resistant strains worldwide

Antibiotics: Mechanisms of Action

- Inhibits synthesis of bacterial cell wall and cell membrane
  - Penicillin family: penicillin, methicillin, nafcillin, oxacillin, amoxicillin, ampicillin, piperacillin, ticarcillin
  - Cephalosporin: cephalexin, cefoxitin, ceftazidime, ceftriaxone; vancomycin, bacitracin
- Inhibits synthesis microbial proteins
  - Chloramphenicol; tetracycline; macrolide: erythromycin, azithromycin, clarithromycin; clindamycin, gentamicin, netilmicin, streptomycin
- Inhibits bacterial metabolic functions
  - Inhibit folic acid synthesis: sulfonamides, trimethoprim
- Inhibits bacterial DNA synthesis
  - ciprofloxacin, norfloxacin, ofloxacin, sparfloxacin
- Competitive inhibition

Notes

Notes

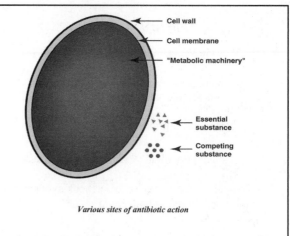

Various sites of antibiotic action

Antibiotics: Adverse Effects

- Toxicity
- Hypersensitivity
- Alteration of normal bacterial flora
- Development of resistant strains
  - 1. Spontaneous mutation
  - 2. Plasmid-acquired resistance
- Mechanisms for circumventing effects of antibiotics
  - Develop enzymes (penicillinase)
  - Change cell wall structure
  - Change internal metabolic machinery

Antibiotic Sensitivity Tests

- Tube dilution: measures the highest dilution inhibiting growth in test tube
- Disk method: inhibition of growth around disk indicates sensitivity to antibiotic

96

Chapter 6

Chlamydiae (1 of 2)

- Gram-negative, nonmotile bacteria
- Form inclusion bodies in infected cells
- Obligate intracellular parasites
- With rigid cell wall and reproduce by a distinct intracellular cycle
- Susceptible to tetracycline and erythromycin
- No vaccine available

Chlamydiae (2 of 2)

- Diseases
  - Psittacosis (pneumonia): inhalation of dried bird feces
  - Trachoma (C. trachomatis A,B, C): chronic conjunctivitis, blindness
  - Non-gonococcal urethritis (men): spread to other areas
  - Cervicitis (women)
    - Lead to salpingitis, PID, infertilty, ectopic pregnancy
  - Neonatal inclusion conjunctivitis:
    - Newborn from infected mom
  - Lymphogranuloma Venereum: sexually transmitted disease

Rickettsiae and *Ehrlichiae* (1 of 2)

- Disease: damage to small blood vessels of skin; leakage of blood into surrounding tissues (rash and edema)
- Rocky Mountain Spotted Fever (ticks)
  - East Coast spring and early summer; flu-like
  - Rash after 2-6 days, hands/feet then trunk, CNS
- Rickettsialpox (mites)
- Typhus: flu-like, rash (epidemic: lice; endemic: fleas; scrub: mites)
- Q Fever (aerosol): pneumonia-hepatitis combination, rash is rare
- Erliochiosis
  - Susceptible to tetracycline or chloramphenicol

Notes

Notes

Rickettsiae and _Ehrlichiae_ (2 of 2)

- Obligate intracellular parasites
- Parasite of insects transmitted to humans
- Transmitted via bite of an arthropod vector (ticks, mites, lice, fleas) except in Q Fever (aerosol)
- _Rickettsiae_ multiply in endothelial cells of blood vessels while _Ehrlichiae_ multiply in neutrophils or monocytes
- Cause febrile illness with skin rash
- Respond to some antibiotics
- Most rickettsial diseases are zoonoses (animal-borne) except epidemic typhus (humans)
- Transmission enhanced by poor hygiene, overcrowding, wars, poverty

Mycoplasma

- Smallest, wall-less, free-living bacteria
  - About the size of a virus (0.3 micrometer)
- With cell membrane (cholesterol), no cell wall
  - Medical implications: Stain poorly
- Penicillin and cephalosporin are not effective
  - Can reproduce outside living cells, can grow on artificial media
- Primary Atypical Pneumonia: Mycoplasma pneumoniae
  - Most common in winter, young adults, outbreaks in groups
  - Cough, sore throat, fever, headache, malaise, myalgia
  - Resolves spontaneously in 10-14 days
  - Responds to antibiotics: tetracycline and erythromycin

Virus (1 of 3)

- Classification
  - Nucleic acid structure: Either DNA or RNA, with an outer envelope made of lipoprotein
  - Size and complexity of genome varies
  - Smaller than cells (20-300 nm diameter)
  - Cannot be seen under a light microscope
- Nucleoid: genetic material, DNA and RNA, not both
- Capsid: protective protein membrane surrounding genetic material

Virus (2 of 3)

- Obligate intracellular parasites
  - Must reproduce or replicate within cells
  - Lack metabolic enzymes; rely on host's metabolic processes for survival
  - Do not have nucleus, ribosomes, mitochondria, and lysosomes; cannot synthesize proteins or generate energy
  - Do not multiply by binary fission or mitosis
- Mode of action
  - Invasion of susceptible cell
    - Asymptomatic latent viral infection
    - Acute cell necrosis and degeneration
    - Cell hyperplasia and proliferation
    - Slowly progressive cell injury
    - Neoplasia
  - Formation of inclusion bodies

Virus (3 of 3)

- Bodily defenses against viral infections
  - Formation of interferon: "broad-spectrum" antiviral agent
  - Cell-mediated immunity
  - Humoral defenses
- Treatment with antiviral agents
  - Block viral multiplication
  - Prevent virus from invading cell
  - Limited application: toxicity and limited effectiveness

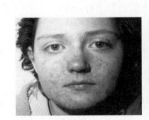

German Measles

Shingles or herpes zoster clusters of vesicles along a segment of skin supplied by a sensory nerve

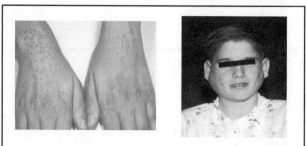

Multiple warts   *Mumps: Parotid glands swelling*

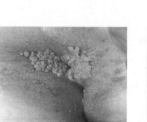 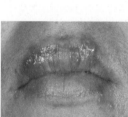

Condylomas   *Oral herpes virus type 1*

Fungi (1 of 2)

- Plantlike organisms without chlorophyll
- Two types: yeasts and molds
- Most are obligate aerobes, opportunistic
- Natural habitat: environment, except Candida
- Cell wall: chitin vs. peptidoglycan
- Cell membrane: ergosterol and zymosterol vs. cholesterol

Fungi (2 of 2)

- Growth factors: high humidity (moist), heat, dark areas with oxygen supply
- Treatment: antifungal drugs
- Other fungi: bread, cheese, wine, beer production
  - Frequently associated with decaying matter
  - Molds: spoilage of foods (fruits, grains, vegetables, jams)
- Infections
  - Superficial fungal infections
  - Mucous membranes (Candida)
  - *Histoplasmosis, Coccidioidomycosis*
  - *Blastomycosis, Cryptococcus*

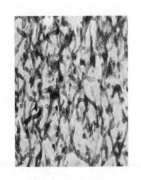

Hyphae – filamentous branching structures

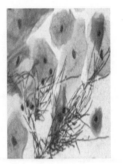

Hyphae in vaginal smear, Candida albicans

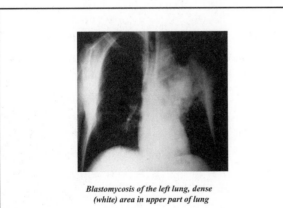

Blastomycosis of the left lung, dense (white) area in upper part of lung

Notes

_____
_____
_____
_____
_____
_____
_____
_____
_____
_____
_____
_____
_____
_____
_____
_____
_____
_____
_____
_____
_____
_____
_____
_____
_____
_____
_____
_____
_____
_____
_____
_____
_____
_____
_____
_____
_____
_____

Discussion

- A young woman receives a course of antibiotics and soon afterward develops a vaginal infection caused by a fungus. Why?
- What factors render a patient susceptible to an infection by a fungus of low pathogenicity?
- How do antibiotics inhibit the growth of bacteria?
- How does penicillin kill bacteria?

Chapter Outline

The chapter outline provides you with an organizational guide to the topics and ideas presented in this chapter of the text.

The Parasite and Its Host
Protozoal Infections
 Malaria
 Amebiasis
 Genital Tract Infections Caused by Trichomonads
 Giardiasis
 Toxoplasmosis
 Cryptosporidiosis
Metazoal Infections
 Roundworms
 Tapeworms
 Flukes
Arthropods

Study Questions

The following questions are provided as a test for comprehension and as a study guide for use with the text chapters. Additional study material is located at http://health.jbpub.com/humandisease/8e, which contains useful tools such as an A&P review, animated flashcards, an interactive online glossary, crossword puzzles, and web links.

Key Terms

Define the following terms:

1. Protozoa _____

2. Metazoa _____

3. *Toxoplasma gondii* _____

4. *Pneumocystis carinii* _____

Fill-in-the-Blank

1. _____ is the large roundworm that lives in the intestinal tract of humans and that is acquired from ingestion of worm eggs.

2. _____ is the small (1 cm long) roundworm that inhabits the colon of infected children and periodically migrates out of the anus at night to deposit eggs on the perianal skin.

3. _____ is the small roundworm that forms cysts in the muscles of infected animals and may cause a serious systemic illness in persons who ingest the cysts contained in incompletely cooked meat.

4. _____ is the long ribbon-like worm that lives in the intestinal tract and that is acquired by eating the flesh of infected animals or fish.

5. _____ is the fluke infestation that causes an itchy skin rash, as a result of swimming in a lake containing the infectious form of the parasite.

6. _____ is the sexually transmitted parasite that causes an intense itching of the pubic skin.

7. _____ is a parasite that infests many birds and animals and that can be transmitted to humans by ingestion of incompletely cooked meat (such as hamburgers) or by contact with infected cats that excrete an infectious form of the parasite in their feces.

Identify

1. Indicate the name of the parasite that causes the following diseases or conditions:

   a. A protozoal disease transmitted by mosquitoes _____

   b. An intestinal infection caused by a pathogenic amoeba _____

   _____

   c. A sexually transmitted infection caused by a small motile parasite that does not form cysts _____

   _____

   d. An intestinal infection caused by a small pear-shaped parasite that causes intestinal cramps and diarrhea

   _____

e. A parasitic infection that may be transmitted from a recently infected pregnant woman to her fetus _____

_____

f. A parasitic infection that may be acquired by contact with cats _____

_____

g. A small parasite that forms highly resistant cysts that may contaminate municipal water supplies, lakes and rivers, and swimming pools; ingestion of the cysts causes cramps and diarrhea _____

_____

h. A small parasite that causes a skin rash _____

2. Identify the three large groups of metazoal parasites.

a. _____

b. _____

c. _____

Matching

Match the parasite in the right column with the clinical manifestation or condition in the left column. Some letters may be used more than once, and some may not be used:

1. ____ "Swimmer's itch"

2. ____ Profuse vaginal discharge

3. ____ Injures the fetus of a pregnant woman

4. ____ Severe life-threatening diarrhea in an immunocompromised person

5. ____ Fever, cough, and pulmonary inflammation

6. ____ Diarrhea from swimming in chlorinated swimming pool

7. ____ Chills and fever

8. ____ Perianal itching awakening a child at night

9. ____ Itching of pubic skin

10. ____ Severe pulmonary infection in an immunocompromised person

A. Pinworms

B. *Plasmodium* species

C. Crab louse

D. *Ascaris* larvae

E. *Trichomonas*

F. *Cryptosporidium*

G. Tapeworm

H. *Toxoplasma*

I. *Schistosomes*

J. *Pneumocystis*

Notes

_____

_____

_____

_____

_____

_____

_____

_____

_____

_____

_____

_____

_____

_____

_____

_____

_____

_____

_____

_____

_____

_____

_____

_____

_____

_____

_____

_____

_____

_____

_____

_____

_____

_____

_____

_____

_____

_____

Chapter 7

Animal Parasites

Learning Objectives

- List common parasitic infections that affect humans.
- Explain mode of transmission
- Describe clinical manifestations and clinical significance

Parasite and Host

- Animal parasites: organisms adapted to living within or on body of another animal (host)
- Not capable of free-living existence
- Have a complex life cycle
- Live within intestinal tract and discharge eggs in feces
- Transmission favored by poor sanitation, high temperature, humidity
- Common in tropical climates, less frequent in cold or temperate climates

Notes

Animal Parasites

- Protozoa
  - One-celled organisms
- Metazoa
  - Multicellular structures
  - Roundworms, tapeworms, flukes
- Arthropods
  - Small insects

Protozoal Infections (1 of 3)

- Microscopic, single-celled organisms
- Diseases: malaria, amoebic dysentery, African sleeping sickness, cryptosporidiosis, toxoplasmosis, giardiasis
- Common in temperate or tropical climates
- Like bacteria, protozoa release toxins and enzymes that destroy cells or interfere with their functions

Protozoal Infections (2 of 3)

- Malaria: caused by various species of Plasmodium
- Amebic dysentery: caused by pathogenic ameba, *Entamoeba histolytica*
- Genital tract trichomonad: caused by *Trichomonas vaginalis*
- Giardiasis: caused by *Giardia lamblia*, infects small intestine; crampy abdominal pain
- Toxoplasmosis: caused by *Toxoplasma gondii*, may infect fetus of pregnant woman and cause congenital malformations

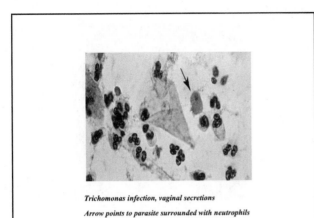

Trichomonas infection, vaginal secretions

Arrow points to parasite surrounded with neutrophils

Protozoal Infections (3 of 3)

- Cryptosporidiosis
  - Caused by a parasite Cryptosporidium parvum; parasitizes the intestinal tract and can cause severe diarrhea
- Pneumocystis pneumonia
  - Caused by Pneumocystis carinii, does not cause disease in immunocompetent persons but causes a severe, sometimes fatal pulmonary infection in persons with HIV/AIDS

Metazoal Infections (1 of 2)

- Roundworm: three most important ones that parasitize human beings:
  - Ascaris: large roundworm that lives within intestinal tract and eggs discharge in feces
  - Pinworms: small roundworm that migrates out of colon through the anus while the infected individual is asleep; deposits its eggs on the perianal skin; frequent in children and spreads through a family
  - Trichinella: small roundworm that parasitizes human and animals; most people become infected by eating improperly cooked pork

Notes

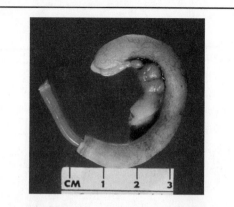

Ascaris in appendix causing symptoms of appendicitis

Metazoal Infections (2 of 2)

- Tapeworms
  - Long, ribbon-like worms that grow to a length of several feet that inhabit the intestinal tract.
  - Humans become infected by eating the flesh of an infected animal that contains the larvae of the parasite.
- Flukes
  - Thick, fleshy, short worms with suckers that attach to the host
  - Some live within the intestinal tract, liver, lungs, venous portal system, some (schistosomes) may infect skin.

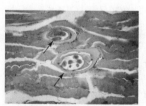 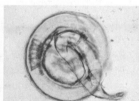

Trichinosis, biopsy of skeletal muscle showing encysted larvae surrounded by fibrous capsules

Trichinosis, higher magnification, unstained coiled larva

Arthropod Infections

- Transmitted by close physical contact and often spread by sexual contact
- Scabies: small parasite burrows in the superficial layers of the skin, where it lays eggs that hatch in a few days
- Crab louse: lives in anal and genital hairs; causes intense itching

Discussion (1 of 2)

- 1. How is malaria transmitted? How does malaria differ from *babesiosis*?
- 2. How do people become infected with pinworms? *Ascaris* infection?
- 3. What are "crabs"? What symptoms do they cause? How are they acquired?

Discussion (2 of 2)

- CASE STUDY
  - Young male, intense itching in pubic area. Small crab lice in pubic hair on exam with numerous eggs on hair shaft. Patient and sexual partner treated with anti-parasitic drug (Kwell)
- CASE STUDY
  - 8 y/o, female, attended a slumber party at neighbor's house. Experienced perianal and vulvar itching that awaken her at night. Mom examined daughter on one such occasion and found 1 cm.-long worm moving around perianal area.

Notes

Chapter Outline

The chapter outline provides you with an organizational guide to the topics and ideas presented in this chapter of the text.

Methods of Transmission and Control
Methods of Transmission
Methods of Control
  Immunization
  Identification, Isolation, and Treatment of Infected Persons
  Control of Means of Indirect Transmission
  Requirements for Effective Control
Sexually Transmitted Diseases
  Syphilis
  Gonorrhea
  Herpes
  Genital Chlamydial Infections
Human Immunodeficiency Virus Infections and AIDS
  HIV and Its Target
  Early Manifestations of HIV Infection
  Late Manifestations of HIV Infection
  Measurements of Viral RNA and CD4 Lymphocytes as an Index of Disease Progression
  Complications of AIDS
  Prevalence of HIV Infection and AIDS in High-Risk Groups
  Prevention and Control of HIV Infection
  Treatment of HIV Infection

Study Questions

The following questions are provided as a test for comprehension and as a study guide for use with the text chapters. Additional study material is located at http://health.jbpub.com/humandisease/8e, which contains useful tools such as an A&P review, animated flashcards, an interactive online glossary, crossword puzzles, and web links.

Key Terms

Define the following terms:

1. Communicable disease _____

2. Chlamydia _____

3. HIV _____

4. AIDS _____

5. Opportunistic infections _____

True/False

Tell whether each statement is true or false. If false, explain why the statement is incorrect.

1. Currently, about 18 percent of all AIDS cases occur in women. _____

_____

2. Among young persons ages 13 to 19 years, most HIV infections occur in males.

_____

3. The drug zidovudine (ZDV), when given to a pregnant HIV-infected mother, significantly reduces the risk of mother-to-infant HIV transmission. _____

_____

4. A newborn infant born to an HIV-infected mother is also treated with ZDV for several weeks after delivery. _____

_____

5. A newborn infant born to an HIV-infected mother may be breastfed because the virus cannot be transmitted by breast milk.

_____

6. Delivery of an HIV-infected mother by cesarean section reduces the risk of mother-to-infant HIV transmission.

_____

Identify

1. Identify the four major sexually transmitted diseases. Indicate in tabular form the major clinical manifestations of each disease and method of treatment.

Disease	Manifestation	Treatment
a.		
b.		
c.		
d.		

2. Identify the three major classes of drugs used to treat HIV infection. Indicate briefly how each class acts to interrupt the replication of HIV.

   a. _____

   b. _____

   c. _____

Discussion Questions

1. Describe how communicable diseases are transmitted. _____

   _____

   _____

   _____

2. Describe how communicable diseases are controlled. _____

   _____

   _____

   _____

3. A woman has been infected with the genital herpes virus (type 2). Describe how she can reduce the risk of transmission of the infection to her sexual partner. _____

   _____

   _____

   _____

4. An HIV-infected woman wishes to become pregnant. What steps can she take to minimize the risk of transmitting the infection to her infant when she becomes pregnant? _____

   _____

   _____

   _____

5. A woman had a test performed for a chlamydial infection, and the test was positive. She is concerned about the consequences of the infection. What would you tell her about the consequences of the infection, the risk of infecting her partner, and steps she should take to eradicate the infection? _____

   _____

   _____

   _____

6. Can an HIV infection be treated? Can it be cured? _____

   _____

   _____

   _____

7. What should an HIV-infected person do to slow the progression of the infection and to prevent transmission of the infection to other persons? _____

_____

_____

8. An HIV-positive woman is considering becoming pregnant. What factors should she consider when she makes a decision as to whether to undertake a pregnancy? _____

_____

_____

9. What are the initial and late manifestations of HIV infection? _____

_____

_____

10. What groups are at high risk of HIV infection? _____

_____

_____

11. How can HIV transmission be reduced or prevented? _____

_____

_____

12. Explain whether each of the following descriptors applies to AIDS. Why or why not?

a. Occurs frequently in homosexual females _____

_____

b. Occurs frequently in homosexual males _____

_____

c. Often fatal as a result of opportunistic infections _____

_____

d. Caused by a virus that damages the immune system _____

_____

e. May be contracted by blood transfusions _____

_____

f. Usually responds to corticosteroids, which stimulate the immune system _____

_____

13. Explain whether each of the following descriptors applies to herpes infection of the genital tract. Why or why not?

    a. A sexually transmitted disease _____

    _____

    b. Initial attack confers permanent immunity _____

    _____

    c. May predispose to cervical carcinoma _____

    _____

    d. Patient may transmit herpes infection from the oral cavity to the genital tract by autoinoculation _____

    _____

    e. Infected woman may transmit virus to her infant during childbirth _____

    _____

    f. Cannot be transmitted to sexual partner unless active lesions present in the genital tract _____

    _____

Notes

Chapter 8

Communicable Diseases

Learning Objectives (1 of 2)

- Explain mode of transmission and control of communicable disease
- Describe herpes infection
  - Symptoms in men and women
  - Effects on sexual partners, fetus, newborn infant
- Describe HIV
  - Pathogenesis, groups affected, effects on immune system
  - Clinical manifestations, test results, methods of prevention

---

Learning Objectives (2 of 2)

- Describe sexually transmitted diseases
  - Major clinical manifestations
  - Complications
  - Methods of treatment

Communicable Diseases

- Communicable disease: disease transmitted from person to person
- Endemic: communicable disease in which a small number of cases are continually present in the population
- Epidemic: communicable disease concurrently affecting large numbers of people in a population

Methods of Transmission

- Communicable disease perpetuates with continuous transmission of infectious agent from person to person by either direct or indirect methods.
- Direct transmission
  - Direct physical contact (sex)
  - Droplet spread (coughing, sneezing)
- Indirect transmission through an intermediary mechanism
  - Contaminated food or water
  - Insects

Methods of Control (1 of 3)

- Must break transmission to eradicate or control disease
- Immunization
  - To reduce number of susceptible persons in the population
    - Disease eventually dies out due to lack of susceptible hosts
    - Smallpox and poliomyelitis have been eliminated due to widespread immunization
  - To protect persons traveling to a geographic area where a disease is endemic

Methods of Control (2 of 3)

- Identification, isolation, and treatment
  - Primary methods of control when immunization is not available
  - Promptly carried out to shorten time in which others may be infected (person-to-person transmission)
  - Isolation: prevents contact with susceptible persons and stops spread
  - If infection is not obvious, disease may not be not recognized and treated, and will continue to spread and be difficult to control (TB, STDs, etc.)

Methods of Control (3 of 3)

- Controlling indirect transmission
  - For contaminated food or water
    - Chlorination of water supplies
    - Effective sewage treatment facilities
    - Standards for handling, manufacturing, and distributing commercially prepared foods
    - Eradication and/or control of animal sources and vectors

Requirements for Effective Control

- Requires knowing cause of disease and methods of transmission
- Otherwise, control measures will be ineffective
- During the bubonic plague or "black death"
  - People did not know that the disease was carried by rodents and the bacterium is transmitted to people by insects
  - May also be spread via droplets causing a pneumonic plague, fatal pulmonary infection

Examples of Methods of Control

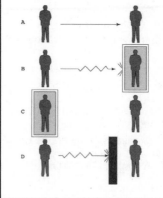

A. **Unimpeded direct or indirect transmission** of a communicable disease from person to person.

B. **Immunization** protects a susceptible person by conferring resistance to infection

C. **Isolation and prompt treatment** of the infected person prevent the spread of disease to susceptible persons.

D. **Control** of means of indirect transmission blocks spread of infectious agent.

Sexually Transmitted Diseases

- Spread primarily by sexual contact
  - Between heterosexual partners
  - Through sexual acts with same sex partner
- Four major STDs
  - Syphilis (*Treponema pallidum*)
  - Gonorrhea (*Neisseria gonorrhoeae*)
  - Herpes (*Herpesvirus*)
  - Chlamydia (*Chlamydia trachomatis*)
- HIV/AIDS: separate class because of high mortality, devastating consequences
  - Spread through heterosexual and homosexual contact
  - Through blood and secretions

Syphilis (1 of 3)

- Treponema pallidum infection
- Major clinical manifestations
- Primary syphilis: chancre
  - Penetrate mucous membranes of genital tract, oral cavity, rectal mucosa, or through break in skin; and multiply rapidly throughout body
  - Forms a chancre: small ulcer at site of inoculation
    - Location: penis, vulva, vagina, oral cavity, or rectum
    - Swarming with treponemas; highly infectious
    - Persists for 4-6 weeks; heals even without treatment
  - Even with healed chancres, treponemas are widely disseminated and continue to multiply

Notes

Syphilis (2 of 3)

- Secondary syphilis: systemic infection with skin rash and enlarged lymph nodes
  - Begins several months after chancre has healed
  - Fever, lymphadenopathy, skin rash, shallow ulcers on mucous membranes of oral cavity and genital tract
  - Persist for several weeks then subsides even without treatment
  - Recurrences subside spontaneously
- Tertiary syphilis: late destructive lesions in internal organs
  - Late manifestations of the disease, may appear 20 years after initial infection; not generally communicable
  - Organisms remain active, causing irreparable organ damage (scarring of aortic valve; degeneration of fiber tracts in spinal cord; mental deterioration; paralysis)

Syphilis (3 of 3)

- Diagnostic tests
  - Microscopic exam
    - Demonstration of treponema from fluid squeezed from chancre
    - Establishes diagnosis several weeks before a blood test becomes positive
  - Serologic tests (antigen-antibody reactions): turns positive soon after chancre appears and remains positive for years
    - Useful for diagnosing disease in asymptomatic individual and in cases where chancre is inaccessible or escapes detection

Congenital Syphilis

- Transmission of disease from mother to child
- May cause death of fetus
- Treatment early in the pregnancy is important as treponemas are less likely to pass through placenta during first few weeks of pregnancy
- During early pregnancy: placental villi are covered by a double layer of epithelium and contain more connective tissue that is less permeable

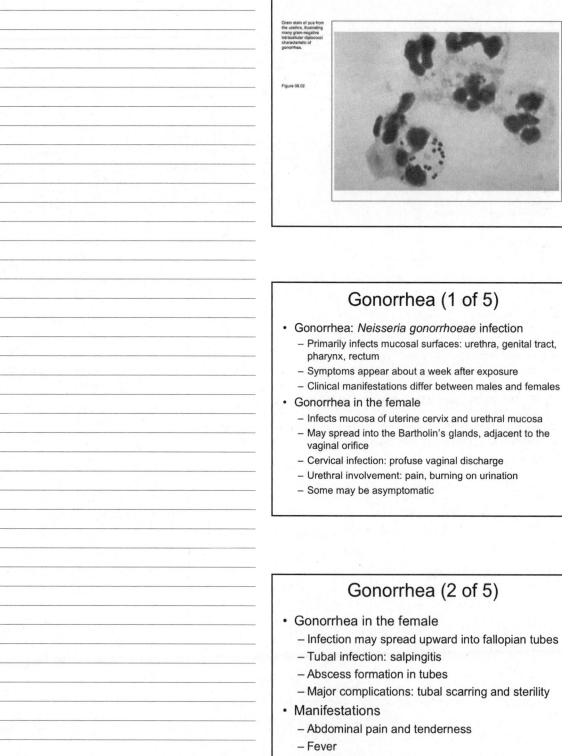

Gram stain of pus from the urethra, illustrating many gram-negative intracellular diplococci characteristic of gonorrhea.

Figure 08.02

Gonorrhea (1 of 5)

- Gonorrhea: *Neisseria gonorrhoeae* infection
  - Primarily infects mucosal surfaces: urethra, genital tract, pharynx, rectum
  - Symptoms appear about a week after exposure
  - Clinical manifestations differ between males and females
- Gonorrhea in the female
  - Infects mucosa of uterine cervix and urethral mucosa
  - May spread into the Bartholin's glands, adjacent to the vaginal orifice
  - Cervical infection: profuse vaginal discharge
  - Urethral involvement: pain, burning on urination
  - Some may be asymptomatic

Gonorrhea (2 of 5)

- Gonorrhea in the female
  - Infection may spread upward into fallopian tubes
  - Tubal infection: salpingitis
  - Abscess formation in tubes
  - Major complications: tubal scarring and sterility
- Manifestations
  - Abdominal pain and tenderness
  - Fever
  - Leukocytosis

Gonorrhea (3 of 5)

- Gonorrhea in the male
  - Acute inflammation of mucosa of anterior urethra
  - Purulent urethral discharge
  - Pain on urination
  - Less likely to be asymptomatic in males than females
- Major complications
  - Spread of infection to posterior urethra, prostate, seminal vesicles, vasa deferentia, and epididymis
  - Sterility: infection in vasa deferentia and epididymis may lead to scarring, blocking the transport of sperm

Gonorrhea (4 of 5)

- Extragenital gonorrhea
  - Rectum: pain and tenderness; purulent bloody mucoid discharge
  - From either anal intercourse or contamination of rectal mucosa from infected vaginal secretions
  - Pharynx and tonsils: oral-genital sex acts
- Disseminated gonococcal infection
  - Organisms gain access into bloodstream and spread throughout body
  - Fever; joint pain; multiple small skin abscesses; infections of the joints, tendons, heart valves; meninges

Gonorrhea (5 of 5)

- Diagnosis and treatment
  - Culture
    - Suspected sites: urethra, cervix, rectum, pharynx
    - Blood in disseminated infections
  - Nucleic acid amplification test: based on identification of nucleic acids in organism
- Treatment: antibiotics
  - Penicillin-resistant strains due to penicillinase enzyme

Notes

Notes

Herpes (1 of 3)

- Herpes: Herpes simplex virus infection
- Two types are not restricted in distribution
- Type 1: infects oral mucous membrane
  - Causes fever blisters, usually infected in childhood, most adults have antibodies to virus
  - May cause genital infections
- Type 2: infects genital tract
  - Infections usually occur after puberty
  - Causes 80% of infections
  - 20% from type 1 due to oral-genital sexual practices
  - May infect oropharyngeal mucous membranes

Herpes (2 of 3)

- Vesicles and shallow ulcers following sexual exposure
- Men: glans or shaft of penis
- Women: extensive involvement
  - Vulva: usually painful
  - Vagina, cervix: little discomfort
- Vesicles: small, painful blisters on external genitalia and genital tract; rupture and form shallow ulcers that coalesce
- Contain large quantities of virus and are infectious to sexual contacts
- Regional lymph nodes are enlarged and tender
- Virus persists in infected tissues causing recurrent infections

Herpes (3 of 3)

- Diagnosis
  - Intranuclear inclusions in infected cells
  - Viral cultures from vesicles or ulcers most reliable diagnostic test
  - Serologic tests in some cases
- Treatment
  - Antiviral drug shortens course and reduces severity, but do not eradicate virus (orally, per IV, or topically)
  - Cold compress and pain relievers
- Major complication: spread from infected mother to infant through active herpetic lesions in mother's genital tract
- Delivery should be by cesarean section

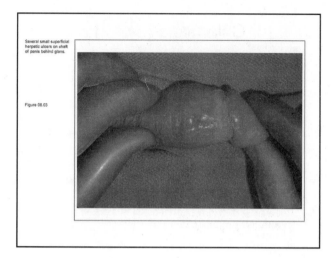

Several small superficial herpetic ulcers on shaft of penis behind glans.

Figure 08.03

Vaginal smear illustrating clusters of herpes-infected epithelial cells containing intranuclear inclusions.

Figure 08.05

Chlamydia (1 of 2)

- *Chlamydia trachomatis* infection; most common STD
- Rise in cases:
  - 3-4 million cases/year
  - From increased recognition due to availability of new diagnostic tests
- Clinical manifestations: similar to gonorrhea
- Women: cervicitis and urethritis
  - Involves uterine cervix, urethra; moderate vaginal discharge
- Men: Non-gonococcal urethritis: an acute urethral inflammation with frequency and burning on urination
- Major complications: sterility in women; epididymitis in men

Chlamydia (2 of 2)

- Tests for diagnosis
  - Detection of Chlamydial antigens in cervical/urethral secretions
  - Fluorescence microscopy
  - Cultures
  - Nucleic acid amplification tests: based on Chlamydial nucleic acids
- Cases
  - 10% to 20%: among young sexually active females attending family planning clinics
  - 17% to 46% among clients in STD clinics
- Treatment: antibiotics

TABLE 8-1

Comparison of four major sexually transmitted diseases

	SYPHILIS	GONORRHEA	HERPES	CHLAMYDIA
Organism	Treponema pallidum	Gonococcus (Neisseria gonorrhoeae)	Herpes virus	Chlamydia trachomatis
Major clinical manifestations	Primary: chancre. Secondary: systemic infection with skin rash and enlarged lymph nodes. Tertiary: late destructive lesions in internal organs	Urethritis. Cervicitis. Pharyngitis. Infection of rectal mucosa (proctitis)	Superficial vesicles and ulcers on external genitalia and in genital tract. Regional lymph nodes often enlarged and tender	Cervicitis. Urethritis
Tests used to establish diagnosis	Demonstration of treponemas in chancre. Serologic tests	Culture of organisms from sites of infection. Nonculture tests also available	Demonstration of intranuclear inclusions in infected cells. Virus cultures. Serologic tests in some cases	Detection of chlamydial antigens in cervical/urethral secretions. Fluorescence microscopy. Cultures. Nonculture tests also available
Major complications	Damage to cardiovascular system and nervous system in tertiary syphilis may be fatal	Disseminated bloodstream infection. Tubal infection with impaired fertility. Spread of infection to prostate and epididymides	Spread from infected mother to infant	Tubal infection with impaired fertility. Epididymitis
Treatment	Antibiotics	Antibiotics	Antiviral drug shortens infection but not curative	Antibiotics

---

Sexually Transmitted Diseases

- Other common but less serious STDs
  - Condylomas: anal and genital warts
  - Vaginitis: *Gardnerella*
  - Trichomonal vaginitis: *Trichomonas vaginalis* infection
  - Scabies and crabs
  - Hepatitis

HIV/AIDS

- Cripples body's immune system
- Attacks and destroys T lymphocytes increasing susceptibility to infections and malignant tumors
- AIDS: end stage and most serious manifestation
- Causes
  - HIV-1: causes AIDS in most parts of the world
  - HIV-2: causes AIDS in Western Africa
- 1981: First AIDS case identified in a small group of homosexual men with an unusual opportunistic lung infection
- 1983: HIV case identified
- 1985: blood test to detect HIV infection

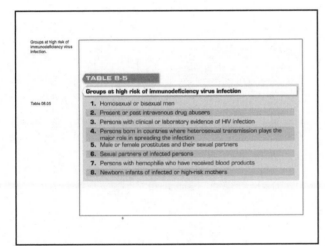

Groups at high risk of immunodeficiency virus infection.

Table 08.05

TABLE 8-5

Groups at high risk of immunodeficiency virus infection

1. Homosexual or bisexual men
2. Present or past intravenous drug abusers
3. Persons with clinical or laboratory evidence of HIV infection
4. Persons born in countries where heterosexual transmission plays the major role in spreading the infection
5. Male or female prostitutes and their sexual partners
6. Sexual partners of infected persons
7. Persons with hemophilia who have received blood products
8. Newborn infants of infected or high-risk mothers

HIV and Its Target

- Target: CD4 protein on cell membranes of helper T lymphocytes, monocytes, macrophages, macrophage-like cells in skin, lymph nodes, and CNS
- CD4 functions as a receptor for virus
  - HIV: an RNA-containing retrovirus
  - Core contains RNA and enzyme reverse transcriptase contained within a protein coat or capsid
  - Core surrounded by a double-layered lipid envelope acquired from the cell membrane of infected cell when virus buds out from cell

Notes

Viral Replication

- Virus binds to cell, viral envelope fuses with cell membrane and virus enters cell
- Once inside cell, virus makes a DNA copy of its RNA genetic material (reverse transcriptase enzyme)
- DNA copy inserted into cell's genetic material (HIV integrase enzyme)
- Viral genes direct synthesis and assembly of more virus particles
- Viral protein assembled into small segments around viral RNA and bud out of cells coated with the cell membrane of infected cells (HIV protease enzyme)

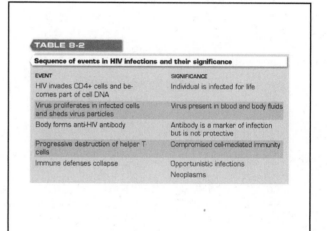

TABLE 8-2

Sequence of events in HIV infections and their significance

EVENT	SIGNIFICANCE
HIV invades CD4+ cells and becomes part of cell DNA	Individual is infected for life
Virus proliferates in infected cells and sheds virus particles	Virus present in blood and body fluids
Body forms anti-HIV antibody	Antibody is a marker of infection but is not protective
Progressive destruction of helper T cells	Compromised cell-mediated immunity
Immune defenses collapse	Opportunistic infections Neoplasms

Clinical Manifestations (1 of 2)

- Virus attacks and kills helper T cells and monocytes
- Monocytes survive but virus continues to replicate in monocytes and transports virus throughout body and brain
- Patient susceptible to opportunistic infections and cancer due to resulting immunodeficiency
- Early stage
  - Large amount of virus detected in blood and body fluids
  - Large numbers of infected lymphocytes in lymph nodes
  - Mild febrile illness
  - Body responds by forming anti-HIV antibodies (in 1 to 6 months after initial infection) and cytotoxic T cells
  - Amount of virus declines but body's defenses cannot eliminate virus

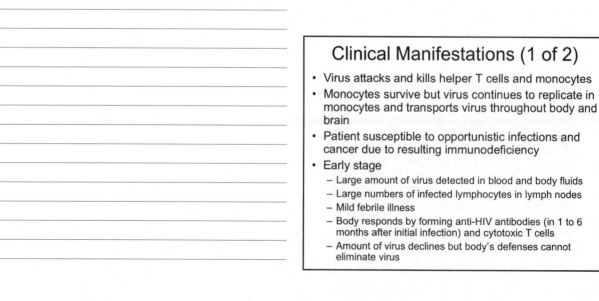

Clinical Manifestations (2 of 2)

- NO latent or dormant phase where virus remains inactive
- Large numbers of virus produced continuously that infect and destroy CD4 cells and circulate in bloodstream
- Amount of virus correlates with magnitude of infection
- Chronic stage
  - Eventually rate at which CD4 cells are replaced cannot keep up with rate of destruction
  - Some strains of HIV may be aggressive, others benign
  - Current anti-viral drugs can suppress proliferation and damage but CANNOT completely eliminate the virus, which persists indefinitely in infected tissues of host

Antibody Response to HIV (1 of 2)

- Antibody response to HIV
  - Antibodies are formed within 1-6 months
  - Detection of antibodies provides evidence of HIV infection
  - Antibodies do not eradicate virus
  - Virus is detectable only by laboratory tests
- Signs and symptoms of AIDS
  - After a high-risk exposure and inoculation, infected person usually experiences a mononucleosis-like syndrome that may be attributed to flu or another virus
  - Infected person may remain asymptomatic for years
  - At early stage, only sign of HIV infection is laboratory evidence of sero-conversion

Antibody Response to HIV (2 of 2)

- Symptoms take many forms
  - Persistent generalized lymphadenopathy caused by impaired function of CD4 cells
  - Nonspecific symptoms: weight loss, fatigue, night sweats, fevers related to altered function of CD4 cells
  - Immunodeficiency
  - Infection of other CD4 antigen-bearing cells
  - Neurologic symptoms resulting from HIV encephalopathy and infection of neuroglial cells

Notes

Early and Late Manifestations of HIV Infection

- Early
  - Asymptomatic
  - Mild febrile illness
- Late
  - Generalized lymph node enlargement
  - Non-specific symptoms
  - Fever, weakness, chronic fatigue, weight loss, thrombocytopenia
  - AIDS

Index of Disease

- Measurement of viral RNA and CD4 lymphocytes
- Viral replication: measure amount of viral RNA in blood
  - Virus replicates in lymph nodes but amount of viral RNA in blood reflects extent of viral replication in lymphoid tissue
- Damage to immune system: measure number of CD4 lymphocytes in blood
  - Normal level: 800-1200
  - Number declines progressively as disease advances
  - Below 500: risk of opportunistic infections
  - Below 200: risk of major HIV complication

Complications of AIDS

- Opportunistic infections from organisms not normally pathogenic or of limited pathogenicity
  - *Pneumocystis carinii* pneumonia
  - *Mycobacterium avium-intracellulare*
  - Parasitic infections: toxoplasmosis; cryptosporidiosis
  - Rapidly progressive tuberculosis or histoplasmosis
- Malignant tumors in AIDS patients
  - Kaposi's sarcoma: human herpes virus 8
  - Malignant tumors of B lymphocytes
  - Cancers of oral cavity, rectum, uterine cervix

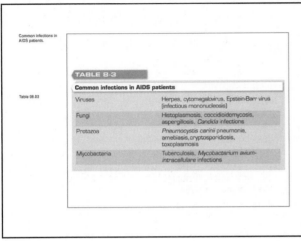

Common infections in
AIDS patients.

Table 08.03

TABLE 8-3	
Common infections in AIDS patients	
Viruses	Herpes, cytomegalovirus, Epstein-Barr virus (infectious mononucleosis)
Fungi	Histoplasmosis, coccidioidomycosis, aspergillosis, *Candida* infections
Protozoa	*Pneumocystis carinii* pneumonia, amebiasis, cryptosporidiosis, toxoplasmosis
Mycobacteria	Tuberculosis, *Mycobacterium avium-intracellulare* infections

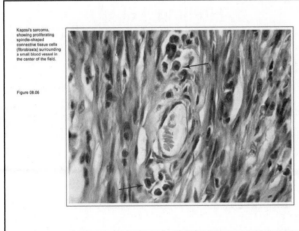

Kaposi's sarcoma,
showing proliferating
spindle-shaped
connective tissue cells
(fibroblasts) surrounding
a small blood vessel in
the center of the field.

Figure 08.06

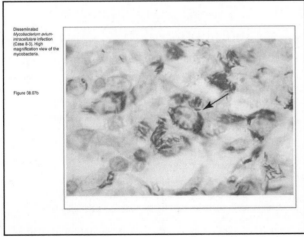

Disseminated
*Mycobacterium avium-
intracellulare* infection
(Case 8-3). High
magnification view of the
mycobacteria.

Figure 08.07b

Notes

_____
_____
_____
_____
_____
_____
_____
_____
_____
_____
_____
_____
_____
_____
_____
_____
_____
_____
_____
_____
_____
_____
_____
_____
_____
_____
_____
_____
_____
_____
_____
_____
_____
_____

HIV Transmission

- HIV virus may enter body by any of several routes
  - Sexual contact
  - Blood and body fluids
  - Mother to infant
- Transmission by blood and blood products
  - Direct inoculation: intimate sexual contact, linked to mucosal trauma from rectal intercourse
  - Transfusion: contaminated blood or blood products, lessened by routine testing of all blood products
  - Sharing of contaminated injection needles
  - Transplacental or postpartum transmission via cervical or blood contact at delivery and in breast milk
- Not transmitted by casual household or social contacts

Treatment of HIV Infections/AIDS (1 of 3)

- No cure for AIDS
- Primary therapy includes use of various combinations of three different types of antiretroviral agents to maximally inhibit HIV viral replication with fewer adverse reactions
- Treatment schedules revised as new drugs are developed and as advantages and side effects of various drug combinations are recognized

Treatment of HIV Infections/AIDS (2 of 3)

- Drugs given in combination to target different phases of the virus life cycle.
- Main groups
  - Non-nucleoside reverse transcriptase inhibitors
  - Nucleoside reverse transcriptase inhibitors (nucleoside analogs)
  - Protease inhibitors
  - Another class of drugs (integrase inhibitors) is under development
- Additional treatment:
  - Supportive therapy, nutritional support, fluid and electrolyte replacement therapy, pain relief, psychological support

Treatment of HIV Infections/AIDS (3 of 3)

- Protease inhibitors: block action of viral protease in viral replication; cut viral protein into short segments to assemble around viral RNA to form infectious particles
  - Drugs reduce number of new virus particles produced
- Reverse-transcriptase inhibitors interfere with copying of viral RNA into DNA by the enzyme reverse transcriptase
  - Drugs substitute a nucleoside analog that resembles normal nucleosides used by virus to construct DNA
  - Virus cannot distinguish between analog and normal nucleoside interrupting viral DNA synthesis

Discussion

- CASE STUDY
  - 39-year-old homosexual male with multiple sexual partners and a positive HIV test had been treated on several occasions for *Candida* infections of the mouth and intermittent chronic diarrhea. He recently developed a red vascular nodule in the oral cavity that was biopsied.
  - Given the patient's history, what is the clinical implication of the tumor in his mouth?
  - What organism is known to cause this tumor?

Notes

Chapter Outline

The chapter outline provides you with an organizational guide to the topics and ideas presented in this chapter of the text.

Causes of Congenital Malformations
Chromosomal Abnormalities
    Sex Chromosome Abnormalities
    Autosomal Abnormalities
Genetically Determined Diseases
    Autosomal Dominant Inheritance
    Autosomal Recessive Inheritance
    Codominant Inheritance
    X-Linked Inheritance
Intrauterine Injury
    Harmful Drugs and Chemicals
    Radiation
    Maternal Infections
Multifactorial Inheritance
Prenatal Diagnosis of Congenital Abnormalities

Study Questions

The following questions are provided as a test for comprehension and as a study guide for use with the text chapters. Additional study material is located at http://health.jbpub.com/humandisease/8e, which contains useful tools such as an A&P review, animated flashcards, an interactive online glossary, crossword puzzles, and web links.

Key Terms

Define the following terms:

1. Sex chromosome body _____

2. Chromosome nondisjunction _____

3. Chromosome translocation _____

4. Chromosome deletion _____

5. Trisomy 21 _____

Fill-in-the-Blank

1. _____ is a hereditary blood disease or condition transmitted by codominant inheritance.

2. _____ is a hereditary disease in which transmission follows an autosomal recessive inheritance pattern.

3. _____ is a hereditary disease in which transmission follows an autosomal dominant inheritance pattern.

4. _____ is a hereditary disease in which the mutant gene is transmitted on the X chromosome.

5. The incidence of congenital malformations in aborted embryos and fetuses is approximately _____.

6. Absence of chromosome 21 is called _____.

7. Most cases of Down syndrome result from _____.

True/False

Tell whether each statement is true or false. If false, explain why the statement is incorrect.

1. Some congenital abnormalities (such as congenital absence of the kidneys) may be incompatible with life after delivery. _____

_____

2. Chromosomal abnormalities in the fetus can usually be determined by amniocentesis. _____

_____

3. Cleft palate often results from interaction of genetic and environmental factors. _____

_____

4. German measles acquired by the mother during pregnancy leads to *chromosomal* abnormalities in the fetus.

_____

5. Infants born with Down syndrome usually have an extra X chromosome. _____

_____

6. Patients born with genetically determined defects (such as phenylketonuria) have normal chromosome karyotypes. _____

7. Fertilized ova contain 23 chromosomes. _____

8. Spermatozoa usually have more chromosomes than do unfertilized ova. _____

9. Most persons with Turner's syndrome have only a single X chromosome (45,X). _____

10. A pregnant woman with phenylketonuria does not need to adhere to a phenylalanine-restricted diet because the high concentration of phenylalanine in the woman's blood does not harm the fetus. _____

11. An increased concentration of alpha fetoprotein in maternal blood or amnionic fluid suggests that the fetus has Down's syndrome.

_____

12. Most infants with Down syndrome are born to mothers who are carriers of chromosome 21, which is attached to another chromosome (translocation carrier). _____

13. A neural tube defect (anencephaly or spina bifida) usually can be identified in an affected fetus by means of an ultrasound examination performed at about 16 weeks, gestation. _____

Identify

1. Identify the four main causes of congenital abnormalities.

   a. _____

   b. _____

   c. _____

   d. _____

2. Identify three maternal infections that may lead to congenital abnormalities in the fetus.

   a. _____

   b. _____

   c. _____

Matching

Match the chromosomal abnormality in the right column with the clinical condition in the left column.

1. ____ Turner syndrome   A. 47,XXX

2. ____ Klinefelter syndrome   B. 45,X

3. ____ Triple X syndrome   C. Trisomy of chromosome 21

4. ____ Down syndrome   D. 47,XXY

Discussion Questions

1. What is the difference between mitosis and meiosis? _____

_____

_____

_____

2. What is the difference between a sex chromosome and an autosome? _____

_____

_____

_____

3. What is a karyotype? How is it determined? _____

_____

_____

_____

4. What is the incidence of congenital abnormalities? _____

_____

_____

_____

5. What is the significance of a reciprocal translocation of chromosome fragments between two nonhomologous chromosomes? (*Hint:* see Case 9-1.) _____

_____

_____

_____

6. What is Down syndrome? Under what conditions may this syndrome occur? _____

_____

_____

_____

7. Describe the role of amniocentesis or chorionic villus sampling in the prenatal diagnosis of Down syndrome.

_____

_____

_____

8. Describe the effect of thalidomide taken by the mother on the development of the fetus. Is this drug still available?

_____

_____

_____

9. Describe how drugs are classified on the basis of possible risk to the fetus when taken by the pregnant woman.

_____

_____

_____

10. What does the term "multifactorial inheritance" mean? Give examples of diseases or conditions transmitted in this way. _____

_____

_____

_____

11. Describe the role of amniocentesis in prenatal detection of fetal abnormalities. Indicate what type of congenital abnormalities can be detected by this method, and indicate in which group of patients the method is most widely used. _____

_____

_____

_____

12. What methods can provide information about the number of X chromosomes possessed by an individual? _____

_____

_____

_____

13. What syndromes and conditions result from an abnormal number of sex chromosomes? _____

_____

_____

_____

14. Explain whether each of the following conditions or situations affecting the mother may lead to congenital malformations in the developing fetus.

a. Heavy cigarette smoking _____

_____

b. Heavy alcohol consumption _____

_____

c. Ingestion of a tetracycline antibiotic _____

_____

d. Penicillin tablets (ampicillin) given to a mother to treat a urinary tract infection _____

_____

e. Dilantin taken by the mother to prevent epileptic seizures _____

_____

f. Excessive use of chewing gum _____

_____

g. Maternal infection by virus of German measles _____

_____

h. Maternal *Toxoplasma* infection _____

_____

i. Excessive consumption of egg salad sandwiches _____

_____

Notes

Chapter 9

Congenital and Hereditary Diseases

Learning Objectives (1 of 2)

- Describe
  - Common causes of congenital malformations and their incidence
  - Abnormalities of sex chromosomes and manifestations
  - Common genetic abnormalities and transmission
- Compare phenylketonuria versus hemophilia in terms of transmission and clinical manifestations
- Describe congenital malformations resulting from uterine injury

Learning Objectives (2 of 2)

- Explain
  - Amniocentesis
  - Multifactorial inheritance
  - Example of multifactorial defect and relevant factors
- List causes and clinical manifestations of Down syndrome
- Discuss reasons for identifying 14/21 chromosome translocation carrier
- Explain methods for diagnosing congenital abnormalities.

Hereditary and Congenital Malformations

- Congenital disease: abnormality present at birth, even though it may not be detected until some time after birth
- Hereditary or genetic disease: resulting from a chromosome abnormality or a defective gene

Genetics (1 of 5)

- Genetics: study of heredity; transmission of physical, biochemical, and physiologic traits from biological parents to their children
- Disorders can be transmitted by gene mutations that can result in disability or death
- Genetic information is carried in genes strung together on strands of DNA to form chromosomes
- Except reproductive cells, every normal human cell has 46 chromosomes

Genetics (2 of 5)

- Chromosomes: composed of double coils of DNA
- Genes: segments of DNA chains
- Genome: sum total of all genes contained in a cell's chromosomes; the same in all cells
- In human beings, normal chromosome component:
  - 22 pairs of autosomes
  - 1 pair of sex chromosomes (XX in females and XY in males)
- Karyotype: a representation of a person's set of chromosomes

Genetics (3 of 5)

- In somatic cells: chromosomes exist in pairs, one member of each pair is derived from male parent and other from female parent
  - With 22 pairs called autosomes
  - Except for the sex chromosomes, members of the pair are similar in size, shape, and appearance (homologous chromosomes)
- Mitosis: cell division of somatic cells
  - Each of two new cells or daughter cells receives the same chromosomes as the parent cell

Genetics (4 of 5)

- Not all genes are expressed in all cells and not all genes active all the time
- Meiosis: cell division that occurs during development of egg and sperm
  - Number of chromosomes is reduced
  - Daughter cells receive only half of chromosomes possessed by the parent cell
- DNA ultimately controls formation of essential substances throughout the life of every cell in the body through the genetic code (precise sequence of AT and CG pairs on the DNA molecule)

Genetics (5 of 5)

- Genes control
  - Hereditary traits, cell reproduction, and daily functions of all cells
  - Cell function, through structures and chemicals made within the cell
  - RNA formation that controls formation of specific proteins; most are enzymes that assist in chemical reactions in cells

Notes

Notes

Trait Predominance (1 of 2)

- Each parent contributes 1 set of chromosomes (or a set of genes) so that every child has two genes for every locus on the autosomal chromosomes
- Some characteristics or traits of the child are determined by 1 gene that may have many variants (e.g. eye color)
- Polygenic traits require interaction of ≥ 1 genes
  - Environmental factors may affect how genes are expressed
- Alleles: variations in a particular gene
- Homozygous: has identical alleles on each chromosome
- Heterozygous: alleles are different

Trait Predominance (2 of 2)

- Children will express a dominant allele when one or both chromosomes in a pair carry it
- A recessive allele is expressed only if both chromosomes carry the recessive alleles
- For example, a child may receive a gene for brown eyes from one parent and a gene for blue eyes from the other parent
  - Gene for brown eyes is dominant
  - Gene for blue eyes is recessive
  - The dominant gene is more likely to be expressed and child is more likely to have brown eyes

Autosomal Inheritance

- For unknown reasons, on autosomal chromosomes, one allele may be more influential than the other in determining a specific trait
- The more powerful or dominant gene is more likely to be expressed than the recessive gene

Sex-Linked Inheritance

- X and Y chromosomes are not literally a pair, as X is much larger than the Y chromosome
- One X chromosome is inactivated (Lyon Hypothesis)
  - In males: one copy of most genes is on the X chromosome
  - Inheritance of these genes is called X-linked
  - A man will transmit one copy of each X-linked gene to his daughters and none to his sons
  - A woman will transmit one copy to each daughter or son

Multifactorial Inheritance

- Environmental factors can affect the expression of some genes
- Example: child's height will be within the range of height of both parents, but environmental factors such as nutritional patterns and health care also influence development
  - The better nourished, healthier children of two short parents may be taller than either

Genetically Determined Diseases

- Result from abnormalities of individual genes on the chromosomes
- Chromosomes appear normal.
- Some defects arise spontaneously.
- Others may be caused by environmental teratogens (agents or influences that cause physical defects in the developing embryo)
- **Mutation**: permanent change in genetic material that may occur spontaneously or after exposure of a cell to radiation, certain chemicals, or viruses

Factors in Congenital Malformations

- Genetic or hereditary disorders or diseases caused by abnormalities in an individual's genetic material (genome)
- Congenital disease or malformation: any abnormality present at birth
- Four factors in congenital malformations
  - 1. Chromosomal abnormalities
  - 2. Abnormalities of individual genes
  - 3. Intrauterine injury to embryo or fetus
  - 4. Environmental factors

Causes of Congenital Malformations

- 2-3% of all newborn infants have congenital defects
- Additional 2-3% defects: NOT recognized at birth; developmental defects demonstrated later as infants grow older
- 25% to 50% spontaneously aborted embryos, fetuses, and stillborn infants have major malformations

Chromosomal Abnormalities

- Nondisjunction: failure of homologous chromosomes in germ cells to separate in first or second meiotic division
  - May involve either sex chromosomes or autosomes
  - Causes abnormalities in distribution of chromosomes between germ cells
  - One of two germ cells has an extra chromosome while the other lacks a chromosome
- Monosomy: absence of a chromosome in a cell
- Trisomy: presence of an extra chromosome in a cell
- Deletions: chromosome breaks during meiosis and broken piece is lost
- Translocations: misplaced chromosome or part of it attaches to another chromosome

Sex Chromosome Abnormalities
(1 of 3)

- Variations in normal number of sex chromosomes are often associated with some reduction of intelligence
  - Y chromosome: directs masculine sexual differentiation, associated with male body configuration regardless of number of X chromosomes present
  - Extra Y: no significant effect as it mainly carries genes concerned with male sexual differentiation
  - Absent Y: body configuration is female
  - Extra X in female: has little effect (one X chromosome is inactivated)
  - Extra X in male: has adverse effects on male development

Sex Chromosome Abnormalities
(2 of 3)

- Two most common ones in the female
  - 1. Turner's Syndrome: absence of one X chromosome
  - 2. Triple X Syndrome: extra X chromosome
- Two most common ones in the male
  - 1. Klinefelter's Syndrome: extra X chromosome
  - 2. XYY Syndrome: extra Y chromosome

Sex Chromosome Abnormalities
(3 of 3)

- Fragile X Syndrome (x-linked mental deficiency)
- Not related to either excess or deficiency of sex chromosomes
- Associated with a characteristic abnormality of the X chromosome
- Second to Down syndrome as a major cause of mental deficiency

TABLE 9-1

Syndromes resulting from an abnormal complement of sex chromosomes

	USUAL GENOTYPE	APPROXIMATE INCIDENCE	UNUSUAL NUMBER OF BARR BODIES	UNUSUAL NUMBER OF Y FLUORESCENT BODIES	FERTILITY
Turner's syndrome	45,X	1:2500 females	0	0	Sterile
Triple X syndrome	47,XXX	1:850 males	2	0	Usually not impaired
Klinefelter's syndrome	47,XXY	1:750 males	1	1	Usually sterile
XYY syndrome	47,XYY	1:850 males	0	2	Usually not impaired

Autosomal Abnormalities (1 of 3)

- Absence of an autosome results in the loss of several genes that development is generally not possible and the embryo is aborted.
- Deletion of a small part of an autosome may be compatible with development but usually results in multiple severe congenital abnormalities.
- **Down syndrome: most common chromosomal abnormality**, an autosomal trisomy

Autosomal Abnormalities (2 of 3)

- With trisomy of small chromosome 21
- Many fetuses are aborted early in pregnancy (70%)
- Those who live have Down syndrome
  - Nondisjunction during oogenesis occurs in 95% of cases
- Increased frequency with advancing maternal age: 1 in 50 if mother is > 40 years old
- Extra chromosome 21 acquired as part of the translocation chromosome

Autosomal Abnormalities (3 of 3)

- Nondisjunction occurring in zygote
  - Most common chromosomal abnormality: 1:600 births
  - Manifestations: mental deficiency, cardiac malformation, major defects in other organ systems
- Trisomy of chromosome 13: Cleft lip and palate; abnormal development of skull, brain, and eyes; congenital heart defect; polydactyly
- Trisomy of chromosome 18:
- Both 13 and 18 trisomies are usually fatal in the neonatal period or in early infancy

Notes

Down Syndrome

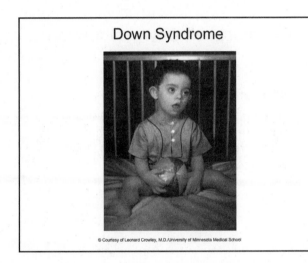

© Courtesy of Leonard Crowley, M.D./University of Minnesota Medical School

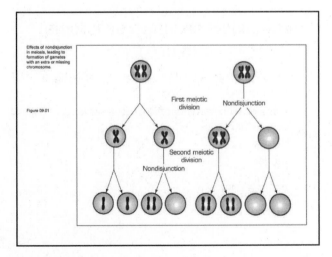

Effects of nondisjunction in meiosis, leading to formation of gametes with an extra or missing chromosome.

Figure 09.01

Translocation Down syndrome (1 of 3)

- Occurs in small number of persons with Down syndrome
- Extra chromosome: chromosome 21 fused with chromosome 14 or another chromosome
- Total number of chromosomes not increased but genetic material is equivalent to 47 chromosomes
- Causes
  - Normal chromosomes in cells of both parents
    - Translocation occurred accidentally during gametogenesis in the germ cells of one of the parents
  - 14/21 carrier in one of the parents
    - Carrier parent has only 45 chromosomes because one is the fusion of chromosome 21 with 14

Translocation Down syndrome (2 of 3)

- 14/21 carrier in one of the parents
- Carrier parent is capable of transmitting abnormal chromosome to his or her children resulting in translocation Down syndrome

Translocation Down syndrome (3 of 3)

- Possible outcomes of pregnancy involving a female carrier
  - Translocation chromosome is nor always transmitted
  - Normal
  - Carrier
  - Nonviable
  - Down Syndrome

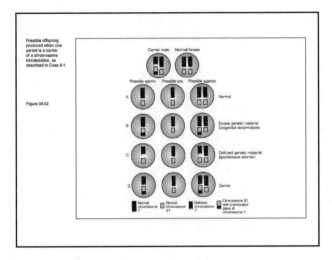

Possible offspring produced when one parent is a carrier of a chromosome translocation, as described in Case 9-1.

Figure 09.02

Transmission of Genetically Determined Diseases

- Autosomal dominant inheritance
- Autosomal recessive inheritance
- Codominant inheritance
- X-linked inheritance
- Most hereditary diseases are transmitted on autosomes
- Few are carried on sex chromosomes

TABLE 9-2

Mode of inheritance, pathogenesis, and major manifestations of some common genetic diseases

ABNORMALITY	MODE OF INHERITANCE	DEFECT	MANIFESTATIONS
Phenylketonuria	Recessive	Phenylalanine hydroxylase deficiency	Mental retardation
Tay-Sachs disease	Recessive	Hexosaminidase A deficiency	Mental retardation, motor weakness, blindness
Cystic fibrosis of pancreas	Recessive	Dysfunction of mucous and sweat glands; thick mucus obstructs bronchioles, pancreatic ducts, and bile ducts	Chronic broncho-pulmonary infections as a result of bronchial obstruction by mucus; pancreatic and liver dysfunction as a result of thick mucous obstruction of excretory ducts
Achondroplasia	Dominant	Disordered bone growth at ends of long bones (epiphyses)	Dwarfism with disproportionately short limbs
Congenital polycystic kidney disease (one type)	Dominant	Maldevelopment of nephrons and collecting tubules causes formation of multiple cysts in kidneys	Renal failure
Multiple neurofibromatosis	Dominant	Multiple tumors arise from peripheral nerves	Disfigurement and deformities caused by tumors; predisposition to malignant change in tumors
Sickle cell trait	Codominant	Red cells contain mixture of normal (A) and sickle (S) hemoglobin	None
Sickle cell anemia	Codominant	Red cells contain no normal hemoglobin	Severe anemia and obstruction of blood flow to organs by means of sickled red cells
Hemophilia	X-linked recessive	Deficiency of protein required for normal coagulation of blood	Uncontrolled bleeding into joints and internal organs after minor injuries

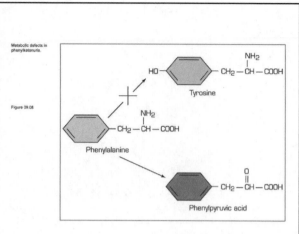

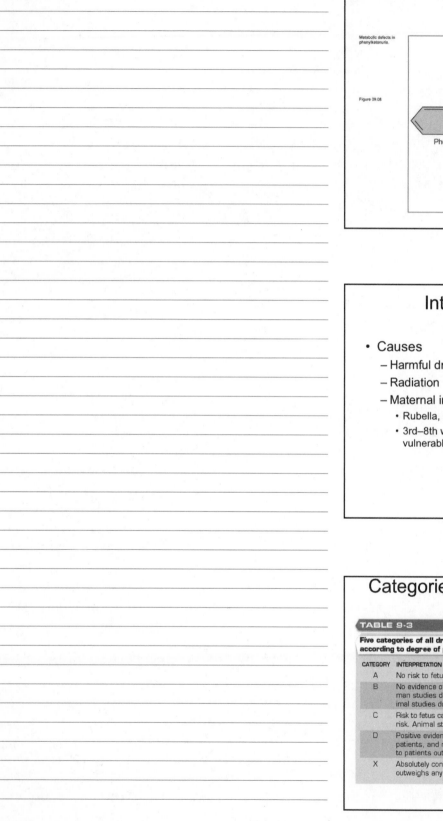

Intrauterine Injury

- Causes
  - Harmful drugs and chemicals (Table 9-3)
  - Radiation
  - Maternal infections (Figure 9-11)
    - Rubella, cytomegalovirus, *Toxoplasma gondii*
    - 3rd–8th week after conception: embryo is most vulnerable to injury as organ systems are forming

Categories of Drugs Harmful to Fetus

TABLE 9-3

Five categories of all drugs used in the United States rated by the FDA according to degree of possible risk to the fetus

CATEGORY	INTERPRETATION
A	No risk to fetus demonstrated in well-controlled studies in humans.
B	No evidence of risk to fetus. Either animal studies show risk but human studies do not or there are no adequate human studies but animal studies do not indicate risk.
C	Risk to fetus cannot be ruled out. No human studies available to assess risk. Animal studies either are not available or indicate possible risk.
D	Positive evidence of risk to fetus; however, drug is needed to treat patients, and no safer alternative drug is available. Potential benefit to patients outweighs risk to fetus.
X	Absolutely contraindicated in pregnancy. Severe risk to fetus greatly outweighs any possible benefit to patients.

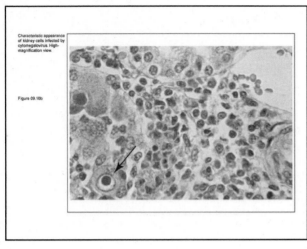

Characteristic appearance of kidney cells infected by cytomegalovirus. High-magnification view.

Figure 09.10b

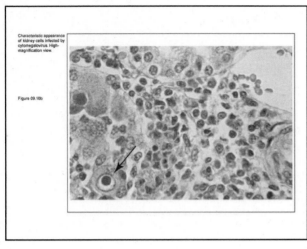

Cytomegalovirus infection in newborn

Multifactorial Inheritance

- Combined effect of multiple genes interacting with environmental agents
- Congenital abnormalities
  - Cleft lip, cleft palate, cardiac malformations, clubfoot, dislocation of hip, anencephaly, spina bifida

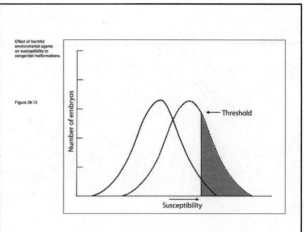

Effect of harmful
environmental agents
on susceptibility to
congenital malformations.

Figure 09.13

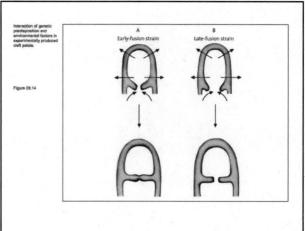

Interaction of genetic
predisposition and
environmental factors in
experimentally produced
cleft palate.

Figure 09.14

Prenatal Diagnosis of Congenital Abnormalities (1 of 2)

- Examination of fetal cells: determination of biochemical abnormalities in fetal cells
  - Chromosomal abnormalities
  - Biochemical abnormalities
  - Analysis of DNA
- Examination of amnionic fluid: products secreted into fluid by fetus that may indicate fetal abnormality

Prenatal Diagnosis of Congenital Abnormalities (2 of 2)

- Ultrasound examination: detection of major structural abnormalities
  - Major structural abnormalities of nervous system (anencephaly; spina bifida)
  - Hydrocephalus
  - Obstruction of urinary tract
  - Failure of kidneys to develop
  - Failure of limbs to form normally
- Fetal DNA analysis: determination of biochemical abnormalities by analysis of DNA of fetal cells
  - Amniocentesis
  - Chorionic villus sampling

Amniocentesis

- Alpha fetoprotein: high concentration in amniotic fluid is suggestive of a neural tube defect
- Amniotic fluid for study: transabdominal amniocentesis
  - Usually performed between the 14th and 18th week of pregnancy
  - Primary use: prenatal detection of chromosomal abnormality in women over age 35 due to higher incidence of Down syndrome in infants born to older women

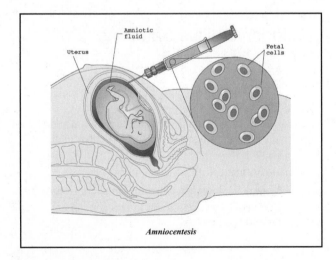

Amniocentesis

Notes

Indications for Amniocentesis

TABLE 9-4

Main indications for amniocentesis or chorionic villus sampling

1. Maternal age over 35 years
2. Previous infant born with Down syndrome or other chromosomal abnormality
3. Known translocation chromosome carrier, or other chromosome abnormality in either parent
4. Risk of fetal genetic disease that can be detected by fetal cell biochemical or DNA analysis
5. Maternal blood tests (triple screen) indicating increased risk of fetal chromosome abnormality

Chorionic Villus Sampling (1 of 2)

- Chorionic villi: frond-like structures that form part of placenta and attach to lining of uterus
  - Fetal cells are obtained for evaluation using chorionic villi sample
  - Amniotic fluid not used for analysis
  - Small catheter inserted through cervix to the site where villi are attached on the uterus
  - Small area is suctioned

Chorionic Villus Sampling (2 of 2)

- Advantages
  - Can be performed earlier than amniocentesis (8th to 10th week)
  - Carries less risk from abortion if parent decides to terminate pregnancy in case of congenital abnormality
- Disadvantages
  - More difficult technically than amniocentesis
  - Complications: spontaneous abortion, limb deformities in fetus

Discussion

- What are the consequences of chromosome nondisjunction?
- What is the karyotype of an individual with Down syndrome? Why does this happen? What are the possible outcomes of a pregnancy involving a 14/21 translocation chromosome?
- What are the causes of congenital abnormalities and their approximate incidences?
- What are the indications for amniocentesis?

Notes

Chapter Outline

The chapter outline provides you with an organizational guide to the topics and ideas presented in this chapter of the text.

Tumors: Disturbed Cell Growth
Tumors
    Classification and Nomenclature
    Comparison of Benign and Malignant Tumors
    Benign Tumors
    Malignant Tumors
    Variations in Terminology
    Necrosis in Tumors
    Noninfiltrating (In Situ) Carcinoma
    Precancerous Conditions
Etiologic Factors in Neoplastic Disease
    Viruses
    Gene and Chromosomal Abnormalities
    Failure of Immunologic Defenses
    Heredity and Tumors
Diagnosis of Tumors
    Early Recognition of Neoplasms
    Cytologic Diagnosis of Neoplasms
    Frozen-Section Diagnosis of Neoplasms
    Tumor-Associated Antigen Tests
Treatment of Tumors
    Surgery
    Radiotherapy
    Hormone Therapy
    Anticancer Drugs
    Adjuvant Chemotherapy
    Immunotherapy
Leukemia
    Classification of Leukemia
    Clinical Features and Principles of Treatment
    Precursors of Leukemia: The Myelodysplastic Syndromes
Multiple Myeloma
Survival Rates in Neoplastic Disease

Study Questions

The following questions are provided as a test for comprehension and as a study guide for use with the text chapters. Additional study material is located at http://health.jbpub.com/humandisease/8e, which contains useful tools such as an A&P review, animated flashcards, an interactive online glossary, crossword puzzles, and web links.

Key Terms

Define the following terms:

1. Teratoma _____

2. Lymphoma _____

3. Precancerous condition _____

4. In situ carcinoma _____

5. Adjuvant chemotherapy _____

6. Carcinoma _____

7. Nevus _____

8. Melanoma _____

9. Multiple myeloma _____

10. Leukemia _____

True/False

Tell whether each statement is true or false. If false, explain why the statement is incorrect.

1. Some neoplasms in humans may be caused by viruses. _____
_____

2. A mutation is a cancer-causing chemical. _____
_____

3. A Pap smear is a screening test used to detect cervical cancer. _____
_____

4. A tumor-associated antigen is a carbohydrate–protein complex secreted by tumor cells that can be used to monitor tumor growth. _____
_____

5. A hormone-dependent tumor is one that produces sex hormones. _____
_____

6. Anticancer drugs injure normal cells as well as cancer cells. _____
_____

7. Adjuvant chemotherapy is used in an attempt to prevent late recurrences of cancer by destroying small foci of metastatic carcinoma before they grow to large size. _____
_____

8. Some types of acute leukemia can be cured by chemotherapy. _____

   _____

9. Myeloma is often associated with small areas of bone destruction. _____

   _____

10. Some chemotherapy drugs impede tumor cell growth by blocking growth factor receptors on the tumor cells so that the tumor cells are unable to respond to the growth factors that stimulate cells to divide. _____

   _____

Identify

1. Give an example for each of the following:

   a. In situ carcinoma _____

   b. Teratoma _____

   c. Precancerous condition _____

2. In this list of common prefixes used to name tumors, write the meaning of the prefix after the name:

   a. Adeno _____

   b. Angio _____

   c. Chondro _____

   d. Fibro _____

   e. Lipo _____

   f. Myo _____

   g. Neuro _____

   h. Osteo _____

   i. Lymphangio _____

   j. Hemangio _____

3. Three large groups of genes play important roles in regulating cell functions, and dysfunctions of these genes may lead to tumors. Identify these three groups of genes.

   a. _____

   b. _____

   c. _____

4. Identify four methods used to treat tumors.

   a. _____

   b. _____

   c. _____

   d. _____

5. How would you name the following neoplasms?

   a. A benign tumor of fibrous connective tissue _____

   b. A malignant tumor of fat cells _____

   c. A benign tumor of pigment-forming cells in the skin _____

   d. A neoplasm of plasma cells _____

   e. A malignant tumor of mature lymphocytes _____

   f. A malignant tumor of blood vessels _____

   g. A malignant tumor of lymph vessels _____

   h. A tumor of lymph nodes containing Reed-Sternberg cells intermixed with lymphocytes, plasma cells, and eosinophils _____

   i. A noninvasive malignant tumor of cervical squamous epithelium _____

   _____

   j. A malignant tumor of lymphocytes _____

   k. A leukemia in which the circulating cells are immature lymphocytes _____

   _____

   l. A benign tumor of the ovary composed of many different types of mature tissues _____

   _____

   m. A benign tumor of cartilage _____

   n. A benign pedunculated tumor arising from the epithelium of the colon _____

   _____

   o. A malignant noninvasive tumor arising from the squamous epithelium of the cervix _____

   _____

Discussion Questions

1. What are the major differences in growth rate, circumscription, cell differentiation, and spread between benign and malignant tumors? Give your comparison in tabular form.

	Benign Tumor	Malignant Tumor
Growth rate		
Cell differentiation		
Growth characteristics		
Spread (metastasis)		

2. Describe how tumors are named. _____

   _____

   _____

   _____

3. What is a Pap smear? What is its application to the early diagnosis of tumors? What is the significance of a Pap smear containing atypical cells? _____

_____

_____

_____

4. What are tumor suppressor genes? What happens if one member of the pair of tumor suppressor genes fails to function normally? _____

_____

_____

_____

5. What is the Philadelphia chromosome? With what conditions is it associated? _____

_____

_____

_____

6. Describe the role of heredity in tumors. _____

_____

_____

_____

7. The eye tumor retinoblastoma is caused by mutations of both members of the paired RB genes within a single retinal cell. Explain the difference between a hereditary retinoblastoma and a sporadic retinoblastoma. (*Hint:* see Fig. 10-22.) _____

_____

_____

_____

8. Describe a simple classification of leukemia based on cell type and maturity of the leukemic cells. How is leukemia classified? _____

_____

_____

_____

9. How does our immune system protect us from cancer? _____

_____

_____

_____

10. What is the significance of an abnormal cervical Pap smear in a 32-year-old woman? What further diagnostic or therapeutic measures would you recommend? _____

_____

_____

_____

11. What clinical, hematologic, and radiologic abnormalities often occur in persons with multiple myeloma? What abnormal laboratory test results often occur? _____

_____

_____

_____

12. A patient has a blood disease characterized by a greatly increased white blood cell count consisting of mature lymphocytes, with anemia and thrombocytopenia. What is the most likely diagnosis? _____

_____

_____

_____

Notes

_____
_____
_____
_____
_____
_____
_____
_____
_____
_____
_____
_____
_____
_____
_____
_____
_____
_____
_____
_____
_____
_____
_____
_____
_____
_____
_____
_____
_____
_____
_____
_____
_____
_____
_____
_____
_____
_____
_____

Chapter 10

Neoplastic Disease

Learning Objectives (1 of 2)

- Compare benign versus malignant tumors; discuss naming of tumors and exceptions to standard terminology
- Summarize principal types of lymphoma
- Differentiate infiltrating versus in situ carcinoma; role of Pap smear in early diagnoses of neoplasms
- Explain classification and clinical manifestation of leukemia
- Differentiate leukemia versus multiple myeloma
- Explain mechanism of body's immunologic defenses against tumor

Learning Objectives (2 of 2)

- Summarize modalities and side effects of cancer treatment
- Describe applications and limitations of tumor-associated antigens
- Compare incidence and survival rates for various malignant tumors
- Explain role of late recurrence and role of adjuvant therapy
- Understand role of oncogenes and disturbance in suppressor gene function in the pathogenesis of tumors

Notes

Definition

- **Neoplasm:** *NEO* = new + *PLASM* = growth
- **Cancer**: any type of malignant growth
  - Unrestrained growth and spread
  - Cells do not respond to control mechanisms that normally regulate cell growth and differentiation
  - Serves no useful purpose
  - Terms *neoplasm* and *tumor* may be used interchangeably

Warning Signs for Cancer

- **C**hange in bowel/bladder habits or function
- **A** sore that does not heal
- **U**nusual bleeding or discharge
- **T**hickening or lump in breast or elsewhere
- **I**ndigestion or difficulty swallowing
- **O**bvious change in wart or mole
- **N**agging cough or hoarseness

Benign Versus Malignant

- BENIGN
  - Growth rate: slow
  - Growth character: expansion
  - Tumor spread: remains localized
  - Cell differentiation: well-differentiated cells
- MALIGNANT
  - Growth rate: rapid
  - Growth character: infiltration
  - Tumor spread: metastasis by bloodstream or lymphatic channels
  - Cell differentiation: poorly differentiated cells

Benign Tumors

- Named by adding suffix -oma to the name of the cells of origin
  - Adenoma: from glandular epithelium
  - Angioma: from blood vessels
  - Chondroma: from cartilage
  - Polyps or papilloma: benign tumor on stalk arising from an epithelial surface

Malignant Tumors (1 of 2)

- Start from a single cell that has sustained damage to its genome, causing it to proliferate abnormally
- Clone of identical cells is formed; if unchecked, eventually develops into a distinct tumor
- Exhibit behavior different from that of normal cells
- Do not respond to normal growth regulatory signals
- Proliferate unnecessarily

Malignant Tumors (2 of 2)

- May secrete growth factors to stimulate their own growth, allowing tumors to flourish at the expense of surrounding normal cells
- Secrete enzymes that break down normal cell and tissue barriers, allowing them to
  - Infiltrate into adjacent tissues
  - Invade lymphatic channels and blood vessels
  - Spread throughout the body
- Tumor cells do not normally "wear out" as normal cells, but become "immortal" and can proliferate indefinitely

Notes

Notes

Tumor Classification (1 of 2)

- Carcinoma: involves epithelial tissue
  - Most common: 85% of all tumors found in skin, large intestine, glands, stomach, lungs, prostate
  - Metastasis: principally through lymph vessels
  - Subtypes:
    - Adenocarcinoma (internal organ or gland)
    - Squamous cell carcinoma (skin)

Tumor Classification (2 of 2)

- Sarcoma: arising from connective tissues such as fat, bone, cartilage, muscle
  - Less common, but spreads more rapidly
  - Little differentiation; anaplasia (lack of form)
  - Metastasis: bloodstream
- Leukemia: neoplasm of blood cells
  - Usually do not form solid tumors
  - Instead, proliferates diffusely within bone marrow, overgrow and crowd out normal blood-forming cells
  - Neoplastic cells "spill over" into the bloodstream and large number of abnormal cells circulate in the peripheral blood

Naming of Tumors

- Tumors are named and classified according to their cells and tissues of origin
- Tumor nomenclature: not completely uniform, but certain generalizations are possible
- Exceptions encountered in naming of
  - Lymphoid tumors
  - Skin tumors arising from pigment-producing cells within the epidermis
  - Certain tumors of mixed cellular components
  - Certain types of tumors composed of primitive cells seen in children

Principles of Naming Tumors

TABLE 10-3

General principles of naming tumors

GENERAL TERM	MEANING
Polyp, papilloma	Any benign tumor projecting from surface epithelium.
___ + oma (suffix)	A benign tumor. The prefix designates primary tissue of origin.
Carcinoma	Malignant tumor arising from surface, glandular, or parenchymal epithelium (but not endothelium or mesothelium).
Sarcoma	Malignant tumor of any primary tissue other than surface, glandular, and parenchymal epithelium.
Leukemia	Neoplasm of blood cells.

Common Prefixes in Tumor Names

TABLE 10-2

Common prefixes used to name tumors

PREFIX	MEANING
Adeno-	Gland
Angio-	Vessels (type not specified)
Chondro-	Cartilage
Fibro-	Fibrous tissue
Hemangio-	Blood vessels
Lymphangio-	Lymph vessels
Lipo-	Fat
Myo-	Muscle
Neuro-	Nerve
Osteo-	Bone

Lymphoma (1 of 2)

- Neoplasm of lymphoid tissue
  - Usually malignant
  - Term "lymphoma" without classification refers to a malignant, not a benign tumor
  - To avoid confusion, the term "malignant lymphoma" maybe used
- Two major classifications
  - Hodgkin's lymphoma (Hodgkin's disease)
  - Non-Hodgkin's lymphoma
- Classification: often with poor correlation between histologic type and biologic behavior (growth rate and response to therapy)

Notes

Lymphoma (2 of 2)

- Basis of classification
  - Diffuse infiltration of lymph nodes
  - Prognosis
    - Low-grade: patients have a favorable prognosis
    - Intermediate-grade: patients do not do nearly as well
    - High-grade: patients do poorly
  - Type of cells giving rise to tumor (T cells, B cells, NK cells, histiocytes) and maturity of cells
    - 75% arise from B lymphocytes
    - Remainder mostly from T lymphocytes

Hodgkin and Non-Hodgkin Lymphoma (1 of 2)

- Hodgkin disease: variable histologic appearance consisting of large cells called Reed-Sternberg cells intermixed with lymphocytes, plasma cells, eosinophils, and fibrous tissues
  - Reed-Sternberg cell: large cell with abundant cytoplasm containing two nuclei appearing as mirror images
    - Some have a single nucleus
    - Each nucleus contains large nucleolus surrounded by clear halo
  - Four different histologic types of Hodgkin disease that differ in clinical behavior and prognosis

Hodgkin and Non-Hodgkin Lymphoma (2 of 2)

- Non-Hodgkin lymphoma: all other lymphoma are generally grouped together under this category
  - Variable in appearance and behavior
  - Classification system based on size, shape, growth pattern of malignant cells, and shape of nuclei and nuclear membranes

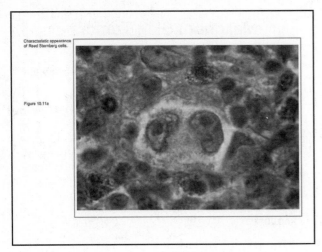

Characteristic appearance
of Reed Sternberg cells.

Figure 19.11a

Skin Tumors (1 of 2)

- Most skin tumors arise from keratinocytes or melanocytes
- Keratinocytes: keratin-forming cells
- Basal cells: deepest layer of keratinocytes adjacent to the dermis
- Squamous cells: upper layer of cells that arise from the proliferation of basal cells
- Melanocytes: (interspersed among keratinocytes) skin cells that normally produce pigment and are responsible for normal skin color; produce melanin, dark-brown pigment

Skin Tumors (2 of 2)

- Melanocytes
  - Benign: nevus ("birthmark" in Latin); common benign pigmented skin lesion derived from melanin-producing cells
  - Malignant: melanoma; malignant tumor of melanocytes
- Keratinocytes
  - Benign: keratoses
  - Malignant: basal cell carcinoma, squamous cell carcinoma

Malignant Skin Tumors

- Basal cell carcinoma
  - Composed of clusters of infiltrating cells that resemble the normal basal cells of the epidermis
  - Indolent, slowly growing tumor that can be locally destructive but rarely metastasizes
- Squamous cell carcinoma
  - Composed of abnormal infiltrating squamous cells
  - More aggressive tumor that sometimes metastasizes
- Both types can be cured by surgical excision with a very good prognosis
- Excessive sunlight exposure predisposes to all types of skin cancer, including melanoma and keratoses

Teratoma

- Tumor arising from cells that can differentiate into many different types of tissues: bone, muscle, glands, epithelium, brain tissue, hair
- Has mixed components, poorly organized
- Frequently occurs in reproductive tract, but may develop in other areas
- Must specify as benign or malignant based on maturity of cells

Primitive Cell Tumors

- Arise from persistent groups of primitive cells and may arise in children
  - Brain
  - Retina
  - Adrenal gland
  - Kidney
  - Liver
  - Genital tract
- Named after site of origin with suffix "-blastoma" added
  - Example: tissue of origin (retina) + blastoma = retinoblastoma

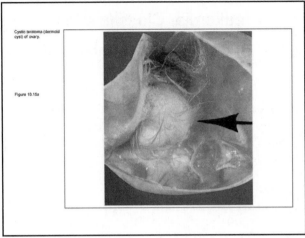

Cystic teratoma (dermoid cyst) of ovary.

Figure 10.15a

Large bulky teratoma of the sacral region in a female infant.

Figure 10.14

Leukemia

- A neoplasm of hematopoietic tissue
- Leukemic cells **diffusely infiltrate the bone marrow and lymphoid tissues**, spill over into the bloodstream, and infiltrate throughout various organs of the body
- Cells may be mostly mature or extremely primitive
- Overproduction of white cells demonstrated in the peripheral blood by a very high white blood count
- **Aleukemic leukemia**: condition in which white cells are confined to the bone marrow such that their number in the peripheral blood is normal or decreased

Leukemia: Classification

- Any type of hematopoietic cells can give rise to a leukemia, but the most common types are:
  - Granulocytic
  - Lymphocytic
  - Monocytic
- Basis for Classification of Leukemia
  - Cell type
    - Granulocytic, lymphocytic, monocytic
  - Maturity of leukemic cells
    - Acute if immature cells
    - Chronic if mature cells

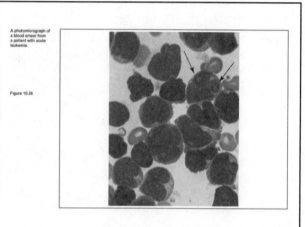

A photomicrograph of a blood smear from a patient with acute leukemia.

Figure 10.26

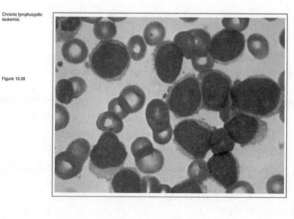

Chronic lymphocytic leukemia.

Figure 10.28

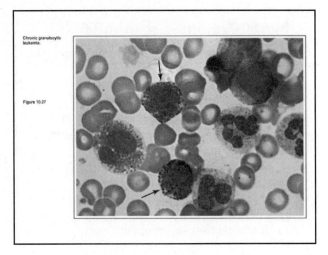

Chronic granulocytic leukemia.

Figure 10.27

Leukemia: Clinical Features (1 of 2)

- Manifestations caused by impairment of bone marrow function
- Leukemic cells crowd out normal cells causing:
  - Anemia: inadequate red cell production
  - Thrombocytopenia: causes bleeding
  - Infections from inadequate number of normal white cells

Leukemia: Clinical Features (2 of 2)

- Caused by infiltration of organs by leukemic cells causing:
  - Splenomegaly: enlarged spleen
  - Hepatomegaly: enlarged liver
  - Lymphadenopathy: enlarged lymph nodes
- In chronic leukemia: evolution of disease proceeds at a relatively slow pace and often can be controlled
- In acute leukemia: a rapidly progressive disease, more difficult to control

Myelodysplasia (Preleukemia)

- A disturbed growth and maturation of marrow cells
  - Anemia: reduced number of erythrocytes
  - Leukopenia: reduced number white cells
  - Thrombocytopenia: reduced number of platelets
- Although called preleukemia, not all patients develop leukemia
- Recently grouped together under the general term myelodysplastic syndromes
- In general, the more severe the maturation disturbance in the bone marrow, the greater the likelihood that leukemia will occur

Multiple Myeloma

- Neoplasm from plasma cells within the bone marrow
- Resembles leukemia, but cell proliferation is confined to the bone marrow and organ infiltration is unusual
- Outpouring of large number of plasma cells into the peripheral blood is also uncommon
- Abnormal plasma cells either infiltrate the bone marrow diffusely or form discrete tumors that weaken the bone
- Leads to spontaneous fractures, pain, and disability

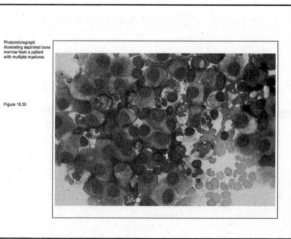

Photomicrograph illustrating aspirated bone marrow from a patient with multiple myeloma.

Figure 10.30

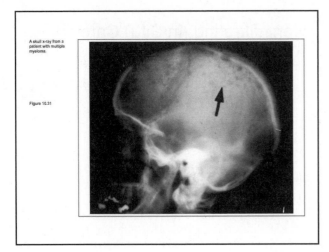

A skull x-ray from a patient with multiple myeloma.

Figure 10.31

Notes

Tumor Blood Supply and Necrosis (1 of 2)

- Tumors derive blood supply from tissues they invade
- Malignant tumors frequently induce new blood vessels to proliferate in adjacent normal tissues to supply the demands of the growing tumor (angiogenesis factor)
- Malignant tumor may outgrow its blood supply; the part of the tumor with the poorest blood supply undergoes necrosis
- Depending on the location of the tumor, the blood supply will be rich or poor

Tumor Blood Supply and Necrosis (2 of 2)

- In tumors in the lung, blood supply is best at the periphery of the tumor and poorest at the center
- If tumor is growing outward from an epithelial surface such as the colon, the best blood supply is at its base and poorest at the surface
- Often, small blood vessels are exposed in the ulcerated base of a tumor that blood may ooze continuously from vessels leading to anemia from chronic blood loss
- An ulcerated tumor may be the source of a severe hemorrhage

Noninfiltrating (in Situ) Carcinoma

- Arises from the surface epithelium
- Remains localized within the epithelium for many years
- Can occur in many locations of the body
  - Cervix
  - Breast
  - Urinary tract
  - Colon
  - Skin

Precancerous Conditions (1 of 2)

- Nonmalignant condition with a tendency to become malignant
  - Actinic keratoses: small, crusted, scaly patches that develop on sun-exposed skin; may develop into cancer if untreated
  - Lentigo maligna: freckle-like proliferation of melanin-producing cells that may develop on sun-exposed skin; may transform later into melanoma
  - Leukoplakia: thick white patches in the mucous membranes of the mouth from exposure to tobacco tars from pipe or cigar smoking or use of smokeless tobacco (snuff or chewing tobacco)

Precancerous Conditions (2 of 2)

- Leukoplakia may give rise to squamous cell cancers of the oral cavity
- Precancerous conditions should always be treated appropriately to prevent malignant change, which occurs in many but not in all cases

Etiologic Factors in Neoplastic Disease (1 of 2)

- Viruses
- Gene and chromosomal abnormalities
- Failure of immunologic defenses
- Heredity
- Viruses: cause some cancers in humans
  - Leukemia and lymphoma: T cell leukemia-lymphoma virus (HTLV-1) that is related to the AIDS virus
  - Kaposi's sarcoma: human herpesvirus 8 (HHV-8)
  - Condylomas: papilloma virus; predisposes to cervical carcinoma
  - Chronic viral hepatitis: hepatitis B and C virus
  - Nasopharyngeal carcinoma: Epstein-Barr virus also causes infectious mononucleosis

Etiologic Factors in Neoplastic Disease (2 of 2)

- Gene and chromosomal abnormalities
- Three large groups of genes play an important role in regulating cell functions
- Mutations in these genes are associated with tumor formation
  - Proto-oncogenes
  - Tumor-suppressor genes
  - DNA repair genes

Proto-oncogenes

- Normal "growth genes" in the human chromosomes that promote some aspects of cell growth, differentiation, or mitotic activity
- Becomes an oncogene if mutation occurs or genes are translocated to another chromosome
- **Oncogene**: abnormally functioning gene that stimulates cell growth excessively, leading to unrestricted cell proliferation

Tumor Suppressor Genes

- Normally suppress cell proliferation
- Loss of function by mutation may lead to unrestrained cell growth
- Exist **in pairs** at corresponding gene loci on homologous chromosomes
- Both suppressor genes must cease to function before cell malfunctions

DNA Repair Genes

- Regulate processes that monitor and repair any errors in DNA duplication during cell division; DNA damage from radiation, chemicals, or other environmental agents
- Mutation: any change in the normal arrangement of DNA nucleotides on the DNA chain
- Failure in function of DNA repair genes increase the likelihood of DNA mutations within the cell

Gene mutations that disrupt cell function.

Table 10.04

TABLE 10-4

Gene mutations that disrupt cell function

GENE	NORMAL FUNCTION	MALFUNCTION
Proto-oncogene	Promotes normal cell growth	Point mutation, amplification, or translocation forms an oncogene, resulting in unrestrained cell growth
Paired tumor suppressor genes	Inhibit cell proliferation	Both genes inactivated in same cell promotes cell proliferation
Paired DNA repair genes	Correct errors in DNA duplication	Gene inactivation increases mutation rate

Failure of Immunologic Defenses (1 of 2)

- Cancers usually arise from multiple genetic "insults" to the genome rather than single gene mutations
- Characterized by activation of oncogenes and loss of function of ≥ 1 tumor suppressor genes
- Followed by additional random genetic changes in tumor cells that indicate instability of tumor cell genome

Failure of Immunologic Defenses (2 of 2)

- Mutant cell produces cell proteins not present in a normal cell; these proteins are recognized as abnormal by the immune system and are destroyed
- Immune system destroys abnormal cells via cell-mediated and humoral mechanisms
- Tumor: a reflection of the failure of the body's immune defenses

Heredity and Tumors (1 of 2)

- Predisposition apparently results from multifactorial inheritance pattern
- Individual at risk has inherited set of genes that influence hormonal or enzyme-regulated biochemical process in the body that can increase susceptibility to a specific cancer
- Example: breast cancer
  - 80% to 90%: no family history of the disease
  - 10% linked to gene mutations

Notes

Notes

_____
_____
_____
_____
_____
_____
_____
_____
_____
_____
_____
_____
_____
_____
_____
_____
_____
_____
_____
_____
_____
_____
_____
_____
_____
_____
_____
_____
_____
_____
_____
_____
_____
_____
_____
_____
_____
_____
_____
_____
_____
_____
_____
_____

Heredity and Tumors (2 of 2)

- Inheritance of certain genetic alterations:
  - Breast cancer susceptibility genes BRCA1 and BRCA2 (5%)
  - Philadelphia (Ph1) chromosome
  - Multiple polyposis of colon
  - Neurofibromatosis
  - Multiple endocrine adenomatosis

Diagnosis of Tumors (1 of 2)

- Recognize early warning signs and symptoms
- Complete medical history and physical examination
- Laboratory procedures
  - Examination of rectum and colon
  - Vaginal examination and Pap smear in women
  - Examination of esophagus and stomach
  - X-ray studies
  - Abnormal smear: slides of abnormal cells shed from surface of tumors
  - Cytologic diagnosis: from smears, needle aspiration, biopsy
  - Frozen section: slides prepared and stained for rapid histologic diagnosis

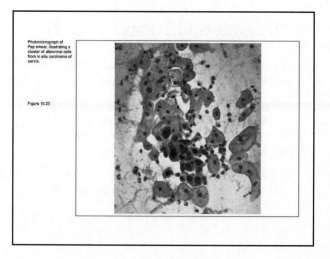

Photomicrograph of Pap smear, illustrating a cluster of abnormal cells from in situ carcinoma of cervix.

Figure 10.23

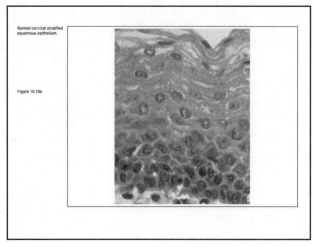

Normal cervical stratified squamous epithelium.

Figure 10.19a

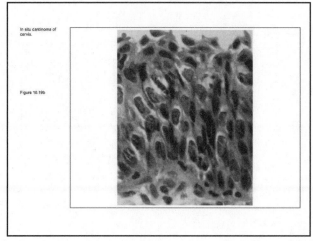

In situ carcinoma of cervix.

Figure 10.19b

Diagnosis of Tumors (2 of 2)

- Tumor associated antigen tests: some cancers secrete substances that can be detected in the blood by lab tests
- CEA (carcinoembrionic antigen): present in amounts related to the size of tumor and its possible spread
  - Produced by most malignant tumors of the GI tract, pancreas, breast
- Alpha fetoprotein: normally produced by fetal tissues in the placenta but not adult cells; elevated in primary carcinoma of the liver
- Human chorionic gonadotropin: normally produced by placenta; elevated in testicular carcinoma
- Acid-phosphatase: normally produced by prostate epithelial cells, may be elevated in prostate cancer

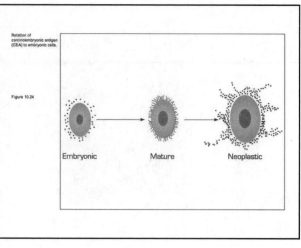

Relation of carcinoembryonic antigen (CEA) to embryonic cells.

Figure 10.24

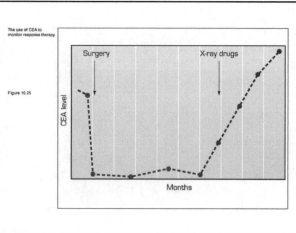

The use of CEA to monitor response therapy.

Figure 10.25

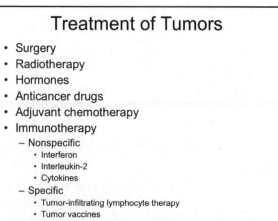

Treatment of Tumors

- Surgery
- Radiotherapy
- Hormones
- Anticancer drugs
- Adjuvant chemotherapy
- Immunotherapy
  - Nonspecific
    - Interferon
    - Interleukin-2
    - Cytokines
  - Specific
    - Tumor-infiltrating lymphocyte therapy
    - Tumor vaccines
    - Tumor antibody therapy

Chemotherapy

- Eliminates cells that divide frequently
- Cancer cells + rapidly dividing normal cells found in the:
  - Mouth, skin, hair, bone marrow, digestive tract, kidneys, bladder
  - Lungs, nervous system, reproductive system
- Normal cells recover quickly, side effects disappear gradually
- How soon the patient will feel better depends on overall health, types of anticancer drugs used

Side Effects of Chemotherapy (1 of 2)

- Anemia: extreme fatigue, weakness, tiredness, paleness, dizziness experienced by more than half of patients; reduces bone marrow's ability to make red blood cells
- Constipation: drugs, decrease in physical activity, unbalanced diet
- Depression: physical and emotional stress
- Diarrhea: drugs affect cells that line intestines
- Fatigue

Side Effects of Chemotherapy (2 of 2)

- Hair loss (alopecia)
- Infection due to reduced ability of bone marrow to produce white blood cells
- Loss of appetite (anorexia)
- Mouth, gum, and throat problems; sores
- Nausea and vomiting
- Sexual problems
  - Males: affect sperm cells; temporary/permanent infertility
  - Women: irregular menstrual periods; vaginal infections; menopause-like symptoms

Notes

Survival Rates in Cancer (1 of 2)

- Vary from 4% to more than 95%
- Survival rates:
  - Thyroid cancer, 95% 5-year survival rate
  - Pancreatic cancer, 4% 5-year survival rate
- Cancer second to heart disease as most common cause of death in the US
- 1 in every 4 people will eventually develop cancer
  - Lung cancer: most common cancer affecting males
  - Breast cancer: most common cancer affecting females
- Early diagnosis and treatment may enhance survival
- Chances for survival significantly reduced once tumor has metastasized to the regional lymph nodes or to distant sites

Survival Rates in Cancer (2 of 2)

- 5-year survival does not indicate cure; some types recur, prove fatal
- Tumor may have already spread by time of diagnosis and initial treatment, but metastatic deposits held in check by immune defense mechanisms
- Recurrence: failure of body's defenses, reactivation of tumor; some malignant tumors recur and prove fatal many years after initial treatment
- Breast cancer and malignant melanoma prone to late recurrences
- Breast cancer: 65% 5-year survival rate and 50% 10-year survival rate

Malignant neoplasms: 5-year survival rates.

Table 10.06

TABLE 10-6

Malignant neoplasms: 5-year survival rates

TYPE OF NEOPLASM	5-YEAR SURVIVAL (%) WHITE	5-YEAR SURVIVAL (%) BLACK	TYPE OF NEOPLASM	5-YEAR SURVIVAL (%) WHITE	5-YEAR SURVIVAL (%) BLACK
Thyroid	96	93	Kidney	62	60
Melanoma	89	66	Non-Hodgkin's lymphoma	56	46
Uterus, cervix	72	60	Ovary	53	53
Uterus, body	86	61	Multiple myeloma	30	33
Breast	88	73	Leukemia	47	39
Bladder	82	65	Stomach	21	20
Larynx	66	54	Lung	15	12
Prostate	98	93	Esophagus	15	8
Hodgkin's disease	85	77	Pancreas	4	4
Colon-rectum	63	53			

Cases diagnosed 1992 to 1998. Survival for all ages with survival for whites and blacks listed separately. Average survival for both sexes used when neoplasm occurs in both sexes.
Source: CA: A Cancer Journal for Clinicians. 2003, 53:24.

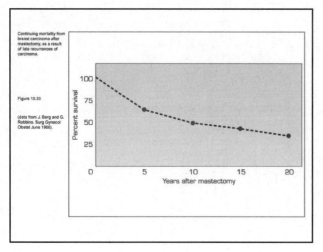

Continuing mortality from breast carcinoma after mastectomy, as a result of late recurrences of carcinoma.

Figure 10.33

(data from J. Berg and G. Robbins. Surg Gynecol Obstet June 1966).

Discussion

- How does leukemia differ from multiple myeloma?
- How is a frozen section used in the diagnosis of tumors?
- What is the difference between a nevus and a melanoma?
- What are the clinical implications of late tumor recurrences and the 5-year survival rate?

Chapter Outline

The chapter outline provides you with an organizational guide to the topics and ideas presented in this chapter of the text.

Study Questions

The following questions are provided as a test for comprehension and as a study guide for use with the text chapters. Additional study material is located at http://health.jbpub.com/humandisease/8e, which contains useful tools such as an A&P review, animated flashcards, an interactive online glossary, crossword puzzles, and web links.

Key Terms

Define the following terms:

1. Hemostasis _____

2. Platelets _____

3. Blood coagulation _____

4. Hemophilia A _____

5. Von Willebrand's disease _____

6. Thrombocytopenia _____

7. Hemorrhage _____

8. Coagulation factors _____

9. Thromboplastin _____

Identify

1. Identify the four factors required for normal hemostasis.

   a. _____

   b. _____

   c. _____

   d. _____

Discussion Questions

1. Construct a simple system to describe the sequence of events involved in normal blood coagulation. (*Hint:* see Fig. 11-1.)

2. Describe the role of platelets in blood coagulation. _____

   _____

   _____

   _____

3. Describe the characteristic appearance of the bleeding associated with platelet deficiency. _____

_____

_____

4. Describe the differences between hemophilia A and von Willebrand's disease. _____

_____

_____

_____

5. What is the disseminated intravascular coagulation syndrome? _____

_____

_____

_____

6. What factors initiate the disseminated intravascular coagulation syndrome? _____

_____

_____

_____

7. List some of the readily available laboratory tests commonly used to evaluate the functions of the various factors involved in blood coagulation. Indicate what each test measures. _____

_____

_____

_____

8. What is the consequence of liberation of thromboplastic material into the circulation? _____

_____

_____

_____

9. What types of diseases produce abnormalities in the first phase of blood coagulation? _____

_____

_____

_____

10. What conditions lead to disturbances in the second phase of blood coagulation? _____

_____

_____

_____

11. What types of diseases are associated with thrombocytopenia? _____

_____

_____

_____

12. What are the major types of blood coagulation disturbances? _____

_____

_____

_____

13. A 5-year-old male child experiences frequent areas of hemorrhage into joints and muscles after minor trauma. Laboratory tests reveal a reduced concentration of a plasma coagulation factor that is concerned with the early stage of the coagulation mechanism (formation of thromboplastin). What is the most likely diagnosis?

_____

_____

_____

Notes

Chapter 11

Abnormalities of Blood Coagulation

Learning Objectives

- Describe functions of blood vessels and platelets in controlling bleeding
- Explain three phases of coagulation and the respective factors involved
- Describe laboratory tests for evaluating hemostasis
- Describe common clinically significant disturbances of hemostasis and their clinical manifestations

Hemostasis

- Arrest of bleeding caused by activation of the blood coagulation mechanism
- Factors concerned with hemostasis
    - 1. Integrity of small blood vessels
    - 2. Adequate numbers of platelets
    - 3. Normal amounts of coagulation factors
    - 4. Normal amounts of coagulation inhibitors
    - 5. Adequate amounts of calcium ions in the blood

Factors Concerned with Hemostasis (1 of 2)

- 1. Integrity of small vessels
  - Small vessels are first line of defense in the body
  - Constrict on injury to facilitate closure by a clot
  - Exposure of underlying connective tissue of the endothelium activates coagulation mechanism
- 2. Adequate number of platelets to accumulate and adhere to injury area

Factors Concerned with Hemostasis (2 of 2)

- Platelets: small fragments of cytoplasm from large precursor cells called megakaryocytes
- Average survival in the circulation is 10 days, removed by macrophages spleen
- Three important platelet functions
  - PLUG defect in the vessel wall
  - Liberate vasoconstrictors and compounds causing platelets to AGGREGATE
  - Release substances (phospholipids) that INITIATE coagulation

Blood Coagulation Process (1 of 2)

- Highly complex chain reaction
- Phase 1: Formation of thromboplastin by either interaction of
  - Intrinsic factors in blood (platelets and plasma factors)
  - Extrinsic factors from components outside circulatory system
- Phase 2: Conversion of prothrombin into thrombin
  - After thromboplastin interacts with other substances to form prothrombin activator

Blood Coagulation Process (2 of 2)

- Phase 3: Conversion of fibrinogen into fibrin by thrombin
  - Thrombin splits off a part of the fibrinogen → forms smaller molecules, fibrin monomers
  - Fibrin monomers join end-to-end into long strands of fibrin and linked side to side
  - Fibrin stabilizing factor strengthens bonds between fibrin molecules to increase strength of fibrin clot
- Blood clot: end stage of clotting process
- Made up of an interlacing meshwork of fibrin threads with plasma, red cells, white cells, and platelets

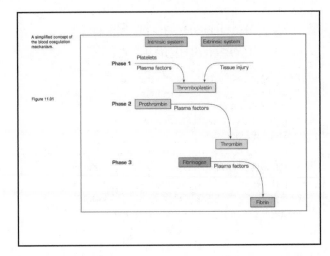

Notes

_____

_____

_____

_____

_____

_____

_____

_____

_____

_____

_____

_____

_____

_____

_____

_____

_____

_____

_____

_____

_____

_____

_____

_____

_____

_____

_____

_____

_____

_____

_____

_____

Disturbances of Blood Coagulation (1 of 7)

- Classification: Four categories
  - Abnormalities of small blood vessels
  - Abnormality of platelet formation
  - Deficiency of one or more plasma coagulation factors
  - Liberation of thromboplastic material into circulation

Disturbances of Blood Coagulation (2 of 7)

- Abnormality of small blood vessels
  - Abnormal bleeding resulting from failure of small blood vessels to contract after tissue injury
  - Abnormality of platelet formation
  - Thrombocytopenia
- 1. Injury or disease of bone marrow damaging the megakaryocytes (precursors of platelets)
- 2. Infiltration of bone marrow by leukemic cells or cancer cells that have spread to the skeletal system, crowding out the megakaryocytes

Disturbances of Blood Coagulation (3 of 7)

- 3. Antiplatelet antibodies destroy platelets in peripheral blood
- 4. Abnormal function of platelets despite normal count
- Petechiae
  - Small red or red-blue spots about 1-5 mm
  - Pinpoint-sized hemorrhages of small capillaries in skin or mucous membranes
  - Indicative of defective or inadequate platelets
  - Do not blanch when pressed
  - Petechiae + fever: in infections such as meningococcemia; dengue hemorrhagic disease

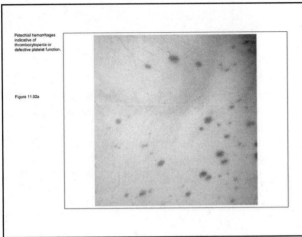

Petechial hemorrhages indicative of thrombocytopenia or defective platelet function.

Figure 11.02a

A large hemorrhage (hematoma) associated with a deficiency of plasma coagulation factors.

Figure 11.02b

Disturbances of Blood Coagulation (4 of 7)

- Phase 1 usually hereditary; relatively rare except
  - Hemophilia A
  - Hemophilia B
  - von Willebrand's disease
- Hemophilia: x-linked hereditary disease affecting males
  - Most common and best known
  - Episodes of hemorrhage in joints and internal organs after minor injury
- Hemophilia A: classic hemophilia = Factor VIII (antihemophilic factor)
- Hemophilia B: Christmas disease (after affected patient) = Factor IX (Christmas factor)

Disturbances of Blood Coagulation (5 of 7)

- von Willebrand disease: von Willebrand factor
  - Large protein molecule produced by endothelial cells required for platelets to adhere to vessel wall at site of injury
  - vWF adheres to the damaged vessel wall, forms a framework that allows platelets and coagulation factors to adhere, interact, form clot
  - Forms a complex with factor VIII and maintains normal level of factor VIII

Disturbances of Blood Coagulation (6 of 7)

- Phase 2: deficiency of prothrombin or factors required for the conversion of prothrombin into thrombin
- Causes of coagulation disturbance
  - Factors produced in liver
  - Vitamin K required for synthesis of most factors
  - Vitamin K synthesized by intestinal bacteria
  - Bile required for its absorption

Disturbances of Blood Coagulation (7 of 7)

- Administration of anticoagulant drugs
  - Inhibits synthesis of biochemically active vitamin K-dependent factors
- Inadequate synthesis of vitamin K
  - Occurs if the intestinal bacteria have been eradicated with prolonged use of antibiotics
- Inadequate absorption of vitamin K
  - Occurs in blockage of common bile duct by a gallstone or tumor, preventing bile from entering the intestine to promote absorption of vitamin
- Severe liver disease
  - Impairs synthesis of adequate amounts of coagulation factors

Causes of Thrombocytopenia

- Injury or disease of bone marrow
- Leukemic or cancer cells infiltrate bone marrow
- Antiplatelet antibody destroys platelets in peripheral blood

Liberation of Thromboplastic Material into Circulation

- Products of the following events have thromboplastic activity, liberated into circulation, result in intravascular coagulation
  - 1. Diseases associated with shock and tissue necrosis
  - 2. Overwhelming bacterial infections
  - 3. Other causes of tissue necrosis

Disseminated Intravascular Coagulation Syndrome (1 of 2)

- Abnormal bleeding state
- Activation of the coagulation mechanism due to
  - Diseases associated with shock
  - Overwhelming bacterial infection
  - Extensive necrosis of tissue
- Products of tissue necrosis and other substances with thromboplastic activity are liberated into the circulation

Notes

Notes

Disseminated Intravascular Coagulation Syndrome (2 of 2)

- Clotting: platelets and plasma coagulation factors are utilized, causing the levels to drop rapidly in the blood
- Activation of fibrinolysin to defend body from widespread intravascular clotting
  - Clots are dissolved to prevent lethal obstruction of the circulatory system
- Net effect: hemorrhage

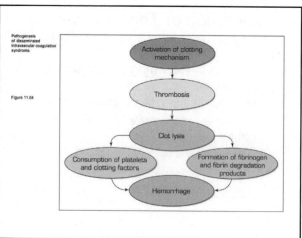

Pathogenesis of disseminated intravascular coagulation syndrome.

Figure 11.04

Activation of clotting mechanism

Thrombosis

Clot lysis

Consumption of platelets and clotting factors

Formation of fibrinogen and fibrin degradation products

Hemorrhage

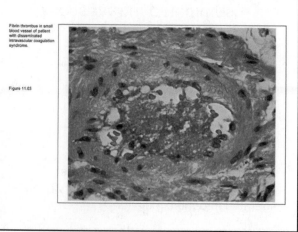

Fibrin thrombus in small blood vessel of patient with disseminated intravascular coagulation syndrome.

Figure 11.03

Laboratory Tests to Evaluate Hemostasis (1 of 2)

- To evaluate overall efficiency of coagulation process
  - Platelet count: examination of blood smear for platelet numbers
  - Bleeding time: time it takes for a small skin lesion to stop bleeding; used to evaluate the function of capillaries in the hemostatic process
  - Clotting time: time it takes for blood to clot in a test tube

Laboratory Tests to Evaluate Hemostasis (2 of 2)

- To evaluate overall efficiency of coagulation process
  - Partial thromboplastin time (PTT): time it takes for blood plasma to clot after a lipid substance is added to the plasma sample; measures time of first phase coagulation
  - Prothrombin time (PT): measures time of combined second and third phases of coagulation

Tests Measuring Phases of the Clotting Mechanism (1 of 3)

- Partial thromboplastin time: measures time it takes for blood plasma to clot after adding lipid and calcium

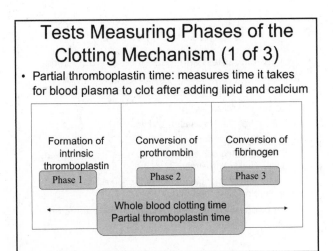

Notes

Tests Measuring Phases of the Clotting Mechanism (2 of 3)

- Prothrombin time: measures time it takes for blood to clot after adding thromboplastin; prolonged time indicates abnormality in second or third phases of coagulation; used to measure effects of coumadin

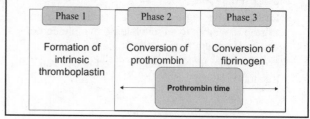

Tests Measuring Phases of the Clotting Mechanism (3 of 3)

- Thrombin time: bypasses the first two phases of blood coagulation, primarily measures the level of fibrinogen

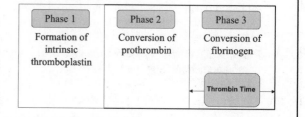

Discussion (1 of 2)

- 55-year-old female admitted for a severe bacterial pneumonia (Staphylococcus aureus) with pus in the left pleural cavity. Patient was given antibiotics.
- On physical exam:
  - Patient has severe nausea and vomiting
  - Unable to eat or drink
  - Bleeding noted per rectum and from the urinary tract after a few weeks of treatment
  - Lab results: Prolonged partial thromboplastin time (PTT) and prothrombin time (PT)
- What phase of coagulation is most likely affected? Explain

Discussion (2 of 2)

- A 10-month-old infant sustained a cut under the lower lip after a fall. The child is bleeding profusely followed by a tarry stool. The child has a history of easy bruising since birth but without previous episodes of bleeding. On physical exam, he has ecchymoses on his chest and left side with a small bruise on abdomen.
- Lab results:
  - Normal prothrombin time (PT)
  - Prolonged partial thromboplastin time (PTT)
  - Low factor VIII and von Willebrand factor (vWF)
- What phase of coagulation is most likely affected? Explain

Notes

Chapter Outline

The chapter outline provides you with an organizational guide to the topics and ideas presented in this chapter of the text.

Study Questions

The following questions are provided as a test for comprehension and as a study guide for use with the text chapters. Additional study material is located at http://health.jbpub.com/humandisease/8e, which contains useful tools such as an A&P review, animated flashcards, an interactive online glossary, crossword puzzles, and web links.

Key Terms

Define the following terms:

1. Edema _____

2. Thrombus _____

3. Embolus _____

4. Infarct _____

Fill-in-the-Blank

1. Reduced capillary osmotic pressure can be caused by _____.

2. Increased capillary permeability can be caused by _____.

3. _____ results in increased capillary hydrostatic pressure.

4. _____ results in obstruction of lymphatic channels.

5. If the capillary hydrostatic pressure exceeds the osmotic pressure, _____ will result.

True/False

Tell whether each of the following statements is true or false. If false, explain why the statement is incorrect.

1. Rapid release of thromboplastic material into the circulation activates the blood coagulation and fibrinolytic systems and leads to a disseminated intravascular coagulation syndrome. _____

   _____

2. Slow release of thromboplastic material into the circulation activates the blood coagulation and fibrinolytic systems and leads to a disseminated intravascular coagulation syndrome. _____

   _____

3. Slow release of thromboplastic material into the circulation activates the blood coagulation and fibrinolytic systems but also causes a compensatory increase in platelets and blood proteins concerned with blood coagulation (coagulation factors), which predisposes the person to intravascular thromboses. _____

   _____

4. Formation of blood clots within leg veins results primarily from slowing or stasis of blood in leg veins. _____

   _____

5. A large pulmonary embolus that completely blocks both pulmonary arteries causes infarction of both lungs.

   _____

Identify

1. Identify the four main causes of edema.

   a. _____

   b. _____

   c. _____

   d. _____

2. Identify the three conditions that may lead to the formation of blood clots within the heart.

   a. _____

   b. _____

   c. _____

3. Identify three diagnostic measures that may assist the clinician in making the diagnosis of a pulmonary infarct.

   a. _____

   b. _____

   c. _____

Matching 1

Several factors predispose to the formation of blood clots within blood vessels:

A. Sluggish blood flow within a blood vessel
B. Damage to the wall of a blood vessel
C. Increased coagulability of the blood

Write the letter of the factor that is of greatest importance in the following situations next to each statement:

1. _____ A thrombus formed in a coronary artery in which the lining (intima) is roughened by accumulation of cholesterol and other lipids in the arterial wall

2. _____ A thrombus formed in an artery of a healthy young woman taking birth control pills

3. _____ A thrombus in a leg vein of a healthy middle-aged man who had recently completed a 10-hour nonstop airplane flight

Matching 2

Match the type of shock with its likely cause:

1. _____ cardiogenic shock

2. _____ anaphylactic shock

3. _____ hypovolemic shock

4. _____ septic shock

a. overwhelming bacterial infection

b. hypersensitivity reaction to a bee sting

c. heart failure following a myocardial infarction (heart attack)

d. large hemorrhage from a gunshot wound

Discussion Questions

1. What factors regulate the flow of fluid into and out of the capillaries? (*Hint:* see Fig. 12-9.) _____

_____

_____

_____

2. Why do some patients with cancer develop blood clots within their circulation because they have a higher than normal level of platelets and blood coagulation factors? _____

_____

_____

_____

3. What is the difference between a thrombus and an embolus? _____

_____

_____

_____

4. What factors predispose a person to venous thrombosis? What are the major complications of a thrombus in a leg vein? _____

_____

_____

_____

5. What factors predispose a person to arterial thrombosis? _____

_____

_____

_____

6. What conditions predispose a person to thrombosis by increasing the coagulability of the blood? _____

_____

_____

_____

7. What is the usual source of pulmonary emboli? _____

_____

_____

_____

8. A 6-year-old child has marked edema of the legs and edema fluid within the abdominal cavity (ascites). The child's blood protein and albumin levels are much lower than normal. The urine contains large amounts of protein. What is the most likely cause of the edema? _____

_____

_____

9. A 58-year-old woman sustains a large pulmonary embolus that completely blocks the main pulmonary artery. Explain whether each of the following descriptors applies to the condition. Why or why not?

   a. Patient experiences severe pleuritic chest pain. _____

   _____

   b. Patient becomes short of breath. _____

   _____

   c. Lung scan is abnormal. _____

   _____

   d. Chest x-ray is abnormal. _____

   _____

   e. Patient had pulmonary infarct. _____

   _____

   f. Patient coughs up blood. _____

   _____

10. What populations have a greater than normal risk of developing thromboembolic disease? _____

_____

_____

_____

11. What factors predispose a person to postoperative venous thromboses? _____

_____

_____

_____

12. What conditions may result from a blood clot that forms in the left ventricle after a myocardial infarction? _____

_____

_____

_____

13. What are the two fundamental circulatory system derangements that lead to shock? _____

_____

_____

_____

Notes

Chapter 12

Circulatory Disturbances

Learning Objectives

- Venous thrombosis: causes and effects
- Pulmonary embolism: pathogenesis, clinical manifestations, diagnostic techniques
- Arterial thrombosis: causes and effects
- Edema and factors regulating fluid circulation between capillaries and interstitial tissue (hydrostatic pressure, capillary permeability, osmotic pressure, open lymphatic channel)
- Hypercoagulable state
- Shock: pathogenesis and treatment

Intravascular Blood Clots

- Normally, blood does not clot within the vascular system
- Pathogenesis of intravascular clotting
  - 1. Slowing or **stasis** of blood flow
  - 2. Blood vessel **wall damage**
  - 3. Increased **coagulability** of blood
- **Thrombus:** an intravascular clot; can occur in any vessel or within the heart
- **Embolus:** a detached clot carried into pulmonary or systemic circulation; plugs vessel of smaller caliber than diameter of clot, blocking blood flow and causing necrosis
- **Infarct:** tissue necrosis from interruption in blood flow

Embolism (1 of 5)

- From blood clots, fat, air, amnionic fluid, and foreign particles
- Fat embolism
  - Following severe bone fracture that disrupts fatty bone marrow and surrounding adipose tissue
  - Emulsified fat globules sucked into veins and carried into lungs, obstructing pulmonary capillaries
  - If it reaches systemic circulation, eventually blocks small vessels in brain and other organs

Embolism (2 of 5)

- Air embolism
  - Large amount of air sucked into circulation from lung injury due to a chest wound
  - May be accidentally injected into circulation
  - Air carried into right heart chambers and prevents filling of heart by returning venous blood
  - Heart unable to pump blood and individual dies rapidly of circulatory failure

Embolism (3 of 5)

- Amnionic fluid embolism
  - Devastating complication of pregnancy
  - Amnionic fluid enters maternal circulation through a tear in fetal membranes
  - Fetal cells, hair, fat, and amniotic debris fluid block maternal pulmonary capillaries causing severe respiratory distress
  - Thromboplastic material in fluid activates coagulation mechanism leading to disseminated intravascular coagulation syndrome

Embolism (4 of 5)

- Foreign particulate matter embolism
  - Various types of particulate material
  - May be injected by substance users that crush and dissolve tablets intended for oral use
  - Material injected intravenously and is trapped within small pulmonary blood vessels
  - Symptoms of severe respiratory distress

Embolism (5 of 5)

- Septic emboli
  - Thrombi form in pelvic vein following uterine infection
  - Bacteria invade thrombi
  - Emboli from infected thrombus travel to lungs, causing pulmonary infarct
  - Bacteria in clot invade pulmonary infarct causing lung abscess

Venous Thrombosis

- Predisposing factors to clot formation in leg veins
  - Prolonged bed rest
  - Cramped position for an extended period
  - Impaired "milking action" of leg musculature that normally promotes venous return resulting in stasis of blood in veins
  - Varicose veins or any condition preventing normal emptying of veins
- Outcome
  - Leg swelling from partial blockage of venous return in leg
  - Pulmonary embolism

Notes

Notes

Pulmonary Embolism (1 of 5)

- Clinical manifestations depend on size of embolus and where it lodges in the pulmonary artery
- Large pulmonary emboli may completely block main pulmonary artery or major branches obstructing blood flow to lungs
- Lung not infarcted due to collateral blood flow from bronchial arteries (from descending aorta) that interconnect with pulmonary arteries via collateral channels
- Cyanosis and shortness of breath due to inadequate oxygenation of blood

Pulmonary Embolism (2 of 5)

- Large pulmonary emboli
  - 1. Right side of heart becomes distended
  - 2. Pulmonary artery becomes overdistended with blood, causing increased pulmonary pressure
  - 3. Left ventricle unable to pump adequate blood to brain and vital organs
  - 4. Systemic blood pressure falls and patient may go into shock

Pulmonary Embolism (3 of 5)

- Small pulmonary emboli
  - Small emboli may pass through main pulmonary arteries, becoming impacted in peripheral arteries supplying lower lobes of the lungs
  - Raises pulmonary pressure and inadequate collateral circulation
  - Affected lung segment undergoes necrosis; wedge-shaped pulmonary infarct
  - If infarct develops: dyspnea, pleuritic chest pain, cough, and expectoration of bloody sputum due to leakage of blood from infarcted lung tissue into bronchi

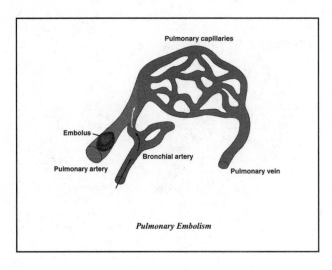

Pulmonary Embolism

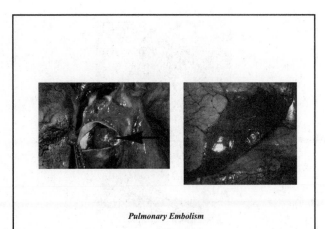

Pulmonary Embolism

Pulmonary Embolism (4 of 5)

- Diagnosis
  - Chest X-ray: detects infarct but not the embolus
  - Radioisotope lung scans: detects abnormal pulmonary blood flow caused by embolus
  - Pulmonary angiogram (gold standard): detects blocked pulmonary artery
  - Computed tomography (CT) scan: detects pulmonary embolus indicated by obstructed flow of contrast medium, information comparable to pulmonary angiography without requiring insertion of catheter in pulmonary artery

Notes

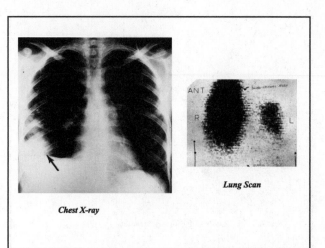

Chest X-ray

Lung Scan

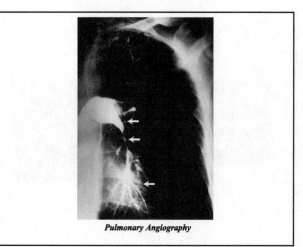

Pulmonary Angiography

Pulmonary Embolism (5 of 5)

- Treatment
  - Anticoagulants: heparin initially followed by coumadin
  - Thrombolytic drugs if with massive embolus
  - Angioplasty (balloon or stent to widen vein)
  - Thrombectomy (clot extraction surgery)
  - General supportive care

Arterial Thrombosis (1 of 2)

- Stasis is not a factor due to rapid blood flow and high intravascular pressure
- Main cause: injury to vessel wall from arteriosclerosis, causing ulceration, roughening of arterial with thrombi formation
- Blocks blood flow
  - Coronary artery: myocardial infarction
  - Major leg artery: gangrene
  - Cerebral artery: stroke

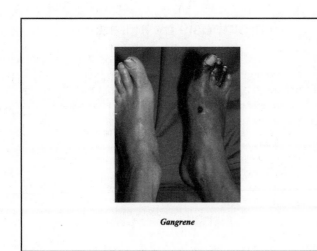

Gangrene

Arterial Thrombosis (2 of 2)

- Intracardiac thrombosis
  - Clot forms
    - Within atrial appendages: heart failure
    - Surfaces of heart valves: valve injury
    - Wall of left ventricle: myocardial infarction
  - May dislodge into systemic circulation and cause infarction: spleen, kidneys, brain

Thrombosis by Increased Coagulability (1 of 2)

- 1. Rise in coagulation factors following surgery or injury
- 2. Estrogen in contraceptive pills stimulates synthesis of clotting factors
- 3. Hereditary gene mutations
  - Mutation of gene that codes for factor V results in abnormal factor V Leiden: more resistant to inactivation, prolonged activity, increased coagulability
  - Mutation of gene regulating prothrombin synthesis
  - Risk for venous thrombosis increases as prothrombin level rises

Thrombosis by Increased Coagulability (2 of 2)

- 4. Thrombosis in patients with cancer, from increased platelets and coagulation factors
  - Predisposes to both arterial and venous thromboses
  - Hypercoagulability due to rapid release of thromboplastic materials into circulation from tumor deposits
  - Platelets and coagulation factors consumed faster than can be replenished, leading to bleeding
  - Large tumors release thromboplastic material slowly but continuously; production of coagulation factors exceeds destruction leading to hypercoagulability

Edema

- Accumulation of fluid in interstitial tissues, first noted in ankles and legs
- Results from disturbance of extracellular fluid circulation between capillaries and interstitial tissues
- Pitting edema: pit or indentation formed when edematous tissue is compressed with the fingertips
- Hydrothorax: fluid accumulates in pleural cavity
- Ascites: fluid accumulates in peritoneal cavity

Pathogenesis of Edema

- Increased capillary permeability
  - Causes swelling of tissues with acute inflammation
  - Increase in capillary permeability from some systemic diseases
- Low plasma proteins
  - Excess protein loss (kidney disease)
  - Inadequate synthesis (malnutrition)
- Increased hydrostatic pressure
  - Heart failure
  - Localized venous obstruction
- Lymphatic obstruction

Factors Regulating Fluid Flow Between Capillaries and Interstitial Tissue

- 1. Capillary hydrostatic pressure: force pushing fluid from capillaries into extracellular space
- 2. Capillary permeability: determines ease of fluid flow through capillary endothelium
- 3. Osmotic pressure: water-attracting property of a solution; exerted by proteins in the blood (colloid osmotic pressure) that attract fluid from interstitial space back into the capillaries
- 4. Open lymphatic channels: collect fluid forced out of the capillaries by the hydrostatic pressure and return fluid into circulation

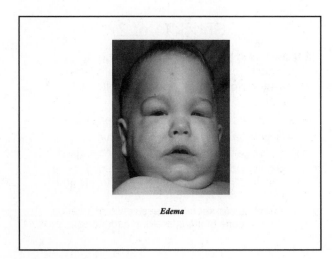

Edema

Notes

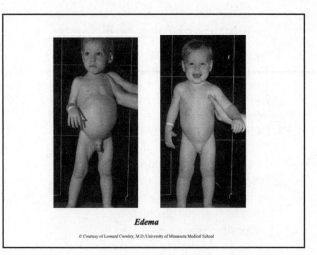

Edema

© Courtesy of Leonard Crowley, M.D./University of Minnesota Medical School

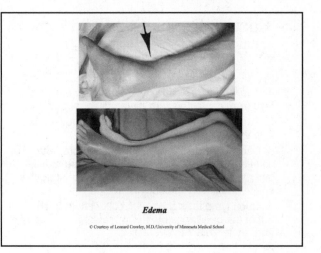

Edema

© Courtesy of Leonard Crowley, M.D./University of Minnesota Medical School

Shock (1 of 2)

- Low blood flow/pressure to adequately supply body with blood; potentially life-threatening; circulating blood volume < capacity of vascular system
- Categories according to pathogenesis
  - Hypovolemic shock: low blood volume
  - Cardiogenic shock: reduced cardiac output
  - Septic shock: excessive vasodilatation secondary to release of microbial toxins and inflammatory mediators
  - Anaphylactic shock: excessive vasodilatation from release of inflammatory mediators

Shock (2 of 2)

- Prognosis depends on early recognition and rapid appropriate treatment
  - Drugs that promote vasoconstriction
  - Use of intravenous fluids or blood to restore blood volume secondary to fluid loss or hemorrhage
  - Treat underlying cause

Notes

Chapter Outline

The chapter outline provides you with an organizational guide to the topics and ideas presented in this chapter of the text.

Cardiac Structure and Function
Normal Cardiac Function
    Cardiac Chambers
    Cardiac Valves
    Blood Supply to the Heart
    Conduction System of the Heart
    Blood Pressure
Heart Disease as a Disturbance of Pump Function
Congenital Heart Disease
    Prevention of Congenital Heart Disease
Valvular Heart Disease
    Rheumatic Fever and Rheumatic Heart Disease
    Nonrheumatic Aortic Stenosis
    Mitral Valve Prolapse
    Serotonin-Related Heart Valve Damage
    Infective Endocarditis
Coronary Heart Disease
    Risk Factors
    Manifestations and Complications
Myocardial Infarction
    Location of Myocardial Infarcts
    Complications of Myocardial Infarcts
    Survival After Myocardial Infarction
    Diagnosis of Myocardial Infarction
    Treatment of Myocardial Infarction
Case Studies
Coronary Artery Disease
    Diagnosis of Coronary Artery Disease
    Treatment of Coronary Artery Disease
    Taking Aspirin to Reduce Risk of Cardiovascular Disease
    Cocaine-Induced Arrhythmias and Myocardial Infarcts
    Blood Lipids and Coronary Artery Disease
    Homocysteine and Cardiovascular Disease
    Chlamydia pneumoniae and Cardiovascular Disease
Hypertension and Hypertensive Cardiovascular Disease
    Cardiac Effects
    Vascular Effects
    Renal Effects
    Cause and Treatment of Hypertension

Study Questions

The following questions are provided as a test for comprehension and as a study guide for use with the text chapters. Additional study material is located at http://health.jbpub.com/humandisease/8e, which contains useful tools such as an A&P review, animated flashcards, an interactive online glossary, crossword puzzles, and web links.

Key Terms

Define the following terms:

1. Bacterial endocarditis _____

2. Dissecting aneurysm _____

3. Stent _____

4. Atherosclerosis _____

5. Rheumatic fever _____

6. Arteriosclerotic aneurysm _____

7. Angina pectoris _____

8. Myocardial infarction _____

9. Lipoprotein _____

Fill-in-the-Blank

1. The _____ valves are open in systole.

2. The _____ valves are open in diastole.

3. A dissecting aneurysm of the aorta is due to _____.

4. One of the important complications of mitral valve scarring due to rheumatic fever is _____.

5. The _____ stage in the formation of an atheromatous plaque is reversible.

True/False

Tell whether each statement is true or false. If false, explain why the statement is incorrect.

1. A coronary artery narrowed by an atheromatous plaque often can be dilated successfully by coronary angioplasty.

   _____

2. A successfully dilated coronary artery may undergo restenosis, but using a stent to keep the vessel open reduces the incidence of restenosis. _____

   _____

3. Stents coated with drugs that suppress the cell proliferation responsible for the restenosis have not been effective and are not recommended to prevent restenosis. _____

   _____

4. The left anterior descending coronary artery supplies the back wall of the heart. _____

   _____

5. Impulses that cause the heart to beat are initiated in the sinoatrial (SA) node. _____

   _____

6. The systolic pressure is a measure of the resistance to blood flow due to constriction of the peripheral arterioles.

   _____

7. The rate of flow through arteries varies directly with the radius of the artery. _____

   _____

8. The systolic pressure is the highest pressure within the vascular system when blood is ejected from the ventricle during systole. _____

   _____

9. A coronary arteriogram (angiogram) may appear normal in some persons with symptoms of coronary artery disease. _____

   _____

10. Isolated systolic hypertension (with normal diastolic pressure) occurs primarily in younger persons and is not harmful._____

    _____

11. A small aortic aneurysm (about 5-cm diameter) can usually be detected by a physical examination, and more detailed diagnostic studies are not required. _____

    _____

Multiple Choice

1. Which of the following conditions IS NOT a characteristic feature of the metabolic syndrome?
   a. hypertension
   b. cyanosis
   c. impaired carbohydrate tolerance
   d. obesity
   e. elevated blood lipids

2. A patient complains of chest pain, and a myocardial infarction is suspected. Which of the following tests or procedures WOULD NOT provide information that would support the diagnosis of a myocardial infarction?
   a. elevation of the ST segment in the electrocardiogram
   b. elevated blood pressure
   c. blood test indicating elevated creatine kinase (CK-MB)
   d. blood test indicating elevated blood troponin.

3. An angiogram performed on a patient with chest pain reveals a recent thrombus blocking a large coronary artery. Assuming that the patient has access to a completely staffed coronary care facility, what would be the most effective way to treat this condition?
   a. bed rest and sedation to alleviate the patient's discomfort
   b. prescribe a low-fat diet
   c. attempt to dissolve the thrombus by thrombolytic therapy
   d. perform a procedure (percutaneous coronary intervention) to remove the thrombus and insert a stent to keep the artery open

4. The main function of the foramen ovale in the fetus is
   a. shunting blood from the left to the right atrium
   b. shunting blood from the right to the left atrium
   c. shunting blood from the pulmonary artery into the aorta
   d. shunting blood from the aorta into the pulmonary artery

5. The main function of the ductus arteriosus is
   a. shunting blood from the left to the right atrium
   b. shunting blood from the right to the left atrium
   c. shunting blood from the pulmonary artery into the aorta
   d. shunting blood from the aorta into the pulmonary artery

Identify

1. Identify the four major factors that are known to increase the risk of coronary heart disease.
   a. _____
   b. _____
   c. _____
   d. _____

2. Identify four complications of an acute myocardial infarction.
   a. _____
   b. _____
   c. _____
   d. _____

3. The term "acute coronary syndrome" includes three different conditions. What are they?
   a. _____
   b. _____
   c. _____

Matching 1

Match the item in the left column with its characteristic or property in the right column.

1. _____ Diastolic heart failure

2. _____ Ejection fraction

3. _____ Stroke volume

4. _____ Systolic heart failure

5. _____ Natriuretic peptide

A. A peptide released from stretched cardiac muscle

B. Impaired ejection of blood from ventricle

C. The percentage of the blood in the ventricle that is ejected during systole

D. Impaired ventricular filling

E. The volume of blood ejected from the ventricle during a systolic contraction

Matching 2

Match the cardiovascular disease or condition in the left column with its manifestations in the right column.

1. _____ Bicuspid aortic valve

2. _____ Coarctation of aorta

3. _____ Patent ductus arteriosus

4. _____ Atrial septal defect

5. _____ Tetralogy of Fallot

a. Narrow segment of proximal aorta obstructs blood flow into distal aorta

b. Predisposes to development of aortic stenosis

c. Cyanosis results from mixing of low-oxygen-content arterial blood with normally oxygenated arterial blood

d. Blood ejected into the aorta mixes with blood in the pulmonary artery

e. Blood in the left atrium mixes with blood in the right atrium.

Discussion Questions

1. Describe how heart valves function to provide unidirectional flow of blood through the heart. _____
   _____
   _____
   _____

2. Describe what happens if the mitral valve doesn't open properly and what happens if it doesn't close properly.
   _____
   _____
   _____

3. What are the structural changes in the mitral valve that lead to mitral valve prolapse? _____
   _____
   _____
   _____

4. What factors predispose a person to calcific aortic stenosis? _____
   _____
   _____
   _____

5. Describe the conditions that predispose a person to infective endocarditis. _____
   _____
   _____
   _____

6. Which patients should have antibiotic prophylaxis prior to dental procedures or surgical procedures? _____
   _____
   _____
   _____

7. What types of diets lower blood lipids? _____

_____

_____

_____

8. Why are cardiac enzyme tests performed on the blood of patients suspected of having a myocardial infarction?

_____

_____

_____

9. A patient complains of chest pain. Clinical examination, enzyme tests, and electrocardiogram reveal a thrombosis of the left anterior descending coronary artery. How should the patient be treated? _____

_____

_____

_____

10. What methods can be used to reestablish blood flow through a blocked coronary artery? _____

_____

_____

_____

11. Describe the effect of high blood pressure on the heart and vascular system. _____

_____

_____

_____

12. Patients at risk for coronary heart disease frequently take low-dose aspirin tablets daily to reduce the risk of heart attacks. What effect does aspirin have? Why is it used? _____

_____

_____

_____

13. What conditions may lead to cardiac valve scarring? _____

_____

_____

_____

14. What diagnostic measures may assist the clinician in making a diagnosis of acute myocardial infarction? _____

_____

_____

_____

15. What is the cause of an aneurysm of the abdominal aorta that occurs in an older individual? How is it treated?

_____

_____

_____

16. What happens during congestive cardiac failure? _____

_____

_____

_____

17. What is C-reactive protein (CRP)? What does an elevated CRP test indicate? _____

_____

_____

_____

Notes

Chapter 13

The Cardiovascular System

Learning Objectives (1 of 2)

- Basic anatomy and physiology
- Causes, effects, and treatment
  - Congenital heart disease
  - Valvular heart disease
- Pathogenesis, risk factors, clinical manifestations, complications, and treatment:
  - Coronary heart disease (CHD)
  - Myocardial infarction (MI)
- Principles of diagnosis and treatment
  - Coronary heart disease (CHD)
  - Myocardial Infarction (MI)

Learning Objectives (2 of 2)

- Dietary effects on coronary heart disease
  - "Good" and "bad" cholesterol
  - Transport of cholesterol by lipoproteins
- Adverse effects, pathogenesis, clinical manifestations, and treatment
  - Hypertension
  - Acute and chronic heart failure
  - Arteriosclerotic and dissecting aneurysms of aorta
  - Diseases affecting veins

Notes

Anatomy and Physiology (1 of 6)

- Function: muscular pump; propels blood through the lungs → tissues
- Heart disease: disturbance of function
- Location: within mediastinum; extends obliquely about 5 inches from second rib to fifth intercostal space; rests on the diaphragm; anterior to vertebral column and posterior to sternum
  - 2/3 of heart mass lies left of midsternal line
  - Apex of heart points downward toward the left hip

Anatomy and Physiology (2 of 6)

- Heart coverings
  - Pericardium (double-walled sac, outer layer of tough connective tissue
  - Epicardium (visceral layer of pericardium covering myocardium)
- Layers of the heart wall
  - Epicardium: outer layer of connective tissue, coronary arteries
  - Myocardium: middle layer, muscular, thickest layer, workhorse of the heart
  - Endocardium: innermost layer, smooth membrane, heart valves part of endocardium

Anatomy and Physiology (3 of 6)

- Chambers: no direct communication bet. right and left halves
  - Right half (right atrium, RA and right ventricle, RV)
    - Pulmonary pump, circulates blood into pulmonary artery, lungs
  - Left half (left atrium, LA and left ventricle, LV)
    - Systemic pump, circulates blood into aorta, organs and tissues

Anatomy and Physiology (4 of 6)

- Atria (singular: atrium) = receiving chambers, thin-walled
- Blood enters RA via three veins:
  - 1. Superior vena cava (from body regions above diaphragm)
  - 2. Inferior vena cava (from body areas below diaphragm)
  - 3. Coronary sinus (collects blood that drains from myocardium)
- Blood enters LA via four pulmonary veins

Anatomy and Physiology (5 of 6)

- Cardiac valves permit flow of blood in only one direction
- Atrioventricular or AV valves: flap-like valves between atria and ventricles; prevent back flow of blood into atria when ventricles contract
  - 1. Tricuspid valve: three flexible flaps; directs blood flow from RA to RV, prevents backflow to RA when RV contracts
  - 2. Bicuspid valve or mitral valve: directs blood flow from LA to LV; prevents backflow to LA when LV contracts

Anatomy and Physiology (6 of 6)

- Semilunar valves
  - Cup-shaped
  - Surround orifices of aorta and pulmonary artery
  - Free margins of valves face upward
  - Prevent backflow of blood into ventricles during diastole
- Pulmonary valve: from RV to pulmonary trunk
- Aortic valve: from LV to aorta

Notes

Pulmonary-Systemic Circulation

- Blood returns to the heart low in oxygen and high in carbon dioxide
- Pulmonary circulation
  - Oxygen-poor blood enters RA → RV through tricuspid valve → pulmonary <u>artery</u> → lungs
- Systemic circulation
  - Freshly oxygenated blood leave lungs through pulmonary <u>veins</u> → LA → LV through mitral valve → aorta → rest of the body

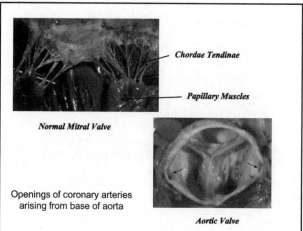

Chordae Tendinae

Papillary Muscles

Normal Mitral Valve

Openings of coronary arteries arising from base of aorta

Aortic Valve

Coronary Circulation (1 of 3)

- Main blood supply of the heart
- Shortest circulation in the body
- Myocardium is too thick for the diffusion of nutrients
- Aorta branches to right and left coronary arteries that carry arterial blood to the heart when relaxed
- Blood passes through capillary beds of myocardium
- Venous blood collected by cardiac veins
- Cardiac veins join together and form the coronary sinus that empties blood into the RA

Notes

Coronary Circulation (2 of 3)

- Blood supply to the heart
  - Right coronary artery, RCA
    - Supplies posterior wall and posterior part of interventricular septum
  - Left coronary artery, LCA and branches
    - Left anterior descending artery, LADA
    - Supplies anterior wall, anterior part of interventricular septum
    - Left circumflex artery, LCA; supplies lateral wall
- Adult cardiac muscle does not proliferate to replace damaged or destroyed muscle fibers
- Most areas of cell death repaired with non-contractile scar tissue

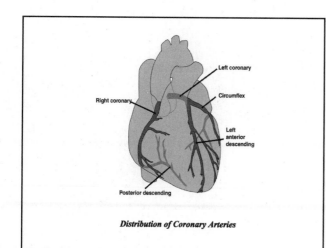

Distribution of Coronary Arteries

Coronary Circulation (3 of 3)

- Angina pectoris
  - Chest pain from temporary reduction in blood flow to cardiac muscles despite increased oxygen demand
  - Causes:
    - Narrowed coronary arteries from arteriosclerosis
    - Stress-induced spasm of coronary arteries
- Prolonged coronary artery blockage can lead to myocardial infarction (MI)

Notes

_____

_____

_____

_____

_____

_____

_____

_____

_____

_____

_____

_____

_____

_____

_____

_____

_____

_____

_____

_____

_____

_____

_____

_____

_____

_____

_____

_____

_____

Conduction System

- A group of specialized muscle cells that initiate electrical impulses
- Impulses are initiated in the SA (sinoatrial node) in RA near opening of the superior vena cava
- Ability of cardiac muscle to depolarize and contract is intrinsic; does not depend on the nervous system

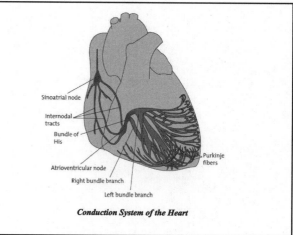

Conduction System of the Heart

Cardiac Cycle

- Consists of all events associated with blood flow through the heart during one complete heart beat
- Atrial systole → atrial diastole → ventricular systole → ventricular diastole
  - Systole: contraction period
  - Diastole: relaxation period
- Cardiac output: typically 5 liters/minute pumped out by each ventricle

Blood Pressure

- Blood flow in the arteries results from the force of ventricular contraction
- Pressure is highest when ventricles contract (systolic pressure)
- Pressure is lowest when ventricles relax (diastolic pressure)

Electrocardiogram, ECG

- Measures electrical activity of heart; diagnostic tool
  - P wave: atrial depolarization, atrial systole
  - QRS complex: ventricular depolarization, ventricular systole
  - T wave: ventricular diastole
  - PR interval: time for depolarization to pass from atria to ventricles via AV bundle
- Detects disturbances in rate, rhythm, conduction, muscle injury, extent of muscle damage

Cardiac Arrhythmias

- Disturbances in heart rate or rhythm
- 1. Atrial fibrillation, AF
  - Atria quiver versus contracting normally
  - Ventricles beat irregularly and fast shortening diastole (pulse deficit)
- 2. Ventricular fibrillation, VF
  - Ventricles unable to contract normally, incompatible with life
- 3. Heart block (complete or incomplete)
  - Delay or interruption of impulse transmission from atria to ventricles, from arteriosclerosis

Notes

Heart Disease—A Disturbance of Pump Function

Mechanical Pump Abnormality	Comparable Heart Diseases
Faulty pump construction	Congenital heart disease
Faulty unidirectional valves	Valvular heart disease
Dirty or plugged fuel line	Coronary heart disease
Overloaded pump	Hypertensive heart disease
Malfunctioning pump	Primary myocardial disease

Congenital Heart Disease

- Causes: German measles, Down syndrome, drugs, genetic factors, undetermined causes
- Presentation
  - 1. Fetal bypass channels fail to close normally
    - Patent ductus ateriosus; patent foramen ovale
  - 2. Atrial, ventricular, or combined septal defects
  - 3. Abnormalities obstructing flow: Pulmonary stenosis, aortic stenosis, coarctation of the aorta
  - 4. Abnormal formation of aorta and pulmonary artery or abnormal connection of vessels: tetralogy of Fallot, transposition of great vessels
- Prevention: protect developing fetus from intrauterine injury

Valvular Heart Disease (1 of 11)

- Rheumatic fever and rheumatic heart disease
- Non-rheumatic aortic stenosis
- Mitral valve prolapse
- Serotonin-related heart valve damage
- Infective endocarditis

Valvular Heart Disease (2 of 11)

- Rheumatic fever
  - Commonly encountered in children
  - NOT a bacterial infection but an immunologic reaction that develops weeks after initial streptococcal infection
  - Complication of group A beta hemolytic streptococcal infection (sore throat and scarlet fever)
  - Fever + inflammation of connective tissue throughout the body, especially heart and joints
  - Acute arthritis (multiple joints) + inflammation of heart

Valvular Heart Disease (3 of 11)

- Rheumatic fever
  - Anti-streptococcal antibodies against strep antigens cross react with similar antigens in tissues
  - Antigen-antibody reaction injures connective tissue and causes fever
  - Clinical outcomes
    - Healing with scarring of tissues (heart valves)
    - Death from severe inflammation and acute heart failure
    - Can recur if another streptococcal infection reactivates hypersensitivity and tissue damage

Valvular Heart Disease (4 of 11)

- Rheumatic heart disease
  - Complication of rheumatic fever
  - Scarring of heart valves following rheumatic inflammation
  - Primarily affects mitral and aortic valves
  - Clinical outcome: valve regurgitation or stenosis → impairs cardiac function, increases strain on heart, eventually leads to heart failure
  - Prevention
    - Treat beta strep infection promptly
    - Prophylactic penicillin throughout childhood and young adulthood to prevent strep infections and reduce risk of recurrent rheumatic fever and further heart valve damage

Notes

Notes

- Non-rheumatic aortic stenosis
  - Occurs in 2% of population
  - Aortic stenosis secondary to bicuspid aortic valve
  - Calcific aortic stenosis
  - Aortic stenosis secondary to bicuspid aortic valve
  - Aortic valve has 2 cusps than usual 3 cusps
  - Functions satisfactorily for a time, then becomes thickened, calcified, and rigid from increased strain on valve, leads to heart failure

- Non-rheumatic aortic stenosis
  - Calcific aortic stenosis
  - Normal 3 cusps, common valvular heart disease
  - Leaflets undergo connective tissue degenerative changes $\rightarrow$ fibrotic, calcified, rigid $\rightarrow$ restricts valve mobility, stenosis
  - Recent studies: also occurs with deposits of lipids and macrophages as in coronary atherosclerosis
  - Clinical outcomes: $\uparrow$ strain $\rightarrow$ left ventricular hypertrophy $\rightarrow$ heart failure
  - Prevention: Control risk factors (high cholesterol, diabetes, hypertension)

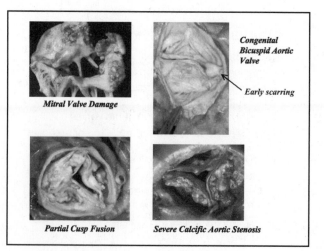

Mitral Valve Damage

Congenital Bicuspid Aortic Valve

Early scarring

Partial Cusp Fusion

Severe Calcific Aortic Stenosis

Valvular Heart Disease (7 of 11)

- Mitral valve prolapse
  - Common but only few develop problems
  - One or both leaflets enlarge, stretch, and prolapse into LA during ventricular systole
  - Prolapsing leaflets may not fit together tightly → blood leaks back into LA; mitral regurgitation
  - On auscultation: "click" sound on systole followed by a "faint systolic murmur" from reflux of blood in between closed valve leaflets
  - Diagnosis: echocardiography
  - Prolapse with mitral regurgitation → give antibiotic prophylaxis prior to dental or surgical procedure

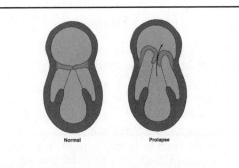

Normal   Prolapse

Mitral valve leaflets are attached to the mitral annulus around valve opening. Normally, valves close at or just below the level of the annulus.

Valvular Heart Disease (8 of 11)

- Serotonin-related heart valve damage
  - Increased serotonin (5-hydroxytryptamine) in blood
  - Produced by neuroendocrine cells in:
    - Secretory and absorptive cells of GIT
    - Epithelium of other organs
  - Released from:
    - 1. Platelets together with histamine
    - 2. Nerve endings; involved in transmitting impulses
    - 3. Neuroendocrine tumors in GIT; also develops thickening of heart valves → impairs cardiac function

Notes

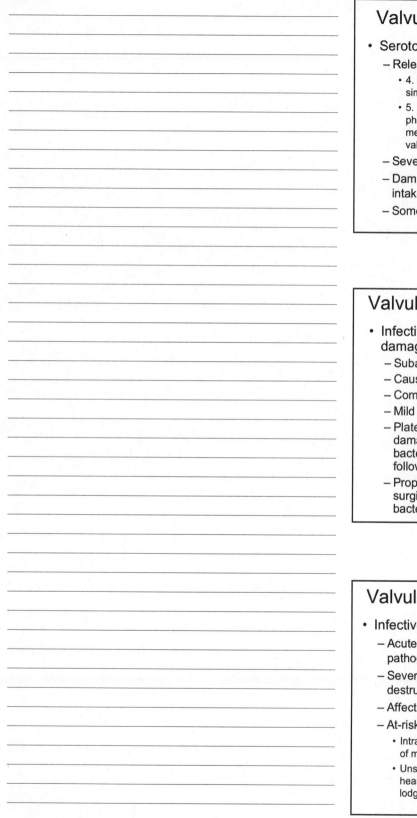

Valvular Heart Disease (9 of 11)

- Serotonin-related heart valve damage
  - Released from:
    - 4. Drugs for treating migraine have chemical structure similar to serotonin; may produce heart valve damage
    - 5. Drugs that suppress appetite (fenfluramine and phentermine, or fen-phen) affect serotonin metabolism in body and are associated with heart valve damage
  - Severity depends on dose and duration of use
  - Damage did not progress after stopping drug intake
  - Some improve over time

Valvular Heart Disease (10 of 11)

- Infective endocarditis: affects abnormal or damaged mitral, aortic valves
  - Subacute infective endocarditis
  - Caused by organisms of low virulence
  - Complication of any valvular heart disease
  - Mild symptoms of infection
  - Platelets and fibrin may deposit on abnormal or damaged valves; then serve as sites for bacteria to implant or for thrombi to form followed by emboli and tissue infarct
  - Prophylactic antibiotics given prior to dental or surgical procedures to prevent transient bacteremia and resulting endocarditis

Valvular Heart Disease (11 of 11)

- Infective endocarditis
  - Acute infective endocarditis caused by highly pathogenic organisms, commonly staphylococci
  - Severe symptoms of infection and valve destruction
  - Affects normal heart valves
  - At-risk groups:
    - Intravenous drug users; affect tricuspid valve instead of mitral or aortic valves
    - Unsterile materials or contaminants enter right side of heart, form large bacteria-laden vegetations on valve, lodge into lungs cause pulmonary infarct

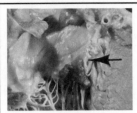

Bacterial Endocarditis,
mitral valve

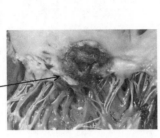

Severe Bacterial Endocarditis
Staphylococcal infection of normal
mitral valve with leaflet destruction
and perforation

Coronary Heart Disease (1 of 2)

- Cause: arteriosclerosis of coronary arteries
  - Narrowing of arteries from lipid deposits (neutral fat and cholesterol) by diffusion from bloodstream
- Pathogenesis: Endothelial injury → cells proliferate in intima
  - Cholesterol and lipids accumulate in cytoplasm (unstable plaques)
  - Cholesterol precipitates as crystals, causing cell necrosis
  - Cholesterol crystals, debris, enzymes leak out
  - Secondary fibrosis, calcification, degenerative changes in arterial wall
  - Formation of atheroma (rough, ulcerated surface predisposed to clot formation)

Coronary Heart Disease (2 of 2)

- Atheroma or atheromatous plaque
  - Irregular mass of yellow, mushy debris encroaching on lumen of artery and extending into muscular and elastic tissues of arterial wall
- Stable plaque
  - Surrounded by fibrous tissue
  - Causes permanent narrowing of vessel

Notes

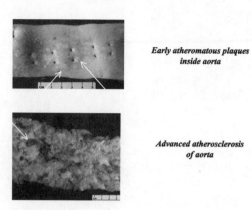

*Early atheromatous plaques
inside aorta*

*Advanced atherosclerosis
of aorta*

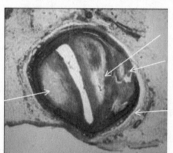

Several stable
atheromatous plaques
surrounded by dense
connective tissue.

Atheromatous deposits reduce lumen of coronary artery
Without excessive demands on heart, 50% or more
arterial narrowing may still supply enough blood to heart,
but is inadequate during exertion.

Coronary Heart Disease Risk Factors

- Most important risk factors
  - Elevated blood lipids
  - High blood pressure
  - Cigarette smoking
  - Diabetes
- Likelihood of coronary heart disease and heart attack
  - 1 risk factor = 2x risk
  - 2 risk factors = 4x risk
  - 3 risk factors = 7x risk
- Other risk factors: obesity; Type A personality

Coronary Heart Disease Manifestations (1 of 2)

- Also referred to as ischemic heart disease
- Due to decreased blood supply to heart muscle from narrowing or obstruction of the coronary arteries (myocardial ischemia)
- Clinical manifestations are variable
  - Asymptomatic (free of symptoms)
  - Angina pectoris, "pain of the chest"
  - Bouts of oppressive chest pain that may radiate into neck or arms; caused by myocardial ischemia

Coronary Heart Disease Manifestations (2 of 2)

- Stable angina: midsternal pressure or discomfort on exertion, subsides with rest or intake of nitroglycerine
- Unstable angina: pain lasts longer, occurs more frequently, and is less completely relieved by nitroglycerine
- Prinzmetal's angina: pain at rest rather than exertion, caused by coronary artery spasm
- More severe and prolonged myocardial ischemia may precipitate an acute episode manifested as:
  - Myocardial infarction: actual necrosis of heart muscle
  - Cardiac arrest: cessation of normal cardiac contractions

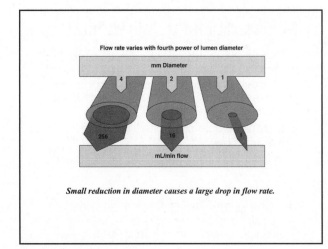

Small reduction in diameter causes a large drop in flow rate.

Notes

Notes

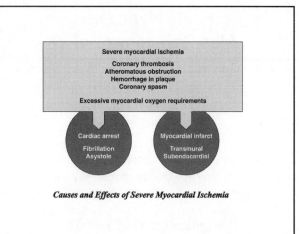

Causes and Effects of Severe Myocardial Ischemia

Myocardial Infarction

- Necrosis of heart muscle from severe ischemia
  - Insufficient blood flow through one of the coronary arteries and inadequate collateral flow into ischemic muscle
- Transmural infarct: full-thickness infarct from endocardium to epicardium, usually from clot in major coronary artery
- Subendocardial infarct: only part of wall undergoes necrosis

Myocardial Infarction–Location

- Often involves muscles of left ventricle and septum
  - Thicker walls require rich blood supply; work harder to pump blood into systemic circulation; rarely involves atria or right ventricle
- Depend on location of obstruction and collateral flow
  - Anterior wall: left anterior descending artery distribution
  - Lateral wall: circumflex artery distribution
  - Posterior wall: right coronary artery distribution
  - Massive anterior and lateral wall: main left coronary distribution, frequently fatal

Myocardial Infarction–Mechanisms

- Basic mechanisms that trigger a heart attack
  - 1. Sudden blockage of a coronary artery from a thrombus or atheromatous debris
  - 2. Hemorrhage into an atheromatous plaque
  - 3. Arterial spasm
  - 4. Sudden greatly increased myocardial oxygen requirements (vigorous physical activities)
- Cardiac arrest may result from
  - 1. Arrhythmia from prolonged or severe myocardial ischemia that disrupts ventricular contraction; most common and rapidly fatal is ventricular fibrillation
  - 2. Asystole: complete cessation of cardiac contractions

Myocardial Infarction–Complications (1 of 2)

- 1. Arrhythmias from irritability of ischemic heart muscle adjacent to the infarct or from conduction disturbance (heart block)
- 2. Heart failure due to badly damaged ventricles
- 3. Intracardial thrombi: mural thrombus forms on ventricular wall; bits of clot embolize into systemic circulation causing infarct in brain, kidneys, spleen
- 4. Pericarditis: infarct extends to epicardial surface, leads to inflammation and fluid accumulation in pericardial sac; may cause chest pain

Myocardial Infarction–Complications (2 of 2)

- 5. Cardiac rupture: blood leaks into pericardial sac from perforation in necrotic muscle, prevents ventricular filling (cardiac tamponade); rupture may occur in ventricular septum or papillary muscle
- 6. Papillary muscle dysfunction: infarcted papillary muscle unable to control mitral valve leaflet resulting in mitral valve prolapse and mitral insufficiency
- 7. Ventricular aneurysm: late complication; outward bulging of healing infarct during ventricular systole; reduces left ventricular function and cardiac output; rather than being ejected, blood fills aneurysm sac

Notes

Notes

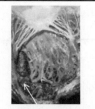

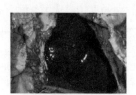

Clotted blood around heart
compressing heart, preventing
ventricular filling

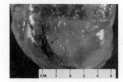

Mural thrombus adherent to
endocardium

Cardiac rupture through a large
transmural infarct

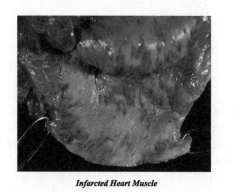

Infarcted Heart Muscle

Myocardial Infarction–Survival

- Factors affecting survival:
  - Size of infarct
  - Age of patient
  - Complications
  - Other diseases
- Mortality rates: 6% for small infarcts without heart failure to ≥ 50% for large infarcts with severe heart failure
- 90% of hospitalized patients survive
- Causes of death following MI: arrhythmia, heart failure, cardiac rupture with tamponade

Myocardial Infarction– Diagnosis (1 of 2)

- Medical history: inconclusive
  - Pain of severe angina may be similar to pain of MI
  - Possible mild symptoms subendocardial infarct
- Physical examination: usually not abnormal unless patient exhibits evidence of shock, heart failure, murmur
- Laboratory data
  - Electrocardiogram, ECG or EKG
  - Enzyme tests; enzymes leak out from necrotic cells after an infarct
  - The larger the infarct, the longer for elevated levels to return to normal

Myocardial Infarction– Diagnosis (2 of 2)

- Enzyme tests
  - Troponin T and troponin I
    - Specific to heart, slight heart damage causes levels to rise
    - Peaks in 24 hours, remains high for 10-14 days
  - Creatine kinase isoenzyme, CK-MB
    - Rises a few hours after MI, peaks in 24 hours
  - Myoglobin
    - Rises rapidly after MI, peaks in few hours, nonspecific
  - Lactic dehydrogenase isoenzyme, LDH
    - Rises more slowly than CK-MB, remains high for 10-14 days

Myocardial Infarction – Treatment (1 of 6)

- Acute coronary syndromes
  - Severe unstable angina
  - Minor myocardial damage
  - Major myocardial infarction
- Immediate treatment: Complete blockage of major coronary artery from a thrombus
  - Chest pain + EKG suggestive of large infarct + high CK-MB, troponin

Notes

Myocardial Infarction–
Treatment (2 of 6)

- Thrombolytic therapy
  - Effective but clot may not dissolve completely
  - Better outcome the sooner clot is dissolved (within 1 hour of first MI symptoms)
  - May cause bleeding problems
  - Angioplasty favored for restoring coronary blood flow
- Streptokinase: fibrinolytic enzyme from beta streptococci; activates plasminogen, reduces blood coagulability, dissolves clots
- Tissue plasminogen activator (TPA): converts plasminogen to plasmin and dissolves clots
- Aspirin: reduces tendency of platelets to aggregate
- Heparin: reduces coagulability of blood, reduces clot formation

Myocardial Infarction–
Treatment (3 of 6)

- Contraindications for thrombolytic therapy:
  - Stroke or diseases of cerebral blood vessels
  - Severe hypertension
  - Recent operation
  - Bleeding disorder or condition (gastric or duodenal ulcer)
- Anticoagulant drugs: reduce coagulability and clot formation
- Beta-blockers: reduce myocardial irritability, complications
- Bed rest advancing to graded activity
- Anti-arrhythmic drugs: reduce irritability of heart muscle
- Cardiac pacemaker: if complete heart block develops

Myocardial Infarction–
Treatment (4 of 6)

- Medical treatment: control or eliminate risk factors
  - 1. Cessation of smoking
  - 2. Control of hypertension
  - 3. Anti-coronary diet: low cholesterol and fat
  - 4. Weight reduction
  - 5. Graduated exercise program
- Evaluate: coronary angiogram to locate and determine degree of obstruction

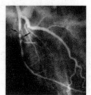

Myocardial Infarction– Treatment (5 of 6)

- Discrepancies in clinical symptoms and apparently normal coronary angiograms:
  - 1. Arteriosclerosis present but angiogram cannot detect it
    - Uniform and diffuse deposits expand outward and not into lumen versus discrete plaques
  - 2. Normal coronary arteries but coronary artery spasm reduces myocardial blood flow from marked sympathetic nervous system vasoconstrictor impulses
    - Prinzmetal's angina and stress-induced coronary vasoconstriction (severe emotional stress → vasospasm)

Myocardial Infarction– Treatment (6 of 6)

- Discrepancies in clinical symptoms and apparently normal coronary angiograms:
  - 3. Normal coronary arteries but abnormal function of coronary arterioles
    - Unable to dilate sufficiently to provide adequate blood flow during exertion

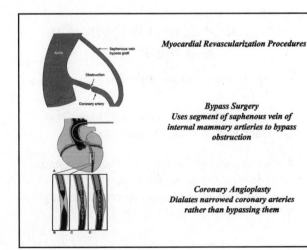

Myocardial Revascularization Procedures

Bypass Surgery
Uses segment of saphenous vein of internal mammary artieries to bypass obstruction

Coronary Angioplasty
Dialates narrowed coronary arteries rather than bypassing them

Discussion

- What is the difference between angina pectoris and myocardial infarction?
- What are the clinical manifestations of myocardial infarction?
- Patients at risk for coronary heart disease frequently take low-dose aspirin tablets to reduce the risk of heart attacks. What effects does aspirin have? Why is it used?

Case Study

- 74-year-old man admitted to ER for severe oppressive chest pain of about 5 hours duration. Two weeks before admission, had less severe chest pain when walking rapidly, but subsided with rest
  - BP: 190/110; lungs clear, normal heart sounds
  - ECG: acute MI on anterior wall of LV
  - Elevated creatine phosphokinase and lactic dehydrogenase
- Which coronary artery is likely involved?
- Why are cardiac enzymes elevated?
- What conditions may follow this man's MI?

Cocaine-Induced Arrhythmias and Infarcts

- Prolongs and intensifies effects of sympathetic nervous system:
  - Increases heart rate: increased oxygen demand
  - Increased muscle irritability: predisposes to arrhythmias
  - Increased peripheral vasoconstriction and coronary artery spasm: high blood pressure
  - Fatal arrhythmias and MI can occur even among those with normal coronary arteries

Blood Lipids and Coronary Artery Disease

- Neutral fat: triglyceride (3 molecules of fatty acid combined with glycerol) from ingested fat, sugar, and carbohydrates
- Trans fat and saturated fat: atherogenic
- Cholesterol: synthesized in body and from diet
- High levels associated with premature atherosclerosis and increased CVD risk; transported by lipoproteins
  - 1. Low density lipoprotein, LDL, "bad cholesterol"
  - 2. High density lipoprotein, HDL, "good cholesterol"
    - Protective; increases with regular exercise, smoking cessation, modest alcohol intake

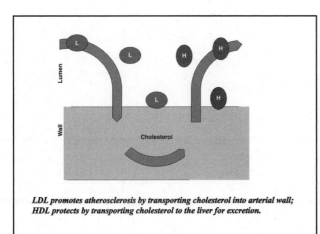

LDL promotes atherosclerosis by transporting cholesterol into arterial wall; HDL protects by transporting cholesterol to the liver for excretion.

Cardiovascular Risk Factors (1 of 2)

- C-reactive protein, CRP
  - Produced in liver and released in response to tissue injury or inflammation
  - High CRP level predicts high CVD risk
  - Detects accumulation of macrophages, lymphocytes, lipids, products of tissue injury in unstable plaques in coronary arteries
- Metabolic syndrome
  - Abdominal obesity, hypertension, abnormal lipids, insulin resistance, impaired glucose tolerance
  - Leads to heart disease and type 2 diabetes

Cardiovascular Risk Factors (2 of 2)

- Homocysteine: sulfur-containing amino acid formed from methionine that is abundant in animal protein
    - Elevated levels in homocysteinuria marked by early onset of severe atherosclerosis
    - High level is a risk factor for cardiovascular disease
    - Metabolism requires vitamins B6, B12, and folic acid and deficiency can cause increase homocysteine levels

Aspirin and Reduced CVD Risk

- Action: Interferes with platelet function by permanently inactivating thromboxane A2 that causes platelets to aggregate and start clotting process
- Rapidly absorbed from stomach and small intestines
- Inhibits platelet function within 1 hour of ingestion
- 30 mg/day can inactivate thromboxane A2 for the entire 10-day life span of platelets
- Reduces risk of cardiovascular disease and stroke
- Increases risk of bleeding in the brain if person has stroke

Hypertension (1 of 2)

- Excessive vasoconstriction of small arterioles resulting in:
    - Increased peripheral resistance; increased diastolic blood pressure
    - Increased force of ventricular contraction
    - Compensatory increase in systolic pressure
- Cardiac effects: increased peripheral resistance → higher workload → heart enlarges → heart failure
- Vascular effects: increased pressure → premature wearing out of vessels; accelerates atherosclerosis; injury to arterioles → rupture and hemorrhage
- Renal effects: narrowed renal arterioles → decreased blood supply to kidneys → injury and degenerative changes in glomeruli and tubules → renal failure

Hypertension (2 of 2)

- Primary or essential hypertension: unknown cause
- Secondary hypertension: from a known disease (chronic kidney disease, pituitary or adrenal tumor, hyperthyroidism)
- Isolated systolic hypertension: mild to moderate rise in systolic pressure but low or normal diastolic pressure
  - Increased rigidity of aorta with age
  - Arteries less able to stretch and absorb force of ejected blood during ventricular contraction
  - Diastolic pressure is normal because of absence of arteriolar vasoconstriction
  - Same harmful effects as primary and secondary hypertension

Primary Myocardial Disease (1 of 2)

- Two types
- 1. Myocarditis: inflammation; injury and necrosis of individual muscle fibers
  - Cause: viruses, parasites (Trichinella), fungi (Histoplasma), or hypersensitivity (acute rheumatic fever); abrupt onset; may lead to acute heart failure
- 2. Cardiomyopathy: no evidence of inflammation
  - Dilated cardiomyopathy: enlargement of heart and dilatation of chambers; impaired ventricular action leads to chronic heart failure; cause uncertain; no treatment
  - Hypertrophic cardiomyopathy: hereditary, transmitted as dominant trait, muscle fibers in disarray with marked hypertrophy of heart muscle

Primary Myocardial Disease (2 of 2)

- Hypertrophic cardiomyopathy
  - Hypertrophy reduces size of ventricles and do not readily dilate in diastole
  - Septal muscles more hypertrophied than rest of myocardium → impedes flow into aorta
  - Thick septum impinges on anterior mitral valve leaflet → intermittently blocks outflow from left ventricle
- Idiopathic hypertrophic subaortic stenosis, IHSS
  - Unknown cause; stenosis below aortic valve
  - Excessive fatigue and lightheadedness on exertion
  - Diagnosis by echocardiogram; use drugs that slow heart rate, beta blockers, calcium channel blockers

Heart Failure

- No longer able to pump adequate amount of blood
- May result from any type of heart disease
- Chronic heart failure: develops slowly and insidiously
- Acute heart failure: rapidly failing heart
  - Forward failure: reduced blood flow to tissues → reduced renal blood flow → salt and water retention to increase blood volume and venous pressure → edema
  - Backward failure: blood "back ups" in veins draining to the heart → increased venous pressure, congestion, edema
  - Both types are present to some degree in patients with heart failure

Heart Failure-Treatment

- 1. Diuretic drugs
  - Promote excretion of excess salt and water by kidneys to lower blood pressure
- 2. Digitalis
  - Increases efficiency of ventricular contraction
- 3. ACE inhibitors
  - Block angiotensin converting enzyme (ACE) that promotes retention of salt and water increasing blood pressure

Acute Pulmonary Edema

- Manifestation of acute heart failure from temporary disproportion in output of blood from ventricles
- Temporary reduction in output from left ventricle "right heart" pumps blood into lungs faster than "left heart" can deliver blood to peripheral tissues
- Rapidly engorges lungs with blood causing:
  - Increased pulmonary capillary pressure
  - Leakage of fluid in alveoli
  - Shortness of breath from fluid accumulation in alveoli and impaired oxygenation

Aneurysms

- Dilatation or outpouching of portion of arterial wall
- Causes: arteriosclerosis (most common); congenital
  - Arteriosclerotic aneurysm: arteriosclerosis causes narrowing, thrombosis, and weakening of vessel wall
    - In aorta: most common in distal part of aorta; may rupture leading to massive and fatal hemorrhage
  - Dissecting aneurysm of aorta: splitting of middle layer consisting of elastic and muscle tissues; degenerative changes cause layers to loose cohesiveness and separate; severe chest and back pain

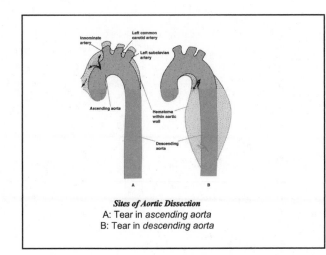

Sites of Aortic Dissection
A: Tear in *ascending aorta*
B: Tear in *descending aorta*

Diseases of the Veins

- 1. Venous thrombosis: blockage by clots
- 2. Phlebitis: inflammation of vein
- 3. Varices or varicosities: excessive dilatation and tortuosity
- Risk of clotting in post-op patients, confined to bed, may lead to pulmonary embolism
- Valves in veins prevent retrograde blood flow; varicose veins result if saphenous veins become dilated and valves become incompetent
- Varicose veins in other locations: hemorrhoids, varicocele, esophageal varices

Chapter 14   The Hematopoietic and Lymphatic Systems

Chapter Outline

The chapter outline provides you with an organizational guide to the topics and ideas presented in this chapter of the text.

Study Questions

The following questions are provided as a test for comprehension and as a study guide for use with the text chapters. Additional study material is located at http://health.jbpub.com/humandisease/8e, which contains useful tools such as an A&P review, animated flashcards, an interactive online glossary, crossword puzzles, and web links.

Key Terms

Define the following terms:

1. Heme _____

2. Globin _____

3. Bilirubin _____

4. Anemia _____

5. Polycythemia _____

6. Hemochromatosis _____

Fill-in-the-Blank

1. The usual survival time of red cells in the circulation is _____.

2. The normal number of reticulocytes in the circulation is approximately _____ percent.

3. _____ is the usual cause of hypochromic, microcytic anemia in a middle-aged man.

4. Some patients have congenital deficiencies of the red cell enzymes that are required to metabolize glucose as a source of energy. These patients often have _____.

5. The disease in which there is an excess of iron in the body is called _____.

6. Infectious mononucleosis is caused by _____.

7. A young red cell is called a _____, and it survives in the circulation about _____ days. Worn-out red cells are destroyed primarily in _____. The hemoglobin is broken down, and its components are recycled.

True/False

1. Tell whether each statement is true or false regarding iron deficiency anemia. If false, explain why the statement is incorrect.

   a. It may result from a bleeding ulcer. _____

   _____

   b. It may result from excessive blood donations. _____

   _____

   c. It may result from a deficiency of vitamins required for efficient blood production. _____

   _____

   d. It may result from excessive menstrual blood loss. _____

   _____

Identification

1. List the five white blood cells in the circulation and indicate their functions.

   a. _____

   b. _____

   c. _____

   d. _____

   e. _____

2. List three laboratory tests that are useful to measure iron stores, iron transport, and iron metabolism.

   a. _____

   b. _____

   c. _____

3. The macrocytic anemia resulting from inability to absorb vitamin B_{12} as a result of atrophy of gastric mucosa is called pernicious anemia. List three other causes of macrocytic anemia caused by inability to absorb or utilize vitamin B_{12}.

   a. _____

   b. _____

   c. _____

4. List four causes of hereditary hemolytic anemia.

   a. _____

   b. _____

   c. _____

   d. _____

5. List two treatments that are suitable for treating a patient with aplastic anemia.

   a. _____

   b. _____

6. List three diseases that are associated with secondary polycythemia.

   a. _____

   b. _____

   c. _____

Discussion Questions

1. Where does bilirubin come from? _____

   _____

   _____

   _____

2. Describe the uptake, transport, utilization, and storage of iron. (*Hint:* see Fig. 14-3.) _____

_____

_____

3. What is the difference between the etiologic and the morphologic classifications of anemia? _____

_____

_____

_____

4. Outline a simple etiologic classification of anemia. _____

_____

_____

_____

5. What are the functions of the spleen? What happens if the spleen is removed? _____

_____

_____

_____

6. What are the clinical manifestations of infectious mononucleosis? How is the disease treated? _____

_____

_____

_____

7. How does primary polycythemia differ from secondary polycythemia? _____

_____

_____

_____

8. What is the difference between polycythemia and thrombocytopenia? _____

_____

_____

_____

9. What is the cause of aplastic anemia? How is it treated? _____

_____

_____

_____

10. What is the difference between aplastic anemia and hemolytic anemia? _____
_____
_____
_____

11. What is hemochromatosis? How is the condition diagnosed? How is it treated? _____
_____
_____
_____

12. What is the lymphatic system? How is it organized? What are the major cells in the lymphatic system? What are the major functions of the lymphatic system? _____
_____
_____
_____

13. List the morphologic features found in aplastic anemia (anemia due to bone marrow failure). _____
_____
_____
_____

14. What conditions are associated with megaloblastic anemia? _____
_____
_____
_____

Notes

Chapter 14

The Hematopoietic and
Lymphatic Systems

Learning Objectives (1 of 2)

- Describe composition and functions of blood, and functions of the lymphatic system
- Explain classification of anemia
- List and describe causes and treatment of hypochromic microcytic anemia and macrocytic anemia
- List causes and treatment of anemia from bone marrow damage and anemia from accelerated blood destruction
- Describe causes and effects of polycythemia and thrombocytopenia

Learning Objectives (2 of 2)

- Describe causes and clinical manifestations of infectious mononucleosis
- List common causes of lymph node enlargement
- Explain role of spleen in protecting the body against infection
- Describe effect of splenectomy on body's defenses

Notes

_____
_____
_____
_____
_____
_____
_____
_____
_____
_____
_____
_____
_____
_____
_____
_____
_____
_____
_____
_____
_____
_____
_____
_____
_____
_____
_____
_____
_____
_____
_____
_____
_____
_____

Composition of Human Blood (1 of 6)

- Transports substances to tissues:
  - O_2, nutrients, hormones, leukocytes, red cells, platelets, antibodies
  - Carbon dioxide and other waste products of cell metabolism to the excretory organs of the body
- Volume of blood: about 5 quarts, but varies according to size of individual
- Almost half of blood consists of cellular elements suspended in plasma (viscous fluid)

Composition of Human Blood (2 of 6)

- Stem cells: precursor cells in bone marrow and differentiate to form red cells, white cells, and platelets
- Cellular elements are:
  - Red cells
  - Leukocytes
    - Neutrophils
    - Monocytes
    - Eosinophils
    - Lymphocytes
    - Basophils
  - Platelets

Composition of Human Blood (3 of 6)

- Red cells
  - Primarily concerned with transport of oxygen
  - Most numerous cells
  - Survive 4 months (120 days)
  - Erythroblast: precursor cell in bone marrow
  - Hemoglobin: oxygen-carrying protein formed by the developing red cell
- Leukocytes
  - Less numerous
  - Different types
  - Survival from several hours to several days, except for lymphocytes

Composition of Human Blood
(4 of 6)

- Lymphocytes may last for several years
- Lymphocytes also produced in the bone marrow but mainly produced in lymph nodes and spleen
- Types of leukocytes
  - Neutrophils
    - Most numerous in adults
    - Make up 70% of total circulating white cells
    - Actively phagocytic
    - Predominant in inflammatory reactions
  - Monocytes
    - Actively phagocytic
    - Increased in certain types of chronic infection

Composition of Human Blood
(5 of 6)

- Eosinophils
  - Increased in allergic reactions
  - Increased in presence of animal-parasite infections
- Lymphocytes
  - Next most common leukocytes in adults
  - Predominant leukocytes in children
  - Mostly located in lymph nodes, spleen, lymphoid tissues
  - Take part in cell-mediated and humoral defense reactions

Composition of Human Blood
(6 of 6)

- Platelets
  - Essential for blood coagulation
  - Much smaller than leukocytes
  - Represent bits of the cytoplasm of megakaryocytes, largest precursor cells in the bone marrow
  - Short survival, about 10 days

Notes

Normal Hematopoiesis (1 of 4)

- Hematopoiesis: formation and development of blood cells
- Bone marrow replenishes the blood cells
- Substances necessary for hematopoiesis
  - Protein
  - Vitamin B_{12}
  - Folic acid (one of the vitamin B group)
  - Iron
- Red cell production: regulated by oxygen content of the arterial blood
- White cell production: not well understood
- Factors that may cause white cell production
  - Products of cell necrosis
  - Hormone secretion by adrenals and endocrine glands

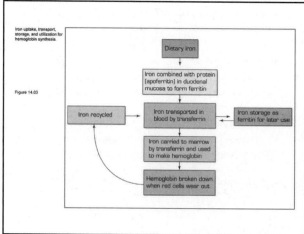

Iron uptake, transport, storage, and utilization for hemoglobin synthesis.

Figure 14.03

Dietary iron

Iron combined with protein (apoferritin) in duodenal mucosa to form ferritin

Iron recycled

Iron transported in blood by transferrin

Iron storage as ferritin for later use

Iron carried to marrow by transferrin and used to make hemoglobin

Hemoglobin broken down when red cells wear out

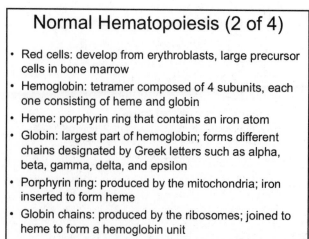

Normal Hematopoiesis (2 of 4)

- Red cells: develop from erythroblasts, large precursor cells in bone marrow
- Hemoglobin: tetramer composed of 4 subunits, each one consisting of heme and globin
- Heme: porphyrin ring that contains an iron atom
- Globin: largest part of hemoglobin; forms different chains designated by Greek letters such as alpha, beta, gamma, delta, and epsilon
- Porphyrin ring: produced by the mitochondria; iron inserted to form heme
- Globin chains: produced by the ribosomes; joined to heme to form a hemoglobin unit

Normal Hematopoiesis (3 of 4)

- Four subunits aggregate to form the complete hemoglobin tetramer
- Red cell accumulates increasing amounts of hemoglobin as it matures
- Nucleus extruded when 80% of total hemoglobin has been synthesized; cell discharged from the marrow into the circulation where it completes its maturation process in the next 24 hours
- Reticulocyte: young red cell without a nucleus but retains some of organelles; identified by special strains
- In 24 hours, reticulocyte matures and survives in the circulation for about 4 months

Normal Hematopoiesis (4 of 4)

- Worn out red cells removed in the spleen
  - Hemoglobin degraded and excreted as bile by liver
  - Porphyrin ring cannot be salvaged
  - Globin chains broken down and used to make other proteins
  - Iron extracted and saved to make new hemoglobin
- Red cell production regulated by O_2 content of arterial blood
  - Reduced O_2 supply stimulates erythropoiesis
  - Reduced O_2 tension does not act directly on bone marrow but mediated by the kidneys, which produce erythropoietin

Anemia: Etiologic Classification (1 of 2)

- Reduction in red blood cells or subnormal level of hemoglobin
- Inadequate production of red cells
- Insufficient raw materials
  - Iron deficiency
  - Vitamin B_{12} deficiency
  - Folic acid deficiency
- Inability to deliver adequate red cells into circulation due to marrow damage or destruction (aplastic anemia), replacement of marrow by foreign or abnormal cells

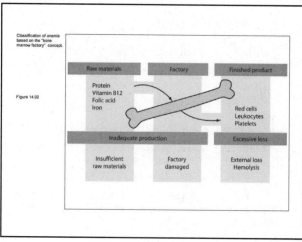

Anemia: Etiologic Classification (2 of 2)

- Excessive loss of red cells
  - External blood loss (hemorrhage)
  - Shortened survival of red cells in circulation
  - Defective red cells: hereditary hemolytic anemia
  - Accelerated destruction of cells from antibodies to red blood cell or by mechanical trauma to circulating red cells

Classification of anemia based on the "bone marrow factory" concept.

Figure 14.02

Raw materials	Factory	Finished product

Protein
Vitamin B12
Folic acid
Iron

Red cells
Leukocytes
Platelets

Inadequate production		Excessive loss

Insufficient raw materials

Factory damaged

External loss
Hemolysis

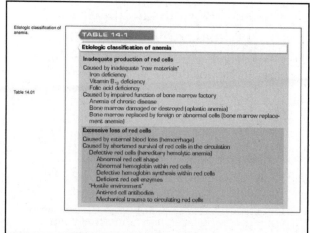

Etiologic classification of anemia.

Table 14.01

TABLE 14-1

Etiologic classification of anemia

Inadequate production of red cells

Caused by inadequate "raw materials"
 Iron deficiency
 Vitamin B$_{12}$ deficiency
 Folic acid deficiency
Caused by impaired function of bone marrow factory
 Anemia of chronic disease
 Bone marrow damaged or destroyed (aplastic anemia)
 Bone marrow replaced by foreign or abnormal cells (bone marrow replacement anemia)

Excessive loss of red cells

Caused by external blood loss (hemorrhage)
Caused by shortened survival of red cells in the circulation
 Defective red cells (hereditary hemolytic anemia)
  Abnormal red cell shape
  Abnormal hemoglobin within red cells
  Defective hemoglobin synthesis within red cells
  Deficient red cell enzymes
 "Hostile environment"
  Anti-red cell antibodies
  Mechanical trauma to circulating red cells

Anemia: Morphologic Classification (1 of 2)

- Classification based on red cell appearance suggests the etiology of the anemia:
  - Normocytic anemia: normal size and appearance
  - Macrocytic anemia: cells larger than normal
    - Folic acid deficiency
    - Vitamin B_{12} deficiency
  - Microcytic anemia: cells smaller than normal

Anemia: Morphologic Classification (2 of 2)

- Hypochromic anemia: reduced hemoglobin content
- Hypochromic microcytic anemia: smaller than normal and reduced hemoglobin content

Iron-Deficiency Anemia (1 of 2)

- Most common type of anemia
- Hypochromic microcytic anemia
- Iron absorbed from duodenum, transferred via transferin, stored as ferritin
- Pathogenesis
  - Inadequate iron intake in diet
  - Infants during periods of rapid growth
  - Adolescents subsisting on inadequate diet
  - Inadequate reutilization of iron present in red cells due to chronic blood loss
- Laboratory tests
  - Serum ferritin
  - Serum iron
  - Serum iron-binding capacity

Notes

Iron-Deficiency Anemia (2 of 2)

- Characteristic laboratory profile
  - Low serum ferritin and serum iron
  - Higher than normal serum iron-binding protein
  - Lower than normal percent iron saturation
- Treatment
  - Primary focus: learn cause of anemia
  - Direct treatment towards cause than symptoms
  - Administer supplementary iron
- Examples
  - Infant with a history of poor diet
  - Adults: common cause is chronic blood loss from GIT (bleeding ulcer or ulcerated colon carcinoma)
  - Women: excessive menstrual blood loss
  - Too-frequent blood donations

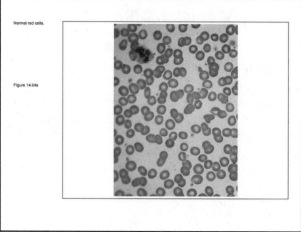

Normal red cells.

Figure 14.04a

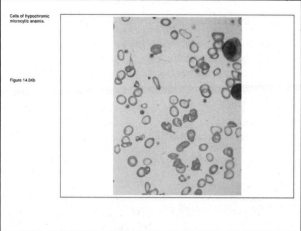

Cells of hypochromic microcytic anemia.

Figure 14.04b

Vitamin B$_{12}$ Deficiency Anemia (1 of 2)

- Vitamin B$_{12}$: meat, liver, and foods rich in animal protein
- Folic acid: green leafy vegetables and animal protein foods
  - Both required for normal hematopoiesis and normal maturation of many other types of cells
  - Vitamin B$_{12}$: for structural and functional integrity of nervous system; deficiency may lead to neurologic disturbances

Vitamin B$_{12}$ Deficiency Anemia (2 of 2)

- Absence or deficiency of vitamin B$_{12}$ or folic acid
  - Abnormal red cell maturation or megaloblastic erythropoiesis with formation of large cells called megaloblasts
  - Mature red cells formed are larger than normal or macrocytes; corresponding anemia is called macrocytic anemia
  - Abnormal development of white cell precursors and megakaryocytes: leukopenia, thrombocytopenia

Pernicious Anemia

- Lack of intrinsic factor results in macrocytic anemia
  - Vitamin B$_{12}$ in food combines with intrinsic factor in gastric juice
  - Vitamin B$_{12}$ intrinsic factor complex absorbed in ileum
- Causes
  - Gastric mucosal atrophy; also causes lack of secretion of acid and digestive enzymes
  - Gastric resection and bypass: vitamin B$_{12}$ not absorbed
  - Distal bowel resection or disease: impaired absorption of vitamin B$_{12}$ intrinsic factor complex
  - May develop among middle-aged and elderly
  - Associated with autoantibodies against gastric mucosal cells and intrinsic factor

Notes

Folic Acid Deficiency Anemia

- Relatively common
- The body has very limited stores, which rapidly become depleted if not replenished continually
- Pathogenesis
  - Inadequate diet: encountered frequently in chronic alcoholics
  - Poor absorption caused by intestinal disease
  - Occasionally occurs in pregnancy with increased demand for folic acid

Diagnostic Evaluation of Anemia

- 1. History and physical examination
- 2. Complete blood count: to assess degree of anemia, leukopenia, and thrombocytopenia
- 3. Blood smear: determine if normocytic, macrocytic, or hypochromic microcytic
- 4. Reticulocyte count: assess rate of production of new red cells
- 5. Lab tests: determine iron, B_{12}, folic acid
- 6. Bone marrow study: study characteristic abnormalities in marrow cells
- 7. Evaluation of blood loss from gastrointestinal tract to localize site of bleeding

Bone Marrow Suppression, Damage, or Infiltration (1 of 2)

- Conditions that depress bone marrow function:
  - Anemia of chronic disease: mild suppression of bone marrow function
  - Aplastic anemia: marrow injured by radiation, anticancer drugs, chemicals; or autoantibodies
  - Marrow infiltrated by tumor or replaced by fibrous tissue

Bone Marrow Suppression, Damage, or Infiltration (2 of 2)

- Treatment depends on cause
  - Blood and platelet transfusions
  - Immunosuppressive drugs
  - Bone marrow transplant in highly selected cases of aplastic anemia
  - In many cases, there are no specific treatment

Hemolytic Anemia (1 of 2)

- Hereditary hemolytic anemia
  - Genetic abnormality prevent normal survival
- 1. Abnormal shape: hereditary spherocytosis
- 2. Abnormal hemoglobin: hemoglobin S (sickle hemoglobin); hemoglobin C; both found predominantly in persons of African descent
- 3. Defective hemoglobin synthesis: thalassemia minor and major; globin chains are normal but synthesis is defective (Greek and Italian ancestry)
- 4. Enzyme defects: glucose-6-phosphatase dehydrogenase deficiency predisposes to episodes of acute hemolysis

Hemolytic Anemia (2 of 2)

- Acquired hemolytic anemia
  - Normal red cells but unable to survive due to a "hostile environment"
  - Attacked and destroyed by antibodies
  - Destruction of red cells by mechanical trauma
  - Passing through enlarged spleen (splenomegaly)
  - In contact with some part of artificial heart valve

Notes

Notes

_____
_____
_____
_____
_____
_____
_____
_____
_____
_____
_____
_____
_____
_____
_____
_____
_____
_____
_____
_____
_____
_____
_____
_____
_____
_____
_____
_____
_____
_____
_____
_____
_____
_____
_____
_____
_____
_____
_____
_____
_____
_____

TABLE 14-2

Inheritance and manifestations of some hereditary hemolytic anemias

ANEMIA	INHERITANCE	CHARACTERISTICS OF RED CELLS	MANIFESTATIONS
Hereditary spherocytosis	Dominant or recessive	Spherocytic	Mild to moderate chronic hemolytic anemia
Hereditary ovalocytosis	Dominant	Oval	Usually asymptomatic; may have mild anemia
Sickle cell anemia	Codominant	Normocytic; cells sickle under reduced oxygen tension	Marked anemia
Hemoglobin C disease	Codominant	Normocytic	Mild to moderate anemia
Sickle cell–hemoglobin C disease	Codominant	Normocytic; cells sickle under reduced oxygen tension	Moderate anemia
Thalassemia minor	Dominant (heterozygous)	Hypochromic-microcytic; total number of red cells usually increased	Mild anemia
Thalassemia major	Dominant (homozygous)	Hypochromic-microcytic	Severe anemia; usually fatal in childhood
Glucose-6-phosphate dehydrogenase deficiency	X-linked recessive	Normocytic; enzyme-deficient cells	Episodes of acute hemolytic anemia precipitated by drugs or infections

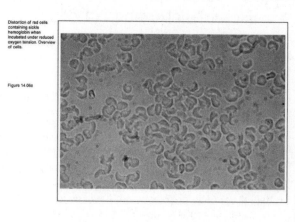

Distortion of red cells containing sickle hemoglobin when incubated under reduced oxygen tension. Overview of cells.

Figure 14.06a

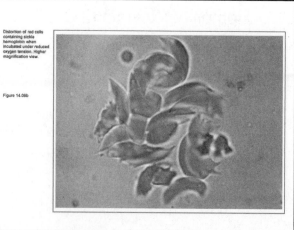

Distortion of red cells containing sickle hemoglobin when incubated under reduced oxygen tension. Higher magnification view.

Figure 14.06b

Chapter 14

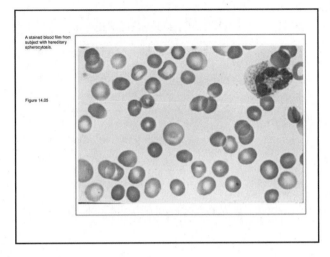

A stained blood film from subject with hereditary spherocytosis.

Figure 14.05

Polycythemia (1 of 2)

- Secondary polycythemia
  - Reduced arterial O_2 saturation leads to compensatory increase in red blood cells (increased erythropoietin production)
  - Emphysema, pulmonary fibrosis, congenital heart disease; increased erythropoietin production by renal tumor
- Primary/Polycythemia vera
  - Manifestation of diffuse marrow hyperplasia of unknown etiology
  - Overproduction of red cells, white cells, and platelets
  - Some cases evolve into granulocytic leukemia

Polycythemia (2 of 2)

- Complications
  - Clot formation due to increased blood viscosity and platelet count
- Treatment
  - Primary polycythemia: treated by drugs that suppress marrow function
  - Secondary polycythemia: periodic removal of excess blood

Hemochromatosis

- Common genetic disease transmitted as autosomal recessive trait
- Iron overload but excreted with difficulty
- Iron accumulation leads to organ damage followed by scarring and permanent derangement of organ function
- Manifestations of disease take years to develop
  - Tan to brown skin
  - Diabetes
  - Cirrhosis
  - Heart failure
- Treatment: periodic removal of blood (phlebotomy) until iron stores are depleted

Thrombocytopenia

- Secondary thrombocytopenic purpura
  - Damage to bone marrow from drugs or chemicals
  - Bone marrow infiltrated by leukemic cells or metastatic carcinoma
- Primary thrombocytopenic purpura
  - Associated with platelet antibodies
  - Bone marrow produces platelets but are rapidly destroyed
  - Encountered in children and subsides spontaneously after a short time
  - Tends to be chronic in adults

Lymphatic System (1 of 2)

- Primary function: provide immunologic defenses against foreign material via cell-mediated and humoral defense mechanisms
- Structure
  - Lymph nodes: bean-shaped structures consisting of a mass of lymphocytes supported by a meshwork of reticular fibers in which are scattered phagocytic cells
  - As lymph flows through the nodes, phagocytic cells filter out and destroy microorganisms and foreign matter
  - Clustered where lymph channels are located

Lymphatic System (2 of 2)

- Spleen: specialized to filter blood
  - Compact mass of lymphocytes and network of sinusoids (capillaries with wide lumens)
  - For antibody formation and phagocytosis of senescent red cells
- Lymphoid tissue: present in thymus, tonsils, adenoids, lymphoid aggregates in intestinal mucosa, respiratory tract, and bone marrow
- Thymus: overlies base of heart; large during infancy and childhood; undergoes atrophy in adolescence
  - Essential in prenatal development of lymphoid system and in formation of body's immunologic defense mechanisms

Lymphatic System Diseases (1 of 2)

- Lymphadenitis: inflamed and enlarged lymph nodes
- Infectious mononucleosis: caused by Epstein-Barr virus, EBV
  - Infection of B lymphocytes causes diffuse lymphoid hyperplasia of spleen, lymph nodes, lymphoid tissues
  - Cytotoxic (CD8+) lymphocytes and antibodies produced by plasma cells destroy most of infected B cells
  - Characterized by enlarged and tender lymph nodes
  - Mostly encountered by young adults transmitted by close contact, usually kissing
  - Avoid body contact sports until spleen is no longer enlarged to avoid risk of splenic rupture
  - Persons with compromised immune system, unrestrained B cell proliferation may give rise to B cell lymphoma

Lymphatic System Diseases (2 of 2)

- Neoplasms
  - Metastatic tumors: breasts, lung, colon, other sites
  - Nodes first affected lie in immediate drainage area of tumor
  - Tumor spreads to more distant lymph nodes through lymphatic channels
- Malignant lymphoma
  - Hodgkin's lymphoma
  - Non-Hodgkin's lymphoma
- Lymphocytic leukemia: from lymphoid precursor cells; acute (primitive forms) or chronic (mature cells)

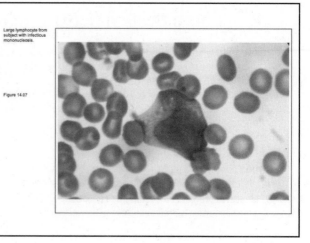

Large lymphocyte from subject with infectious mononucleosis.

Figure 14.07

Spleen

- Phagocytosis
- Antibody formation: prompt elimination of pathogenic organisms
- Reasons for splenectomy
  - Traumatic injury: to prevent fatal hemorrhage
  - Blood diseases: excessive destruction of blood cells in the spleen (hereditary hemolytic anemia)
  - Patients with Hodgkin's disease prior to treatment
- Effects
  - Less-efficient elimination of bacteria
  - Impaired production of antibodies
  - Predisposed to systemic infections
- Treatment: antibacterial vaccines; antibiotic prophylaxis

Discussion

- A patient has an enlarged lymph node
  - What types of diseases could produce lymph node enlargement?
  - How does the physician arrive at a diagnosis when a patient presents with enlarged lymph node?
- What is the EB virus? What is its relationship to infectious mononucleosis? What are the clinical manifestations, complications, and treatment for infectious mononucleosis?

Chapter Outline

The chapter outline provides you with an organizational guide to the topics and ideas presented in this chapter of the text.

Study Questions

The following questions are provided as a test for comprehension and as a study guide for use with the text chapters. Additional study material is located at http://health.jbpub.com/humandisease/8e, which contains useful tools such as an A&P review, animated flashcards, an interactive online glossary, crossword puzzles, and web links.

Key Terms

Define the following terms:

1. Miliary tuberculosis _____

2. Pulmonary fibrosis _____

3. Pneumothorax _____

4. Pulmonary emphysema _____

5. Pneumonia _____

Fill-in-the-Blank

1. Movement of air in and out of the lungs is called _____, and movement of oxygen and carbon dioxide between alveoli and pulmonary capillaries is called _____.

2. Escape of air from the lung associated with collapse of the lung is called a _____.

3. Development of a positive (higher than atmospheric) pressure in the pleural cavity associated with collapse of the lung is called a _____, and this condition is treated by _____.

4. Collapse of part of the lung caused by obstruction of bronchi or bronchioles with absorption of the trapped air into the bloodstream is called _____.

5. The agent that causes severe acute respiratory syndrome (SARS) is _____.

6. Primary atypical pneumonia is caused by _____.

7. The characteristic multinucleated cell associated with the necrosis in tuberculosis is called a _____.

8. The skin test that detects hypersensitivity to the antigens in the tubercle bacillus as an indication of previous exposure to the organism is called the _____ test.

9. Deficiency of surfactant in the lungs of premature infants leads to a condition called _____.

10. The condition characterized by breathing difficulty caused by bronchospasm is called _____.

11. Progressive pulmonary fibrosis caused by inhalation of rock dust is called _____.

12. Pulmonary fibrosis caused by inhalation of asbestos fibers is called _____.

13. The disease caused by exposure to asbestos fibers may predispose a person to development of malignant lung and pleural tumors. The lung tumor is called a _____, and the pleural tumor is called a _____.

14. The disease characterized by chronic bronchitis associated with breakdown of alveolar septa, formation of cystic spaces throughout the lung, and loss of lung elasticity is called _____.

15. The incidence of pulmonary emphysema is _____.

16. _____ is the major factor responsible for the rising incidence of lung carcinoma in women.

17. _____ is a condition characterized by chronic inflammation with dilation of bronchi.

18. Inhalation of a foreign body in the lung may cause _____.

True/False

1. Tell whether each statement is true or false regarding the severe acute respiratory syndrome (SARS). If false, explain why the statement is incorrect.

   a. This highly communicable disease is caused by an unusual coronavirus. _____

   _____

   b. The virus can be transmitted by coughing and sneezing and by the virus-contaminated hands of an infected patient.

   _____

   c. The virus responds to antiviral antibiotics. _____

   _____

   d. The lungs of severely affected SARS patients develop features characteristic of adult respiratory distress syndrome.

   _____

2. Tell whether each statement is true or false regarding the treatment of emphysema by lung volume reduction surgery (LVRS). If false, explain why the statement is incorrect.

   a. LVRS may be suitable for some patients who have emphysema restricted to the upper lobes of the lungs.

   _____

   b. LVRS involves resecting segments of emphysematous upper lobes in an effort to reduce the size of the overinflated lungs so that the less severely affected lower lobes can function more efficiently. _____

   _____

   c. The mortality rate for medically treated patients with emphysema is similar to the mortality rate for surgically treated patients. _____

   _____

   d. Surgical treatment is much more effective than medical treatment in almost all emphysema patients. _____

   _____

3. Tell whether each statement is true or false. If false, explain why the statement is incorrect.

   a. Infants born to mothers with diabetes are at increased risk of developing the neonatal respiratory distress syndrome.

   _____

   b. Infants delivered by cesarean section are at greater risk of neonatal respiratory distress syndrome than are infants delivered vaginally. _____

   _____

   c. Lung volume reduction surgery is a very effective treatment of severe pulmonary emphysema and provides long-term improvement of the disease. _____

   _____

d. Immunocompromised persons who become infected with the tubercle bacillus (*Mycobacterium tuberculosis*) are at a greater risk of developing active progressive pulmonary tuberculosis than are persons with a normal immune system. _____

e. Lung carcinoma is responsible for more deaths in women than breast carcinoma. _____
_____

Identification

1. List three conditions that appear to be related to cigarette smoking.

   a. _____

   b. _____

   c. _____

Discussion Questions

1. How do the lungs function? _____
_____
_____
_____

2. What is the difference between ventilation and gas exchange? _____
_____
_____
_____

3. How is pulmonary function disturbed if the alveolar septa are thickened and scarred? _____
_____
_____
_____

4. How is pneumonia classified? What are its major clinical features? _____
_____
_____
_____

5. How does the tubercle bacillus differ in its staining reaction from other bacteria? _____
_____
_____
_____

6. What factors determine the outcome of a tuberculous infection? _____
_____
_____

7. How does a cavity develop in lungs infected with tuberculosis? Is a person with a tuberculous cavity infectious to other people? _____
_____
_____

8. What type of inflammation is caused by the tubercle bacillus? _____
_____
_____

9. A patient has tuberculosis of the kidney, but no evidence of pulmonary tuberculosis is detected by means of a chest x-ray. How did this happen? _____
_____
_____

10. What is meant by the term "inactive tuberculosis"? Under what circumstances may an old, inactive tuberculous infection become activated? What types of patients are susceptible to reactivation of a tuberculous infection?
_____
_____

11. How does a pneumothorax occur? What is its effect on pulmonary function? _____
_____
_____

12. What factors predispose a person to the development of pulmonary emphysema? How may it be prevented?
_____
_____
_____

13. A 35-year-old man has a pulmonary infiltrate with chills, fever, chest pain, and purulent sputum. What is the most likely diagnosis? _____

_____

_____

_____

14. A postoperative patient with a normal temperature has a pulmonary infiltrate, chest pain, and bloody sputum. What is the most likely diagnosis? _____

_____

_____

_____

15. What is the cause of interstitial pneumonia (primary atypical pneumonia)? _____

_____

_____

_____

Chapter 15   The Respiratory System

Notes

_____

_____

_____

_____

_____

_____

_____

_____

_____

_____

_____

_____

_____

_____

_____

_____

_____

_____

_____

_____

_____

_____

_____

_____

_____

_____

_____

_____

_____

_____

_____

_____

_____

_____

_____

Chapter 15

The Respiratory System

Learning Objectives

- Principles of ventilation and gas exchange
- Causes, clinical effects, complications, and treatment
  - Pneumothorax
  - Atelectasis
  - Tuberculosis
- Differentiate bronchitis vs. bronchiectasis
- COPD, bronchial asthma, RDS: pathogenesis, anatomic and physiologic derangements, clinical manifestations, treatment
- Asbestosis
- Lung carcinoma: types, manifestations, and treatment

Oxygen Delivery: A Cooperative Effort

- Respiratory system oxygenates blood and removes carbon dioxide
- Circulatory system transports gases in the bloodstream

Lung: Structure and Function

- System of tubes conduct air into and out of the lungs
  - Bronchi: largest conducting tube
  - Bronchioles: less than 1 mm
  - Terminal bronchioles: smallest
  - Respiratory bronchioles: distal to terminal bronchiole with alveoli projecting from walls; form alveolar ducts and sacs; transport air and participate in gas exchange
- Alveoli: O_2 and CO_2 exchange; surrounded by alveolar septum; with cells that produce surfactant
- Lung divided into lobes consisting of smaller units or lobules

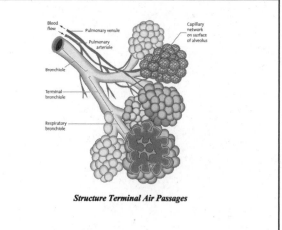

Structure Terminal Air Passages

Gas Exchange (1 of 2)

- Acinus or respiratory unit: functional unit of lung
- Two functions of respiration
- 1. Ventilation: movement of air into and out of lungs
  - Inspiration
  - Expiration
- 2. Gas exchange between alveolar air and pulmonary capillaries
  - Atmospheric pressure, sea level = 760 mmHg
  - Partial pressure: part of total atmospheric pressure exerted by a gas
  - Partial pressure of oxygen, PO_2
  - = 0.20 x 760 mmHg = 152 mmHg

Gas Exchange (2 of 2)

- Gases diffuse between blood, tissues, and pulmonary alveoli due to differences in their partial pressures
  - Alveolar air   Blood (Pulm capillaries)
  - ↑ PO_2 105 mmHg ⟶ PO_2 20 mmHg)
  - ↓ PCO_2 35 mmHg ⟵ PCO_2 60 mmHg
- Requirements for efficient gas exchange
  - 1. Large capillary surface area in contact with alveolar membrane
  - 2. Unimpeded diffusion across alveolar membrane
  - 3. Normal pulmonary blood flow
  - 4. Normal pulmonary alveoli

Pulmonary Function Tests

- 1. Evaluate efficiency of pulmonary ventilation and pulmonary gas exchange
- 2. Tested by measuring volume of air that can be moved into and out of lungs under normal conditions
- Vital capacity: maximum volume of air expelled after maximum inspiration
- One-second forced expiratory volume (FEV_1): maximum volume of air expelled in 1 second
- Arterial PO_2 and PCO_2
- Pulse oximeter

The Pleural Cavity

- Pleura: thin membrane covering lungs (visceral pleura) and internal surface of the chest wall (parietal pleura)
- Pleural cavity: potential space between lungs and chest wall
- Intrapleural pressure: pressure within pleural cavity
  - Normally lesser than intrapulmonary pressure
  - Referred as "negative pressure" or subatmospheric because it is lesser than atmospheric pressure
  - Tendency of stretched lung to pull away from chest creates a vacuum
  - Release of vacuum in pleural cavity leads to lung collapse

Notes

Pneumothorax (1 of 2)

- Escape of air into pleural space due to lung injury or disease
- Stab wound or penetrating injury to chest wall: atmospheric air enters into pleural space
- Spontaneous pneumothorax – no apparent cause; rupture of small, air-filled subpleural bleb at lung apex
- Manifestations
  - Chest pain
  - Shortness of breath
  - Reduced breath sounds on affected side
  - Chest x-ray: lung collapse + air in pleural cavity

Pneumothorax (2 of 2)

- Tension pneumothorax
  - Positive pressure develops in pleural cavity
  - Air flows through perforation into pleural cavity on inspiration but cannot escape on expiration
  - Pressure builds up in pleural cavity displacing heart and mediastinal structures away from affected side
- Chest tube inserted into pleural cavity; left in place until tear in lung heals
  - Prevents accumulation of air in pleural cavity
  - Aids re-expansion of lung

Atelectasis (1 of 2)

- Collapse of lung
- Obstructive atelectasis caused by bronchial obstruction from
  - Mucous secretions, tumor, foreign object
  - Part of lung supplied by obstructed bronchus collapses as air absorbed
  - Reduced volume of affected pleural cavity
  - Mediastinal structures shift toward side of atelectasis
  - Diaphragm elevates on affected side
  - May develop as a postoperative complication

Atelectasis (2 of 2)

- Compression atelectasis
  - From external compression of lung by
    - Fluid
    - Air
    - Blood in pleural cavity
  - Reduced lung volume and expansion

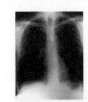

Before atelectasis

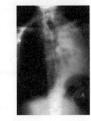

Atelectasisentire left lung
Affected lung appears dense with absorption of air; left half of diaphragm elevated; trachea and mediastinal structures shifted to side of collapse

Pneumonia (1 of 3)

- Inflammation of the lung
  - Exudate spreads through lung
  - Exudate fills alveoli
  - Affected lung portion becomes relatively solid (consolidation)
  - Exudate may reach pleural surface causing irritation and inflammation
- Classification
  - By etiology
  - By anatomic distribution of inflammatory process
  - By predisposing factors

Pneumonia (2 of 3)

- Etiology: most important, serves as a guide for treatment
  - Bacteria, viruses, fungi, *Chlamydia*, *Mycoplasma*, *Rickettsia*
- Anatomic distribution of inflammatory process
  - Lobar: infection of entire lung by pathogenic bacteria
  - Legionnaire's Disease: gram-negative rod
  - Bronchopneumonia: infection of parts of lobes or lobules adjacent to bronchi by pathogenic bacteria
  - Interstitial or primary atypical pneumonia: caused by virus or *Mycoplasma*; involves alveolar septa than alveoli; septa with lymphocytes and plasma cells

Pneumonia (3 of 3)

- Predisposing factors
  - Any condition associated with poor lung ventilation and retention of bronchial secretions
  - Postop pneumonia: accumulation of mucous secretions in bronchi
  - Aspiration pneumonia: foreign body, food, vomit
  - Obstructive pneumonia: distal to bronchial narrowing
- Clinical features of pneumonia
  - Fever, cough, purulent sputum, pain on respiration, shortness of breath

SARS

- Highly communicable pulmonary infection
  - Cause: unusual coronavirus first identified in late 2002
  - No antiviral therapy available against SARS
  - SARS-associated virus not closely related to other coronaviruses
  - Causes lower respiratory infections
- Manifestations
  - Fever, chills
  - Mild respiratory infection
  - Occasional diarrhea
  - Acute respiratory distress 3-7 days from onset: cough, shortness of breath, evidence of pneumonia on x-ray; possibly requiring mechanical ventilation

Pneumocystis Pneumonia

- Cause: *Pneumocystis carinii*, protozoan parasite of low pathogenicity
- Affects mainly immunocompromised persons
  - AIDS, receiving immunosuppressive drugs, premature infants
- Cysts contain sporozoites released from cysts that mature to form trophozoites; sporozoites appear as dark dots at the center of cyst on stained smears
- Organisms attack and injure alveolar lining leading to exudation of protein material into alveoli
- Cough, dyspnea, pulmonary consolidation
- Diagnosis: lung biopsy by bronchoscopy or from bronchial secretions

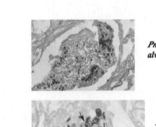

Pneumocystis carinii cysts in alveolar exudate

Pneumocystis carinii cysts
Higher magnification, central dark dots within cysts are clusters of sporozoites

Tuberculosis

- Infection from acid-fast bacteria, *Mycobacterium tuberculosis*
- Organism has a capsule composed of waxes and fatty substances; resistant to destruction
- Transmission: airborne droplets
- Granuloma: giant cell with central necrosis, indicates development of cell-mediated immunity
- Multi-nucleated giant cells: bacteria + fused monocytes + periphery of lymphocytes and plasma cells
  - Organisms lodge within pulmonary alveoli
  - Granulomas are formed
  - Spreads into kidneys, bones, uterus, fallopian tubes, others

Tuberculosis-Outcome

- Infection arrested and granulomas heal with scarring
- Infection may be asymptomatic, detected only by chest x-ray and/or *Mantoux* test
- Infection reactivated: healed granulomas contain viable organisms reactivated with reduced immunity leading to progressive pulmonary TB
- Spread through blood to other organs (extrapulmonary)
  - Secondary focus of infection may progress even if pulmonary infection has healed
- Diagnosis
  - Skin test (*Mantoux*)
  - Chest x-ray
  - Sputum culture

Reactivated and Miliary Tuberculosis

- Reactivated tuberculosis: active TB in adults from reactivation of an old infection; healed focus of TB flares up with lowered immune resistance
- Miliary tuberculosis
  - Multiple foci (small, white nodules, 1-2 mm in diameter) of disseminated tuberculosis, resembling millet seeds
  - Large numbers of organisms disseminated in body when a mass of tuberculous inflammatory tissue erodes into a large blood vessel
  - Extensive consolidation of one or more lobes of lung
  - At-risk: AIDS and immunocompromised individuals

Drug-Resistant Tuberculosis

- Resistant strains of organisms emerge with failure to complete treatment or premature cessation of treatment
- Multiple drug-resistant tuberculosis, MTB
  - TB caused by organisms resistant to at least two of the anti-TB drugs
  - Course of treatment is prolonged,
  - Results less satisfactory
- Extremely drug-resistant tuberculosis, XDR-TB
  - Caused by organisms no longer controlled by many anti-TB drugs
  - Eastern Europe, South Africa, Asia, some cases in the United States

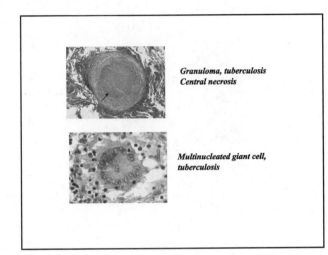

Granuloma, tuberculosis
Central necrosis

Multinucleated giant cell,
tuberculosis

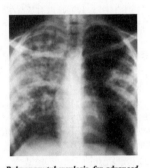

Pulmonary tuberculosis, far-advanced
Extensive consolidation of both lungs

Bronchitis and Bronchiectasis

- Inflammation of the tracheobronchial mucosa
- Acute bronchitis
- Chronic bronchitis: from chronic irritation of respiratory mucosa by smoking or atmospheric pollution
- Bronchiectasis: walls weakened by inflammation become saclike and fusiform
  - Distended bronchi retain secretions
  - Chronic cough; purulent sputum; repeated bouts of pulmonary infection
- Diagnosis: bronchogram
- Only effective treatment: surgical resection of affected segments of lung

Notes

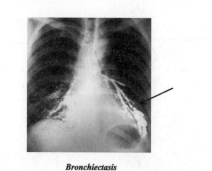

Bronchiectasis
Left, sac-like and fusiform dilatation of bronchi
Right, normal bronchi

Chronic Obstructive Pulmonary Disease (1 of 4)

- Combination of emphysema and chronic bronchitis
- Pulmonary emphysema
  - Destruction of fine alveolar structure of lungs with formation of large cystic spaces
  - Destruction begins in upper lobes eventually affecting all lobes of both lungs
  - Dyspnea, initially on exertion; later, even at rest
- Chronic bronchitis: chronic inflammation of terminal bronchioles; cough + purulent sputum

Chronic Obstructive Pulmonary Disease (2 of 4)

- Three main anatomic derangements in COPD
- 1. Inflammation and narrowing of terminal bronchioles
  - Swelling of bronchial mucosa → reduced caliber of bronchi and bronchioles → increased bronchial secretions → increased resistance to air flow → air enters lungs more readily than it can be expelled → trapping of air at expiration
- 2. Dilatation and coalescence of pulmonary air spaces
  - Diffusion of gases less efficient from large cystic spaces
- 3. Loss of lung elasticity; lungs no longer recoil normally following inspiration

Chronic Obstructive Pulmonary Disease (3 of 4)

- Chronic irritation: smoking and inhalation of injurious agents
- Pathogenesis
  - 1. Inflammatory swelling of mucosa
    - Narrows bronchioles; increased resistance to expiration; causing air to be trapped in lung
  - 2. Leukocytes accumulate in bronchioles and alveoli, releasing proteolytic enzymes that attack elastic fibers of lung's structural support
  - 3. Coughing and increased intrabronchial pressure convert alveoli into large, cystic air spaces, over-distended lung cannot expel air
  - 4. Retention of secretions predisposes to pulmonary infection

Chronic Obstructive Pulmonary Disease (4 of 4)

- Lungs damaged by emphysema cannot be restored to normal
- Management
  - Promote drainage of bronchial secretions
  - Decrease frequency of superimposed pulmonary infections
  - Surgery does not improve survival, initial benefit is short-term

Alpha$_1$ Antitrypsin Deficiency (1 of 2)

- Results in emphysema
  - Antitrypsin normally inactivates enzymes that may injure alveolar septa
  - Low antitrypsin levels correlate with lung disease because it protects lungs from proteolytic enzymes
- Antitrypsin: Alpha$_1$ globulin: prevents lung damage from lysosomal enzymes (trypsin, fibrinolysin, thrombin)
  - Released from leukocytes in lung
  - Concentration in blood under genetic influence
  - Deficiency permits enzymes to damage lung tissue

Notes

Alpha₁ Antitrypsin Deficiency (2 of 2)

- Severe antitrypsin deficiency
  - Digestion of connective tissues of alveolar septa, terminal air passages
  - Develops progressive pulmonary emphysema
  - Manifests in adolescence or early adulthood
  - Tends to affect lower lobes of lungs
  - No associated chronic bronchitis
  - Absent cough and excessive sputum production
- Moderate antitrypsin deficiency
  - Do not develop severe emphysema at early age
  - Susceptible to lung damage from smoking, atmospheric pollution, andrespiratory infections

Bronchial Asthma

- Spasmodic contraction of smooth muscles walls of bronchi and bronchioles
- Dyspnea and wheezing on expiration
- Greater impact on expiration than on inspiration
- Attacks are precipitated by allergens: inhalation of dust, pollens, animal dander, other allergens
- Treatment
  - Drugs that dilate bronchial walls: epinephrine or theophylline
  - Drugs that block release of mediators from mast cells

Neonatal Respiratory Distress Syndrome

- Progressive respiratory distress soon after birth
- Hyaline membrane disease after red-staining membranes lining alveoli
- Pathogenesis: inadequate surfactant in lungs
  - Alveoli do not expand normally during inspiration
  - Tends to collapse during expiration
- At-risk groups
  - Premature infants
  - Infants delivered by cesarean section
  - Infants born to diabetic mothers
- Treatment
  - Adrenal corticosteroids to mother before delivery
  - Oxygen + surfactant

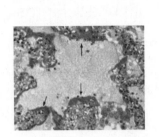

Neonatal Respiratory Distress Syndrome
Leakage of protein rich in fibrinogen that tends to clot and form adherent eosinophilic hyaline membranes impeding gas exchange.

Adult Respiratory Distress Syndrome

- Shock – major manifestation
- Conditions: fall in blood pressure and reduced blood flow to lungs
  - Severe injury (traumatic shock)
  - Systemic infection (septic shock)
  - Aspiration of acid gastric contents
  - Inhalation of irritant or toxic gases
  - Damage caused by SARS
- Damaged alveolar capillaries leak fluid and protein
- Impaired surfactant production from damaged alveolar lining cells
- Formation of intra-alveolar hyaline membrane

Comparison: Neonatal Versus Adult

	Neonatal Respiratory Distress	Adult Respiratory Distress
Groups Affected	Premature infants	Adults sustained direct or indirect lung damage
	Delivery by cesarean section	
	Infant born to diabetic mother	
Pathogenesis	Inadequate surfactant	Direct damage: lung trauma, aspiration, irritant or toxic gases
		Indirect damage: ↓ pulmonary blood flow from shock or sepsis
		Associated condition: surfactant production reduced
Treatment	Corticosteroids to mother before delivery	Support circulation & respiration
	Endotracheal surfactant	Endotracheal tube & respirator
	Oxygen	Positive pressure oxygen

Pulmonary Fibrosis

- Fibrous thickening of alveolar septa from irritant gases, organic and inorganic particles
    - Makes lungs rigid restricting normal respiratory excursions
    - Diffusion of gases hampered due to increased alveolar thickness
    - Causes progressive respiratory disability similar to emphysema
- Collagen diseases
- Pneumoconiosis: lung injury from inhalation of injurious dust or other particulate material
    - Silicosis (rock dust) and asbestosis (asbestos fibers)

Lung Carcinoma

- Usually smoking-related neoplasm
- Common malignant tumor in both men and women
- Mortality from lung cancer in women exceeds breast cancer
- Arises from mucosa of bronchi and bronchioles
- Rich lymphatic and vascular network in lungs facilitates metastasis
- Often referred as bronchogenic carcinoma because cancer usually arises from bronchial mucosa
- Treatment: surgical resection or radiation and chemotherapy for small cell carcinoma and advanced tumors

Lung Carcinoma Classification

- Classification
    - Squamous cell carcinoma: very common
    - Adenocarcinoma: very common
    - Large cell carcinoma: large, bizarre epithelial cells
    - Small cell carcinoma: small, irregular dark cells with scanty cytoplasm resembling lymphocytes; very poor prognosis
- Prognosis
    - Depends on histologic type
    - Generally poor due to early spread to distant sites

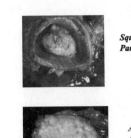

Squamous cell carcinoma, lung
Partially obstructing a major bronchus

Adenocarcinoma, lung
Arising from smaller bronchus at
lung periphery

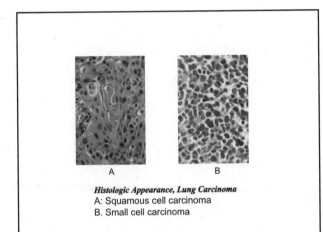

A   B

Histologic Appearance, Lung Carcinoma
A: Squamous cell carcinoma
B. Small cell carcinoma

Discussion

- 1. Differentiate MDR-TB from XDR-TB. What are the clinical and practical implications of these cases?
- 2. What socio-economic factors are associated with the increased prevalence of tuberculosis? Under what circumstances may an old inactive tuberculous infection become activated? What types of patients are susceptible to a reactivated tuberculosis?
- 3. What is the difference between pulmonary emphysema and pulmonary fibrosis? What factors predispose to their development?

Chapter Outline

The chapter outline provides you with an organizational guide to the topics and ideas presented in this chapter of the text.

Structure and Physiology of the Breast
Examination of the Breasts
    Mammograms
Abnormalities of Breast Development
    Accessory Breasts and Nipples
    Unequal Development of the Breasts
    Breast Hypertrophy
    Gynecomastia
Benign Cystic Change in the Breast
Fibroadenoma
Carcinoma of the Breast
    Breast Carcinoma Risk Related to Hormone Treatment
    Breast Carcinoma Susceptibility Genes
    Classification of Breast Carcinoma
    Evolution of Breast Carcinoma
    Clinical Manifestations
    Treatment
Sarcoma of the Breast
A Lump in the Breast as a Diagnostic Problem

Study Questions

The following questions are provided as a test for comprehension and as a study guide for use with the text chapters. Additional study material is located at http://health.jbpub.com/humandisease/8e, which contains useful tools such as an A&P review, animated flashcards, an interactive online glossary, crossword puzzles, and web links.

Key Terms

Define the following terms:

1. Mammogram _____

2. Gynecomastia _____

3. Axilla _____

4. Estrogen _____

5. Progestin _____

6. Mastectomy _____

7. Tamoxifen _____

8. Adjuvant chemotherapy _____

9. Aromatase inhibitor drugs _____

Fill-in-the-Blank

1. Persons with mutations of the tumor suppressor genes *BRCA1* or *BRCA2* have a greatly increased risk of not only breast carcinoma but also _____ carcinoma.

2. A well-circumscribed benign tumor occurring in the breast of a young woman is called a _____.

3. Breast enlargement in the male breast is called _____.

4. Following treatment of an invasive breast carcinoma, most patients are also treated with drugs or hormones. This type of treatment is called _____.

5. When examining axillary lymph nodes from patients with breast carcinoma, it is possible to identify and examine the first lymph node that receives lymphatic drainage from the axilla. This node is called a _____.

True/False

Tell whether each statement is true or false. If false, explain why the statement is incorrect.

1. A mutation of either the *BRCA1* or *BRCA2* gene increases the long-term risk of both breast and ovarian carcinoma.

   _____

2. Long-term treatment of postmenopausal patients with estrogen and progestin increases the risk of breast carcinoma.

   _____

3. When treating breast carcinoma, the long-term results of total mastectomy with axillary lymph node dissection are much better than the results of segmental mastectomy or lumpectomy followed by radiation therapy. _____

   _____

4. An estrogen receptor-positive breast carcinoma has a better prognosis than a breast carcinoma lacking hormone receptors. _____

_____

5. The prognosis of a breast carcinoma in which the *HER-2* gene is amplified is much better than that of a breast carcinoma lacking an amplified *HER-2* gene. _____

_____

6. An axillary lymph node containing metastatic carcinoma is called a sentinel lymph node. _____

_____

7. An estrogen receptor-negative breast carcinoma is usually treated with the drug tamoxifen. _____

_____

8. Adjuvant therapy for most patients with breast carcinoma usually consists of hormonal therapy and/or chemotherapy.

_____

Identify

1. What are the three common conditions that cause a lump in the breast?

   a. _____

   b. _____

   c. _____

2. Name three laboratory tests that are performed on breast carcinoma tissue to assess prognosis and guide treatment.

   a. _____

   b. _____

   c. _____

Discussion Questions

1. Describe the methods used to treat breast carcinoma surgically. _____

_____

_____

_____

2. How can benign breast conditions be distinguished from breast cancer? _____

_____

_____

_____

3. What are the applications and limitations of a mammogram? _____

_____

_____

_____

4. What factors predispose a person to breast carcinoma? _____

_____

_____

_____

5. What is the role of heredity in regard to breast carcinoma? _____

_____

_____

_____

6. A 67-year-old woman has a lump in the breast. Which diagnostic procedures will assist the physician in determining the nature of the lump? _____

_____

_____

_____

Notes

_____

_____

_____

_____

_____

_____

_____

_____

_____

_____

_____

_____

_____

_____

_____

_____

_____

_____

_____

_____

_____

_____

_____

_____

_____

_____

_____

_____

_____

_____

_____

_____

_____

_____

Chapter 16

The Breast

Learning Objectives

- Describe normal structure and physiology of breast and common developmental abnormalities
- Explain applications and limitations of mammography in the diagnosis and treatment of breast disease
- Describe three common breast diseases that present as lump in the breast
- Describe clinical manifestations of breast carcinoma, methods of diagnosis and treatment
- Explain role of heredity in the pathogenesis of breast carcinoma

Breast Structure (1 of 4)

- Breasts: modified sweat glands specialized to secrete milk
- Main function is milk production
- Two main types of tissues
  - Glandular tissues (lobules and ducts)
  - Stromal (supporting) tissues
  - Supporting tissue includes fatty and fibrous connective tissue that give the breast its size, shape, and support
- Two main types of breast changes
  - Benign (non-cancerous)
  - Malignant (cancerous)

Notes

_____

_____

_____

_____

_____

_____

_____

_____

_____

_____

_____

_____

_____

_____

_____

_____

_____

_____

_____

_____

_____

_____

_____

_____

_____

_____

_____

_____

_____

_____

_____

_____

Breast Structure (2 of 4)

- Composed of 20 lobes of glandular tissue
  - Each lobe made up of a cluster of milk-producing glands or lobules
  - Lobules connected by branching ducts or small tubes and converge to the nipple
  - Fat and connective tissue, blood vessels, lymph vessels
- Suspensory ligaments: bands of fibrous tissue extending from skin of breast to the connective tissue covering chest wall muscles

Breast Structure (3 of 4)

- Abundant blood supply and lymphatic drainage
  - Lymph vessels carry lymph fluid instead of blood
  - Most lymph vessels of breast lead to the axillary nodes (supraclavicular and mediastinal nodes)
  - If breast cancer cells reach axillary nodes and continue to grow, nodes swell and cancer more likely to spread to other organs

Breast Structure (4 of 4)

- Puberty: enlarge in response to estrogen and progesterone
- Post-pubertal changes
  - Proliferation of glandular and fibrous tissue
  - Accumulation of adipose tissue
- Variations in breast size depend on amount of fat and fibrous tissue rather than glandular tissue
- Extremely responsive to hormonal stimulation
  - Menstrual cycle: cyclic hyperplasia followed by involution
  - Pregnancy and lactation: hypertrophic glandular and ductal tissues
  - After menopause: sex hormone levels decline, breasts gradually decrease in size

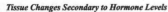

Tissue Changes Secondary to Hormone Levels

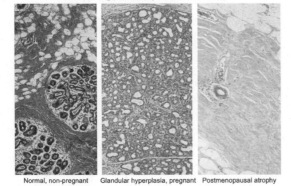

Normal, non-pregnant   Glandular hyperplasia, pregnant   Postmenopausal atrophy

Breast Examination (1 of 3)

- Clinical examination
  - Inspection, palpation, examination of axillary tissues
  - FIRST: arms at the sides
  - NEXT: arms elevated and lowered
  - FINALLY, hands on hips
  - Begin palpation at periphery of breast in a clockwise direction until tissues under the nipples are examined
- Mammogram to identify lesions not detected on clinical examination
  - Baseline: age 35–40
  - Annually: age 40 thereafter

Breast Examination (2 of 3)

- Mammogram
  - Most useful for postmenopausal women, whose breasts contain more fat and less glandular tissue than breasts of younger women
  - Dense tumor in a postmenopausal breast contrasts sharply with the less-dense fatty tissue
  - Younger woman's breast have more glandular and fibrous tissue that are denser and provide less contrast

Breast Examination (3 of 3)

- Mammogram may identify lesions not detected on clinical examination
  - Denser cysts and tumors: white on mammogram
  - Less dense fatty tissue: dark on mammogram
  - Cysts and benign tumors: well circumscribed
  - Malignant tumors
    - Have irregular borders
    - Frequently contain fine flecks of calcium

Mammogram

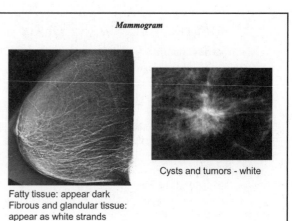

Cysts and tumors - white

Fatty tissue: appear dark
Fibrous and glandular tissue:
appear as white strands

Calcifications

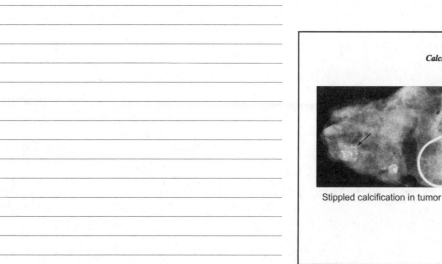

Stippled calcification in tumor

Ductal carcinoma, with
necrosis and calcification

Abnormalities in Breast Development (1 of 2)

- Embryologically, breasts developed from column of cells (mammary ridges) located anteriorly from axilla to upper thighs
- Most of the ridges disappear during prenatal development except for those at the midthoracic area, giving rise to breasts and nipples

Abnormalities in Breast Development (2 of 2)

- Accessory breasts and nipples: most commonly found in the armpits or on lower chest below and medial to the normal breasts
- Unequal development: fully developed breasts are usually similar in size but not identical, sometimes one fails to develop as much as its counterpart
- Breast hypertrophy: at puberty, one or both breasts over-respond to hormonal stimulation; true hypertrophy is from overgrowth of fibrous tissue, not glands or fat
- Gynecomastia: ductal and fibrous tissue of adolescent male breast proliferate affecting one or more breast; from temporary imbalance of female and male hormones (increase in estrogen) in the male at puberty

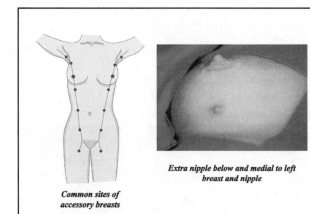

Extra nipple below and medial to left breast and nipple

Common sites of accessory breasts

Benign Cystic Change in the Breast

- Very common benign condition; also called fibrocystic disease
- Focal areas of proliferation of glandular and fibrous tissue
- Irregular cyclic response to hormones during menstrual cycle
- Ultrasound examination helpful in distinguishing a cystic from a solid mass
- Treatment
  - Aspiration of cyst
  - Surgical excision if no aspiration

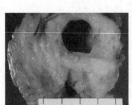 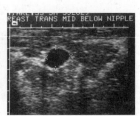

Benign breast cysts, in cross-section, previously filled with fluid

Ultrasound, breast cyst

Fibroadenoma

- Benign
- Well-circumscribed tumor of fibrous and glandular tissue
- Common in young women
- Surgically excised

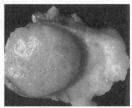

Breast Carcinoma (1 of 4)

- Risk factors
  - Familial tendency (mother or sister with breast cancer)
  - Hormonal factors
  - Birth of first child after age 30
  - Early menarche
  - Late menopause
  - Occurs in both sexes, but rare in men, whose breasts are not subject to stimulation by ovarian hormones
  - Occurs 1 in every 10 women

Breast Carcinoma (2 of 4)

- Hormones have been used for many years to treat menopausal symptoms consisting of estrogen alone or estrogen + progestin
  - Progestin: synthetic compound with progesterone activity
- Combined hormone therapy (estrogen-progestin) increases density of breast tissue, complicating the interpretation of mammograms
- Risk related to hormone treatment
  - Long-term estrogen-progestin use significantly increases risk of breast carcinoma (8%)
  - Long-term use of estrogen without progestin slightly increases risk breast carcinoma (1%)

Breast Carcinoma (3 of 4)

- Inheritance of mutant breast cancer susceptibility genes
- Mutant BRCA1 gene
  - Increases breast and ovarian carcinoma risk
  - Breast cancer risk at 80%
  - Ovarian cancer risk is at 20–40%
  - Large gene with many different mutations
- Mutant BRCA2 gene
  - Breast cancer risk at 80%
  - Lower ovarian carcinoma risk at 10–20%

Notes

Breast Carcinoma (4 of 4)

Clinical Manifestations
- **Lump in the breast**
- **Nipple or skin retraction**

Skin edema (*orange peel sign*)

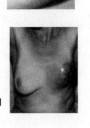

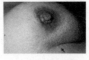

Tumor infiltrates breast and becomes **fixed to chest wall**; metastasis

Classification of Breast Carcinoma

- 1. Site of origin
  - Ductal carcinoma (90%)
  - Lobular carcinomas (10%)
  - Non-infiltrating or in situ cancer
    - Confined initially within the duct or lobule
    - Becomes invasive and extends toward adjacent breast tissue
- 2. Presence or absence of invasion
- 3. Degree of differentiation of tumor cells
  - Well-differentiated: cells that resemble normal breast tissue
  - Poorly-differentiated: bizarre cells arranged haphazardly; immature; very different from normal breast tissue

Evolution of Breast Carcinoma

- Early stages: too small to be detected by breast exam
  - Mammogram can identify carcinoma up to 2 years before detection by breast exam
- Cancer continues to grow, initially in situ; eventually becomes invasive
- Metastasizes to axillary lymph nodes and distant sites
- Problems with late metastases
- Early diagnosis allows prompt treatment and improves the cure rate

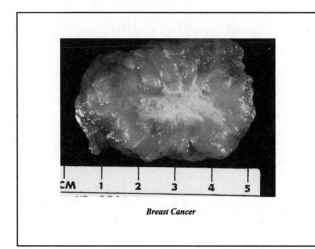

Breast Cancer

Breast Carcinoma Treatment: Surgical Resection

- 1. Modified radical mastectomy
  - Also called total mastectomy with axillary lymph node dissection
  - Resecting entire breast, axillary tissue with lymph nodes; leaves pectoral muscles
  - May be followed by breast reconstruction
- 2. Partial mastectomy: removing only part of breast with the tumor
  - Lumpectomy: removing tumor + small amount of adjacent breast tissue
  - Axillary lymph nodes removed in both lumpectomy and partial mastectomy followed by radiation to eradicate any remaining carcinoma in the breast

Breast Carcinoma Treatment: Adjuvant Therapy

- To eradicate any tumor cells that may have spread beyond the breast
  - Anticancer drugs (adjuvant chemotherapy)
  - Anti-estrogen drugs (adjuvant hormonal therapy)
- Whichever method of treatment is selected, part of tumor obtained is surgically tested to:
  - 1. Detect presence of estrogen and progesterone receptors
  - 2. Detect amplification of HER-2 gene that speeds growth rate of tumor cells; HER-2 positive tumors have less favorable prognosis

Notes

Determining Hormone Receptor Status of Tumor

- 1. Prognosis
  - Estrogen receptors (ER) and progesterone receptors (PR) in breast carcinoma
  - Hormone receptor positive tumors are better differentiated with favorable prognosis
  - Patients with ER positive tumors may receive adjuvant hormonal therapy with antiestrogen drug
- 2. Guide for treatment: tumors with hormone receptors respond to anti-estrogen adjuvant therapy

Recurrent and Metastatic Carcinoma (1 of 2)

- May appear many years after original tumor has been resected
- Tumor no longer curable, treatment is to control growth, relieve symptoms, and improve quality of life
- Methods of treatment depend on the following factors:
  - Hormone receptor status of tumor
  - Age of patient
  - Length that elapsed from initial treatment to appearance of metastasis
  - Pre- and postmenopausal, hormone-receptor positive tumor: use anti-estrogen drugs

Recurrent and Metastatic Carcinoma (2 of 2)

- Methods of treatment
- Hormone-receptor positive tumor
  - Premenopausal: anti-estrogen drugs
  - Postmenopausal: aromatase inhibitor drugs
- Hormone-receptor negative tumor
  - Hormonal manipulation if unresponsive to tamoxifen or aromatase inhibitor
- Radiation
  - To control metastatic deposits in bone and soft tissues

Breast Sarcoma

- Rare in comparison to breast carcinoma
- Arises from fibrous tissue or blood vessels
- Large bulky tumor
- May metastasize widely
- Treatment is by surgical resection of the involved breast

Breast Sarcoma

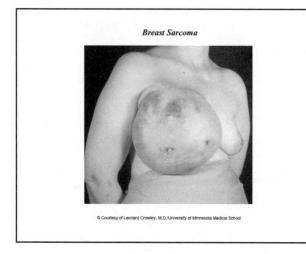

© Courtesy of Leonard Crowley, M.D./University of Minnesota Medical School

A Lump in the Breast

- Diagnostic possibilities
  - 1. Cystic disease
  - 2. Fibroadenoma
  - 3. Carcinoma
- Diagnostic approach
  - Clinical evaluation
  - Mammogram
  - Biopsy

Discussion

- Which statement regarding breast cancer risk is UNTRUE?
    - A. Late menses and early menopause can increase breast cancer risk
    - B. Risk is higher in families with a history of breast cancer
    - C. Hormone use can increase the risk of breast cancer
    - D. The risk is higher for women who have never borne children

Chapter Outline

The chapter outline provides you with an organizational guide to the topics and ideas presented in this chapter of the text.

Study Questions

The following questions are provided as a test for comprehension and as a study guide for use with the text chapters. Additional study material is located at http://health.jbpub.com/humandisease/8e, which contains useful tools such as an A&P review, animated flashcards, an interactive online glossary, crossword puzzles, and web links.

Key Terms

Define the following terms:

1. Endometriosis _____

2. Toxic shock syndrome _____

3. Dysfunctional uterine bleeding _____

4. Dysmenorrhea _____

Fill-in-the-Blank

1. Warty overgrowths of genital tract squamous epithelium are caused by _____ and are called _____.

2. Abnormal, disorderly proliferation of cervical squamous epithelium is called _____.

3. A common benign uterine tumor is called a _____.

4. Cramp-like abdominal discomfort related to menstruation is called _____.

5. The cell that gives rise to a benign cystic ovarian teratoma (dermoid cyst) is _____.

6. An estrogen-producing tumor arising from the follicular cells (granulosa cells) lining an ovarian follicle is called a _____

7. The organism responsible for toxic shock syndrome is _____.

8. The condition in which endometrium is found in locations outside the endometrial lining of the uterus is called _____.

True/False

1. Tell whether each statement is true or false regarding estrogen–progestin contraceptive pills. If false, explain why the statement is incorrect.

   a. These pills prevent ovulation. _____
   _____

   b. They may predispose a woman to tubal pregnancies. _____
   _____

   c. They may promote development of endometriosis. _____
   _____

   d. They may lead to thromboembolic complications in susceptible individuals. _____
   _____

   e. The risk of pill-related complications is lower in cigarette smokers. _____
   _____

2. Tell whether each statement is true or false regarding human papillomavirus (HPV). If false, explain why the statement is incorrect.

   a. Only a few types of HPV can infect the cervix. _____

   _____

   b. Most HPV types are carcinogenic (cancer causing). _____

   _____

   c. Most HPV infections cannot be eradicated by the body's immune defenses and become chronic. _____

   _____

   d. Testing cervical material obtained by a Pap smear for HPV may be a useful supplementary test when atypical cells are identified in the Pap smear. _____

   _____

3. Tell whether each statement related to fertilization and implantation of a fertilized ovum is true or false. If false, explain why the statement is incorrect.

   a. Sperm can survive in a woman's genital tract for 5–6 days after sexual intercourse and are still able to fertilize

   an ovum. _____

   _____

   b. Unprotected sexual intercourse several days before ovulation can result in a pregnancy. _____

   _____

   c. It takes about a week for a fertilized ovum to travel through the fallopian tube and implant in the endometrium.

   _____

   d. Postcoital (after intercourse) contraception (the "morning after pill") is unlikely to prevent conception unless taken within 3 hours after intercourse. _____

   _____

Identify

1. Identify the organisms responsible for the three common causes of vaginitis.

   a. _____

   b. _____

   c. _____

2. A woman consults her physician because of irregular uterine bleeding. Identify five possible causes of uterine bleeding.

   a. _____

   b. _____

   c. _____

   d. _____

   e. _____

Discussion Questions

1. A woman has a human papillomavirus (HPV) infection of her cervical epithelium. What factors influence her risk of developing cervical dysplasia or in situ carcinoma? _____

   _____

   _____

   _____

2. If a woman is 65 years old and has irregular uterine bleeding, what is the likely cause of the bleeding? _____

   _____

   _____

   _____

3. What are the clinical features of toxic shock syndrome in a menstruating woman? _____

   _____

   _____

   _____

4. Describe how contraceptive pills function to prevent pregnancy. _____

   _____

   _____

   _____

5. What are the manifestations and complications of endometriosis? _____

   _____

   _____

   _____

6. What parts of the female genital tract may be involved in gonorrheal infection? _____

   _____

   _____

   _____

7. How does gonorrhea lead to sterility? _____

   _____

   _____

   _____

8. What is the difference between in situ and invasive cervical carcinoma? How is the Pap smear used in the diagnosis of carcinoma? _____

_____

_____

_____

9. Explain whether the following conditions may predispose susceptible individuals to toxic shock syndrome.

   a. Use of tampons _____

   _____

   b. Use of a vaginal (contraceptive) diaphragm _____

   _____

   c. Use of contraceptive sponges _____

   _____

   d. Use of an IUD _____

   _____

   e. Use of contraceptive foam and condoms _____

   _____

10. A patient has dysmenorrhea and endometriosis is suspected. What diagnostic procedures are helpful in establishing a diagnosis of this condition? _____

_____

_____

_____

11. A 62-year-old woman has irregular vaginal bleeding. What conditions could account for this condition? _____

_____

_____

_____

Notes

Chapter 17

The Female Reproductive System

Learning Objectives

- Describe common genital tract infections and relate these to sexually transmitted diseases
- Describe clinical manifestations and complications of endometriosis
- List common causes of irregular uterine bleeding
- Describe common diseases of the cervix, endometrium, myometrium, and vulva
- List common cysts and tumors of the ovary
- Explain pathogenesis, clinical manifestations, treatment of toxic shock syndrome
- Explain methods of artificial contraception and side effects; abnormalities in the genital tract following use of DES in pregnancy

---

Female Genital Tract: Infections (1 of 3)

- Vaginitis: common, causes vaginal discharge, itching, and irritation
    - Candida albicans
    - Trichomonas vaginalis
    - Gardnerella (Hemophilus) vaginalis in conjunction with anaerobic bacteria (nonspecific vaginitis)
- Cervicitis: mild chronic inflammation; common in women who have had children
    - More severe inflammation caused by gonococci or Chlamydia
    - May spread to infect tubes and adjacent tissues (PID)

Female Genital Tract: Infections (2 of 3)

- Salpingitis: tubal infection
- Pelvic inflammatory disease, PID: inflammation of fallopian tubes, along with ovaries at times
- Manifestations and complications
  - Lower abdominal pain and tenderness, fever, leukocytosis
  - Usually secondary to ascending spread of cervical gonorrheal or Chlamydial infection
  - Tubal scarring following healing predisposes to ectopic pregnancy or may cause sterility

Female Genital Tract: Infections (3 of 3)

- Condylomas: venereal warts in genital tract
  - Benign tumor-like overgrowths of squamous epithelium
  - Acquired and transmitted by sexual contact
- Common locations
  - Mucosa of cervix and vagina
  - Around vaginal opening
  - Around anus
- Treatment: to destroy lesions
  - Applying a strong chemical
  - Electrocoagulation
  - Freezing
  - Surgical excision

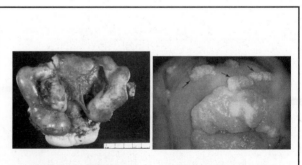

Chronic pelvic inflammatory disease, swollen tubes with occluded fimbriated ends

Multiple condylomas in cervical and vaginal mucosa

Endometriosis (1 of 2)

- Deposits of endometrial tissue outside normal location in endometrial cavity
  - Ectopic sites: uterine wall; ovary; elsewhere in pelvis, appendix; rectum
  - Ectopic endometrium responds to hormonal stimuli and undergoes cyclic menstrual desquamation and regeneration
  - Secondary scarring may obstruct fallopian tubes
- Diagnosis: laparascopy
  - Allows visualization of ectopic deposits followed by removing or destroying these deposits surgically, through drugs, or hormones

Endometriosis (2 of 2)

- Treatment
  - Synthetic hormones with progesterone activity to completely suppress menstrual cycle
  - Oral contraceptives to suppress ovulation: makes endometrium thin and atrophic and menstrual cycles light, which retards progressing of endometriosis and associated scarring
  - Drugs that suppress output of gonadotropin from pituitary gland: leads to decline in ovarian function, allowing deposits of endometriosis to regress by being deprived of cyclic estrogen-progesterone stimulation

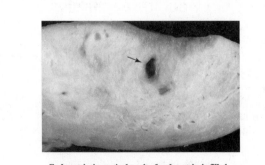

Endometriosis, cystic deposit of endometriosis filled with old blood in uterine wall

Cervical Polyps

- Cervical polyps
  - Benign, arise from the cervix
  - Usually small but may be quite large
  - Erosion of tip may cause bleeding
  - Surgical removal
- Cervical dysplasia: abnormal growth and maturation of cervical squamous epithelium
- Dysplastic changes range from:
  - Mild dysplasia
    - Result of cervical inflammation
    - Regresses spontaneously
  - Severe dysplasia
    - Does not regress
    - May progress to in situ carcinoma
    - May progress to invasive carcinoma

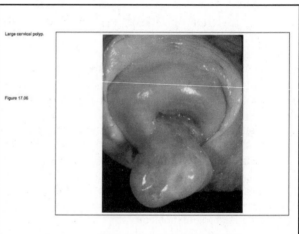

Large cervical polyp.

Figure 17.06

Cervical Intraepithelial Neoplasia (1 of 2)

- Cervical dysplasia and in situ carcinoma considered very closely related
- Constitute different stages in a progressive spectrum of epithelial abnormalities classified as cervical intra-epithelial neoplasia, CIN
  - Grade I: Mild dysplasia
  - Grade II: Moderate dysplasia
  - Grade III: Severe dysplasia
- Some human papilloma virus (HPV) strains that cause cervical condylomas are carcinogenic and predispose to cervical neoplasia

Cervical Intraepithelial Neoplasia (2 of 2)

- HPV genital tract infections are common
  - More than 80 different strains of HPV
  - 40 types can infect genital tract
  - 8 strains are high-risk types and considered carcinogenic
  - Common in young sexually active women
  - > 90% infections resolve spontaneously in 6-12 months
  - Some may have repeated infections
- Diagnosis: HPV test to supplement Pap smear when cytologic changes in Pap smear are inconclusive (atypical squamous cells of undetermined significance)
  - If HPV test is negative, cytologic changes are not significant

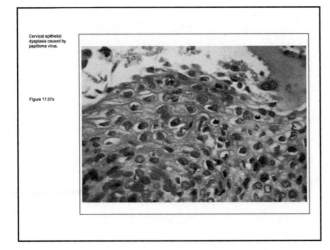

Cervical epithelial dysplasia caused by papilloma virus.

Figure 17.07a

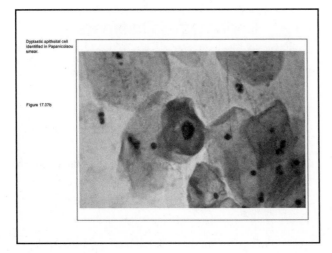

Dysplastic epithelial cell identified in Papanicolaou smear.

Figure 17.07b

Cervical Dysplasia and Carcinoma (1 of 2)

- Squamocolumnar junction or transition zone
- Cervical abnormalities develop first in cells at the junction between squamous epithelium at exterior of the cervix and the columnar epithelium lining cervical canal
- Usually located at the external os
- Pap smear shows abnormal cells
- Colposcopy localizes abnormalities
- Biopsies establish diagnosis

Cervical Dysplasia and Carcinoma (2 of 2)

- Treatment depends on extent of disease
- Dysplasia and in situ carcinoma
  - Cryocautery (freezing)
  - Surgical excision of abnormal area
  - Hysterectomy (removal of uterus)
  - Results are excellent
- Invasive carcinoma
  - Radiation
  - Radical hysterectomy (resection of uterus, fallopian tubes, ovaries, adjacent tissues)
  - Results are less satisfactory

Endometrial Disorders

- Benign endometrial hyperplasia
  - Associated with irregular uterine bleeding
- Benign endometrial polyps
  - Common
  - May bleed if tip is eroded
- Endometrial adenocarcinoma
  - Related to prolonged endometrial stimulation by estrogen use
  - Irregular uterine bleeding or postmenopausal bleeding

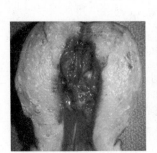
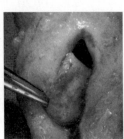

Benign endometrial hyperplasia,
polypoid mass in endometrial cavity

Endometrial polyp in
endometrial cavity

Uterine Myomas

- Benign smooth muscle tumors from uterine wall
  - Approximately 30% of women over 30 years of age have myomas
  - May cause irregular/heavy uterine bleeding
  - Symptoms related to pressure on bladder and rectum

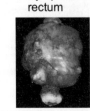
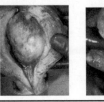

Irregular Uterine Bleeding

- Dysfunctional uterine bleeding:
  - Occurs because follicle fails to mature and no corpus luteum is formed (anovulatory cycle)
  - Disturbance of normal cyclic interaction of estrogen and progesterone on the endometrium
  - Uterus is subjected to continuous estrogen stimulation and responds by shedding and bleeding in an irregular manner instead of shedding all at once as in a normal period (anovulatory bleeding)
- Other causes of uterine bleeding
  - Benign endometrial hyperplasia
  - Endometrial and cervical polyps
  - Uterine myomas
  - Uterine carcinoma

Notes

_____
_____
_____
_____
_____
_____
_____
_____
_____
_____
_____
_____
_____
_____
_____
_____
_____
_____
_____
_____
_____
_____
_____
_____
_____
_____
_____
_____
_____
_____
_____
_____

Normal Cycle

- First half: endometrial glands and stroma proliferate under influence of estrogen from ovarian follicle
- Midcycle: ovulation occurs
  - Follicle discharges its egg, becomes a corpus luteum that produces estrogen and progesterone
  - Progesterone: endometrium undergoes secretory phase to prepare for receiving fertilized ovum
- If no pregnancy occurs
  - Corpus luteum degrades
  - Estrogen-progesterone levels fall
  - Secretory endometrium is shed with blood
- New cycle begins

Dysmenorrhea (1 of 2)

- Primary dysmenorrhea
  - Most common type; pelvic organs are normal
  - Menstrual periods are painless for first two years after menarche because the cycles are anovulatory
  - Dysmenorrhea occurs when regular ovulatory menstrual cycles begin
  - Prostaglandins synthesized under the influence of progesterone during secretory phase of cycle and released from endometrium during menses and stimulate myometrial contractions causing pain

Dysmenorrhea (2 of 2)

- Primary dysmenorrhea
  - Crampy lower abdominal pain that begins just before menstruation
  - Pain lasts for 1-2 days after onset of menstrual flow
  - Treatment: prostaglandin inhibitors, oral contraceptives
- Secondary dysmenorrhea: from various diseases of the pelvic organs, such as endometriosis
  - Treatment: correct underlying cause

Ovarian Cysts (1 of 2)

- Ovarian cysts
  - Arise from ovarian follicles or corpora lutea that have failed to regress normally and converted to fluid-filled cysts
- Functional cysts
  - Follicle and corpus luteum cysts from deranged maturation and involution, regress spontaneously, do not become large
- Endometrial cysts
  - Endometrial deposits in ovary filled with old blood and debris

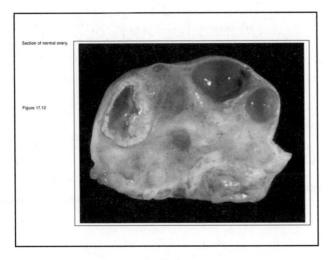

Section of normal ovary.

Figure 17.12

Ovarian Cysts (2 of 2)

- Benign cystic teratoma (dermoid cyst)
  - Arise from unfertilized ova that undergo neoplastic change
  - Contains skin, hair, teeth, bone, parts of gastrointestinal tract, thyroid, and other tissues growing in a jumbled fashion
- Malignant teratoma
  - Very rare

Notes

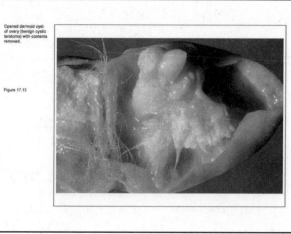

Opened dermoid cyst of ovary (benign cystic teratoma) with contents removed.

Figure 17.13

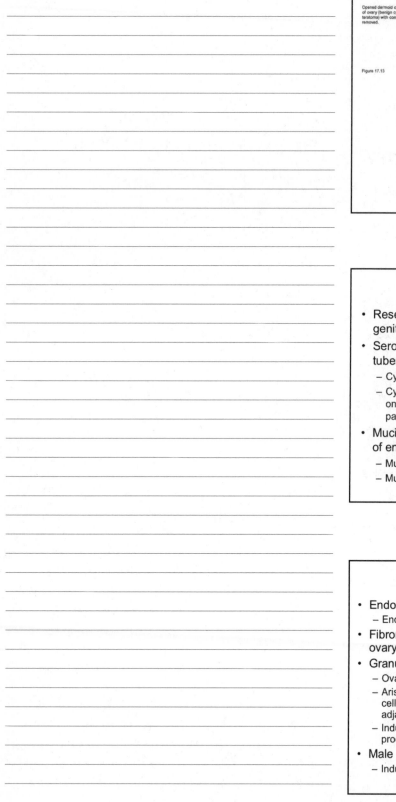

Ovarian Tumors (1 of 2)

- Resemble epithelium found in other parts of the genital tract
- Serous tumor: resembles cells lining fallopian tubes
  - Cystadenoma: benign, cystic serous tumor
  - Cystadenocarcinoma: neoplastic epithelium may extend on the surface of tumor and break off, implanting in other parts: pelvis, peritoneal cavity, omentum
- Mucinous tumor: resembles mucus-secreting tumor of endocervix
  - Mucinous cystadenoma
  - Mucinous cystadenocarcinoma

Ovarian Tumors (2 of 2)

- Endometrioid tumor: resembles endometrial tissue
  - Endometrioid carcinoma
- Fibroma: from fibrous connective tissue cells of ovary
- Granulosa-theca cell tumor
  - Ovarian tumor that produces estrogen
  - Arises from the granulosa cells or estrogen-producing cells that line the follicle or from theca cells located adjacent to follicle cells
  - Induces excessive endometrial stimulation from estrogen produced by tumor
- Male hormone-producing ovarian tumors
  - Induces masculinization

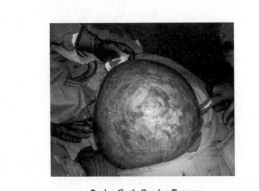

Benign Cystic Ovarian Tumors

Diseases of the Vulva

- Vulvar dystrophy
  - Irregular white patches on vulvar skin (leukoplakia)
  - Intense itching
  - May progress to carcinoma
  - Local treatment usually effective
- Carcinoma of the vulva
  - Found in pre- and post-menopausal women
  - Usually with a preexisting vulvar dystrophy
  - Treated by vulvectomy and excision of inguinal lymph nodes

Toxic Shock Syndrome (TSS) (1 of 2)

- Occurs most commonly in women using high-absorbency tampons
- No tampon can be considered entirely free from risk
- Caused by toxin produced by *Staphylococci* in vagina
- Menstrual blood and secretions serve as good culture medium for bacteria
- Tampons slow drainage of menstruate, may cause superficial erosions on vaginal mucosa allowing absorption of toxin through injured skin

Toxic Shock Syndrome (TSS)
(2 of 2)

- Clinical manifestations
  - Fever, vomiting, diarrhea, muscle aches and pains
  - Erythematous or sunburn-like rash followed by flaking and peeling
- Treatment
  - General supportive measures until effects of toxin wear off
  - Discontinue tampon use; TSS recurrence rate is 30%
  - Antibiotics to eradicate *Staphylococci* do not shorten course of disease
  - TSS also occurs from staphylococcal infections of skin, bones, kidneys, with toxin released in the bloodstream

Contraception

- Natural family planning
  - Avoidance of intercourse at time of ovulation
- Artificial contraception
  - Barrier methods: diaphragms and condoms; effective, no side effects
  - Oral contraceptives: suppress ovulation
    - Side effects: increased tendency for thromboembolic complications, especially among smokers; hypertension
  - Intrauterine contraceptive devices, IUDs: prevent implantation
    - Increased incidence of tubal infections and tubal pregnancies

Emergency Contraception

- Prevents pregnancy following unprotected intercourse or sexual assault
  - Sperm can survive as long as 6 days in genital tract and can still fertilize an ovum
  - Intercourse several days before ovulation can lead to a pregnancy
  - Prevents pregnancy by interfering with ovulation; tubal transport of ovum; and implantation within endometrium
- Effectiveness
  - If taken within 12 hours after intercourse, risk of pregnancy <1% and 3% if taken within 72 hours
  - Some protection is still provided for as long as 5 days

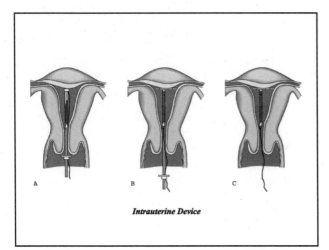

Intrauterine Device

Diethylstilbestrol (DES) (1 of 2)

- Nonsteroidal estrogens used from 1946–1970 to treat mothers prone to spontaneous abortion and other obstetric problems
- Can cause developmental abnormalities in genital tracts among women whose mothers used DES during pregnancy

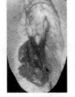

Diethylstilbestrol (DES) (2 of 2)

- Benign lesions
  - Form fibrous bands in upper vagina or cervix with projecting ridges that form either polypoid masses projecting from cervix or as collar-like structures that encircle cervix
  - Adenosis: small foci of columnar epithelium appearing bright red and interspersed with pale pink normal cervical and vaginal squamous epithelium
- Malignant lesion
  - Clear cell adenocarcinoma: cervix or vagina
  - Neoplastic cells have a clear or pale cytoplasm

Discussion

- A 23-year-old female presents with high fever, chills, vomiting, and muscle aches. On examination, patient has a markedly low blood pressure with a rash on her trunk. Search for possible sites of infection pointed to the vaginal area and tampon use. Patient is on the fifth day of her monthly period.
  - A. Vaginitis
  - B. Cellulitis
  - C. Drug reactions
  - D. Vulvar carcinoma
  - E. Toxic Shock Syndrome

Chapter 18 Prenatal Development and Diseases Associated with Pregnancy

Chapter Outline

The chapter outline provides you with an organizational guide to the topics and ideas presented in this chapter of the text.

Case Studies
Hemolytic Disease of the Newborn (Erythroblastosis Fetalis)

Study Questions

The following questions are provided as a test for comprehension and as a study guide for use with the text chapters. Additional study material is located at http://health.jbpub.com/humandisease/8e, which contains useful tools such as an A&P review, animated flashcards, an interactive online glossary, crossword puzzles, and web links.

Key Terms

Define the following terms:

1. Amniotic fluid _____

2. Gestational trophoblast disease _____

3. Placenta _____

4. Rh immune globulin _____

Fill-in-the-Blank

1. In a woman with a regular 28-day menstrual cycle, ovulation normally occurs on day _____.

2. If the egg is fertilized, its implantation occurs _____ days after fertilization occurs.

3. During the _____ period, the developing organism is most vulnerable to injury from drugs, maternal infections, or other factors that disturb prenatal development.

4. The outer sac surrounding the embryo is called the _____, and the finger-like processes projecting from the sac are called _____.

5. In the placenta, the blood circulating through the villi is blood pumped into the placenta by the _____, and the blood flowing around the villi is blood pumped into the placenta by _____.

6. An excess of amnionic fluid is called _____.

7. A reduced volume of amnionic fluid is called _____. This condition may be caused by _____.

8. The condition in which the placenta attaches to the lower part of the uterus and covers the cervix is called _____. This condition is usually treated by _____.

9. Identical twins are formed by separation of the inner cell mass during the early stages of prenatal development. If the separation is incomplete, the result is _____.

10. If the placental circulations of identical twins are interconnected, one twin may become anemic, and the other twin will have an excessive amount of blood. This condition is called _____.

11. The placenta produces two steroid hormones, called _____ and _____. It also produces two protein hormones, called _____ and _____.

12. In the usual case of hemolytic disease caused by Rh incompatibility, the Rh (D) type of the father is _____. The infant's Rh type is _____, and the mother's Rh type is _____.

True/False

Tell whether each statement is true or false. If false, explain why the statement is incorrect.

1. Two Rh-negative parents may have an Rh-positive infant. _____

_____

2. An Rh-negative infant may be born to two Rh-positive parents. _____

_____

3. Rh immune globulin is sometimes administered to Rh-negative mothers during pregnancy. _____

_____

4. Rh hemolytic disease usually occurs in firstborn infants and is usually less severe in subsequent pregnancies.

_____

5. Tell whether each statement is true or false regarding hydatidiform mole. If false, explain why the statement is incorrect.

   a. It occurs less frequently in U.S. and Canadian women than in women living in Asia. _____

   _____

   b. Incomplete removal of a hydatidiform mole may be followed by development of a choriocarcinoma. _____

   _____

   c. A woman who has had a mole evacuated by curettage may attempt another pregnancy as soon as her normal menstrual periods resume after the curettage. _____

   _____

   d. Some moles may exhibit aggressive behavior and invade the uterine wall. _____

   _____

6. Tell whether each statement is true or false regarding Rh immune globulin. If false, explain why the statement is incorrect.

   a. Its administration will usually prevent sensitization of an Rh-negative mother who has given birth to an Rh-positive infant. _____

   _____

   b. Its administration will usually prevent ABO hemolytic disease in group O mothers who have given birth to group A or B infants. _____

   _____

   c. Its administration will reduce the concentration of preexisting Rh antibodies in an Rh-negative mother who has previously been sensitized to the Rh antigen. _____

   _____

   d. It is never given to Rh-positive infants born to Rh-negative mothers. _____

   _____

7. Tell whether each of the following statements is true or false. If false, explain why the statement is incorrect.

a. Choriocarcinoma developing as a complication of a hydatidiform mole is very aggressive and has a very poor prognosis despite appropriate chemotherapy treatment.

_____

_____

b. Most cases of neonatal hemolytic disease result from an Rh-incompatible pregnancy (mother Rh negative; father and fetus Rh positive).

_____

_____

c. ABO hemolytic disease occurs less frequently than does Rh hemolytic disease and is more difficult to treat.

_____

_____

d. Most case of ABO hemolytic disease occur in group O infants born to group A mothers.

_____

_____

e. A high concentration of unconjugated bilirubin in the blood of a newborn infant with neonatal hemolytic disease is hazardous and may cause permanent damage to the infant's nervous system._____

_____

f. Giving immune globulin containing a high concentration of Rh antibodies to an Rh-negative mother who has given birth to an Rh-positive infant greatly reduces the likelihood that the mother will develop Rh antibodies that will complicate future pregnancies in which the infant is Rh-positive.

_____

_____

g. Transfer of fetal Rh-positive red cells into the circulation of an Rh-negative mother usually occurs when the placenta separates and is expelled after delivery. _____

_____

Identify

1. Prenatal development is divided into three separate periods:

a. _____

b. _____

c. _____

2. List the two conditions that may lead to the excess amniotic fluid.

a. _____

b. _____

3. The term "gestational trophoblast disease" includes what three conditions?

a. _____

b. _____

c. _____

Discussion Questions

1. In what part of the genital tract does fertilization of the egg occur? _____

_____

_____

_____

2. Briefly describe how gestational trophoblast disease is treated and how the patient should be managed after the condition is treated. _____

_____

_____

_____

3. Normally, maternal and fetal blood do not intermix in the placenta when the intact placenta remains within the uterus. How does this situation change when the placenta separates from the uterus after the baby has been delivered?

_____

_____

_____

4. Postpartum administration of Rh immune globulin to an Rh-negative woman who has given birth to an Rh-positive infant is recommended and given routinely to such patients. What is the purpose of the injection, and why is it effective? _____

_____

_____

_____

5. Can two Rh (D)-negative parents have an Rh-positive baby? Why or why not? _____

_____

_____

_____

6. Can two Rh (D)-positive parents have an Rh-negative baby? Why or why not? _____

_____

_____

_____

7. Describe how ABO hemolytic disease differs from Rh hemolytic disease. _____

_____

_____

8. Why do spontaneous abortions occur? _____

_____

_____

9. What are the consequences of prolonged retention of a dead fetus within the uterine cavity? _____

_____

_____

10. What is an ectopic pregnancy? What factors predispose a woman to development of an ectopic pregnancy in the fallopian tube? What are the consequences of a tubal pregnancy? _____

_____

_____

11. What conditions are associated with ectopic pregnancies? _____

_____

_____

12. Who should receive the Rh immune globulin injection? When is it given? Why is it given? How does it work?

_____

_____

13. Why do some women develop an elevated blood glucose in the second trimester of pregnancy, which returns to normal postpartum? _____

_____

14. What is preeclampsia? When does it occur? Why does it occur? How is it treated? _____

_____

_____

Notes

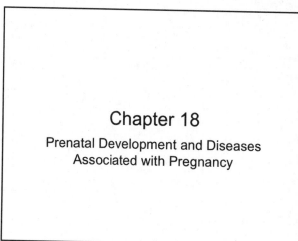

Chapter 18
Prenatal Development and Diseases Associated with Pregnancy

Learning Objectives (1 of 2)

- Explain process of fertilization; implantation; early development of ovum; origin of decidua, fetal membranes, and placenta
- Describe formation and elimination of amnionic fluid; conditions leading to abnormal levels
- Explain causes and effects of spontaneous abortion and ectopic pregnancy
- Identify and explain problems following failure of contraceptive pills or intrauterine device
- Describe mechanism and clinical manifestations associated with abnormal attachment of placenta

Learning Objectives (2 of 2)

- Differentiate: Identical vs. fraternal twins
- Describe determination of zygosity from examination of placenta; disadvantages of a twin pregnancy
- Classify types of gestational trophoblast disease, methods of treatment
- Explain pathogenesis, clinical manifestations, diagnostic criteria, treatment for hemolytic disease of the newborn

Fertilization

- Union of sperm and ovum occurs in fallopian tube
- Sperm travel via own propulsion and by passive transported upward into the fallopian tubes by rhythmic contractions of uterine muscles
- Ovum is expelled from follicle at ovulation
- Fertilization is possible when sperm are present in fallopian tubes at the time egg is expelled at ovulation
- First cell division completed 30 hours after fertilization
- Only 1 sperm can enter egg
- Sperm penetration causes zona pellucida to become impermeable to penetration by other sperm

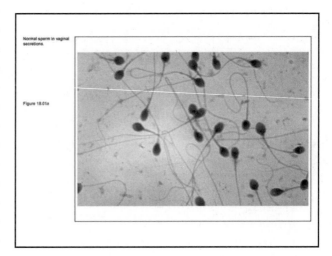

Normal sperm in vaginal secretions.

Figure 18.01a

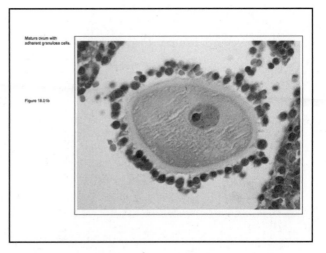

Mature ovum with adherent granulosa cells.

Figure 18.01b

TABLE 18-1

Conception rate based on day of intercourse

DAY OF INTERCOURSE	PERCENTAGE OF CONCEPTIONS
6 days before ovulation	8 percent
5 days before ovulation	10 percent
4 days before ovulation	16 percent
3 days before ovulation	no data
2 days before ovulation	28 percent
1 day before ovulation	32 percent
day of ovulation	36 percent
day after ovulation	none

Based on data from Wilcox, A.J. et al. *New England Journal of Medicine* 333:1517–21.

Conception rate based on day of intercourse.

Table 18.01

Early Development: Fertilized Ovum

- Fertilization occurs in fallopian tube
  - Sperm contain genetic material and enzymes for penetration
  - Zygote develops into a small ball of cells
  - Fluid accumulates to form blastocyst
    - Inner cell mass: forms embryo
    - Trophoblast: forms placenta and membranes
  - Blastocyst begins to differentiate
- Implantation by end of 1st week
  - Blastocyst implants in endometrium
  - Amnionic sac and yolk sac form
  - Small germ disk and yolk sac project into chorionic cavity
  - Organ systems begin to form; embryo becomes cylindrical by 4th week

In Vitro Fertilization and Embryo Transfer

- Some women ovulate normally but are infertile because fallopian tubes obstructed by scarring or removed due to previous ectopic pregnancies
- Patient's follicle is aspirated by laparoscopy
- Ovum is fertilized and allowed to develop outside the body into 8- or 16-cell stage
- Fertilized ovum implanted into uterus
- Low success rate
  - Possibility of chromosomally abnormal embryos
  - Abnormal embryos usually unable to survive and are aborted

Stages of Prenatal Development

- Pre-embryonic period: First 3 weeks after fertilization
  - Blastocyst becomes implanted and inner mass cell differentiates into 3 germ layers to eventually form specific tissues within embryo
- Embryonic period: 3rd through 7th week
  - Begins to assume a human shape
  - All organ systems are formed
  - Very critical period of development
- Fetal period: 8th week to term
  - Fetus continues to grow
  - No major changes in basic structure
  - Subcutaneous fat accumulates; fills body shortly before delivery

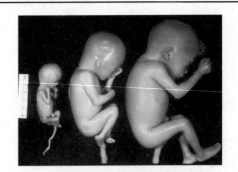

Progressive changes in fetal size,
3.5 months, 4.5 months, and 5.5 months

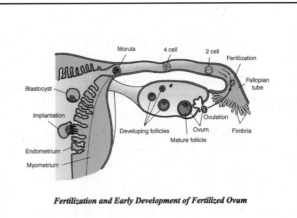

Fertilization and Early Development of Fertilized Ovum

Duration of Pregnancy

- Gestation: total duration of pregnancy from fertilization to delivery
  - Dated from time of conception: 38 weeks
  - Dated from first day of last menstrual period (date of ovulation unknown): 40 weeks
    - First day of the calculation is two weeks before the date of conception
    - May be expressed as 280 days
  - Also expressed as 10 lunar (28-day) months or 9 calendar (31-day) months; divided into 3 periods called trimesters

Decidua, Fetal Membranes, Placenta

- Decidua: endometrium of pregnancy
  - Decidua basalis: under chorionic vesicle
  - Decidua capsularis: over chorionic vesicle
  - Decidua parietalis: lines rest of the uterus
- Chorion laeve: superficial smooth chorion
- Chorion frondosum: bushy chorion
- Amnionic sac: enclosed within chorion, forms a protective environment
- Yolk sac: forms intestinal tract

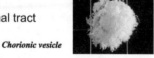

Chorionic vesicle

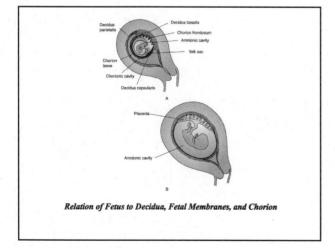

Relation of Fetus to Decidua, Fetal Membranes, and Chorion

Placenta

- Double circulation of blood
  - Fetoplacental circulation: from fetus to villi
  - Uteroplacental circulation: maternal blood circulates around villi
- No actual intermixing of maternal and fetal blood
- Fetus connected to placenta by umbilical cord
- Functions of the placenta
  - Provides O_2 and nutrition for fetus
  - Has endocrine function: synthesizes hormones (estrogen; progesterone; protein hormones)
    - Human placental lactogen, HPL
    - Human chorionic gonadotropin, HCG

Amnionic Fluid (1 of 2)

- Produced by filtration and excretion
  - Filtration from maternal blood early in pregnancy
  - Fetal urine later in pregnancy
- Fetus swallows fluid:
  - Absorbed from fetal intestinal tract into fetal circulation
  - Transferred across placenta into mother's circulation
  - Excreted by mother in her urine
- Balance is maintained in secretion and excretion of amnionic fluid
- Quantity varies with stage of pregnancy

Amnionic Fluid (2 of 2)

- Polyhydramnios: increased volume of amniotic fluid
  - Fetus unable to swallow and fluid accumulates (anencephaly)
  - Fluid is swallowed but not absorbed due to congenital obstruction of fetal upper intestinal tract
- Oligohydramnios: reduced volume of amniotic fluid
  - Fetal kidneys failed to develop and no urine is formed
  - Congenital obstruction of urethra does not allow urine to form amnionic fluid

Gestational Diabetes

- Hyperglycemia: harmful to fetus
- Pregnancy hormones induce maternal insulin resistance
- Diabetes results from inability to increase insulin secretion to compensate for increased insulin resistance
- Diagnosis: similar to non-gestational diabetes
- Diabetes usually relents following delivery

Spontaneous Abortion

- 10-20% of all pregnancies
- Early abortion results from
  - Chromosome abnormalities
  - Defective implantation
  - Maldevelopment of fetus
- Late abortion results from
  - Detachment of placenta
  - Obstruction of blood supply through cord
  - Complication: Disseminated intravascular coagulation
  - Cocaine abuse: disturbs blood flow to placenta and may cause placental abruption and intrauterine fetal death

Small well-formed spontaneously aborted fetus near the end of the first trimester.

Figure 16.06

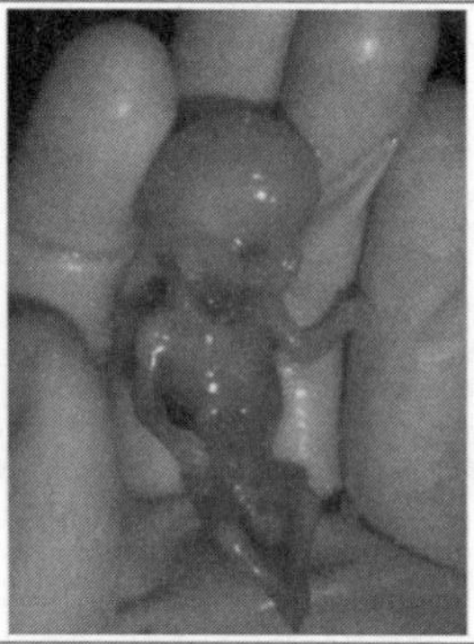

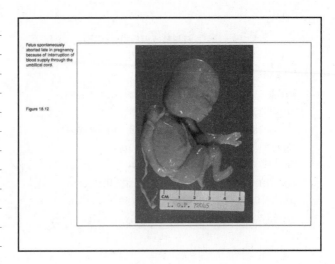

Fetus spontaneously aborted late in pregnancy because of interruption of blood supply through the umbilical cord.

Figure 18.12

Ectopic Pregnancy

- Development of embryo outside the uterine cavity
- Most common site: fallopian tubes
- Predisposing factors
  - Previous infection of fallopian tubes
  - Failure of normal muscular contractions of tubal wall
  - Both fallopian tunes predisposed
- Consequences
  - Rupture of fallopian tube
  - Profuse bleeding from torn vessels
  - Potentially life-threatening to mother

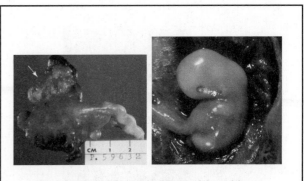

Ectopic Pregnancy, fallopian tube with mass of placental tissue; embryo within intact amnionic sac

Artificial Contraception

- Failure of oral contraceptives
  - Developing embryo exposed to synthetic estrogen and progestin compounds
  - Exposure to estrogen and progestin compounds may induce congenital abnormalities in developing embryo
- Failure of an intrauterine device
  - IUD predisposes pregnant uterus to infection
  - Must be removed as soon as pregnancy is diagnosed

Abnormal Attachment of Umbilical Cord

- Velamentous insertion
  - Cord attached to fetal membranes than placenta
  - May tear or is compressed during labor
  - May be fatal to infant
  - No adverse effect on mother

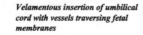
Velamentous insertion of umbilical cord with vessels traversing fetal membranes

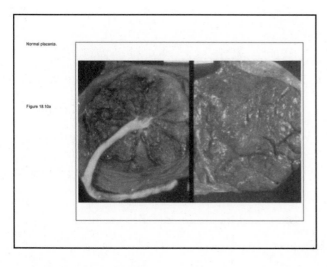

Normal placenta.

Figure 18.10a

Abnormal Attachment of Placenta

- Normally, placenta attaches high on the anterior or posterior uterine wall
- Placenta previa: placenta attached at lower part of uterus; may cover cervix
  - Central placenta previa: placenta covers entire cervix
  - Partial placenta previa: margin of placenta covers cervix
- Causes episodes of bleeding late in pregnancy
- Hazardous to both mother and infant
- Requires delivery by cesarean section

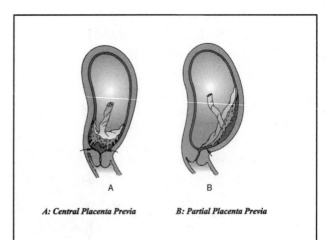

A: Central Placenta Previa   *B: Partial Placenta Previa*

Twins (1 of 2)

- Disadvantages of twinning
  - Twins smaller than single infant at comparable stage of gestation
  - Over-distention of uterus promotes premature onset of labor
    - Delivery of premature infants
    - Reduced chance of survival
  - Congenital malformations occur twice as often in twins

Twins (2 of 2)

- Twin transfusion syndrome
  - Vascular anastomoses connect placental circulations of identical twins
  - One twin is polycythemic and one is anemic
  - Tolerated if minor disproportions in blood, if severe, may be fatal to both twins
- Vanishing twin: one of the twin dies and is resorbed
- Blighted twin: one of the twin dies and persists as degenerated fetus
- Fraternal twins: 2 separate ova fertilized by 2 different sperm
- Identical twins: single fertilized ovum splits
- Conjoined twins: variable union between identical twins

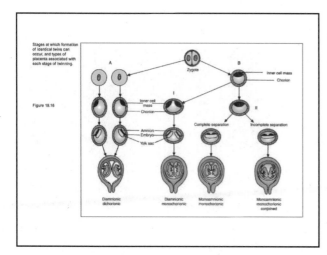

Stages at which formation of identical twins can occur, and types of placenta associated with each stage of twinning.

Figure 18.16

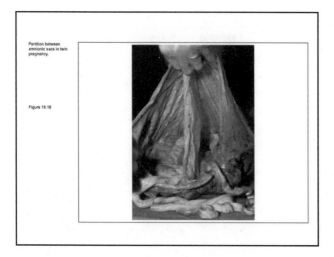

Partition between amnionic sacs in twin pregnancy.

Figure 18.18

Notes

_____
_____
_____
_____
_____
_____
_____
_____
_____
_____
_____
_____
_____
_____
_____
_____
_____
_____
_____
_____
_____
_____
_____
_____
_____
_____
_____
_____
_____
_____
_____
_____
_____
_____

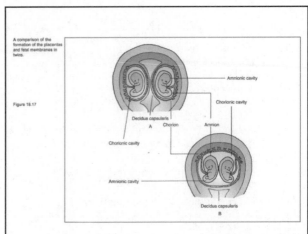

A comparison of the formation of the placentas and fetal membranes in twins.

Figure 18.17

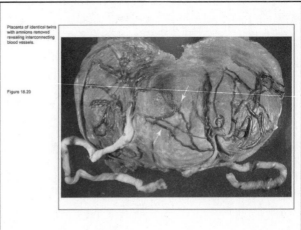

Placenta of identical twins with amnions removed revealing interconnecting blood vessels.

Figure 18.20

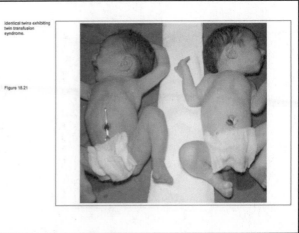

Identical twins exhibiting twin transfusion syndrome.

Figure 18.21

Triplet placenta.

Figure 18.22

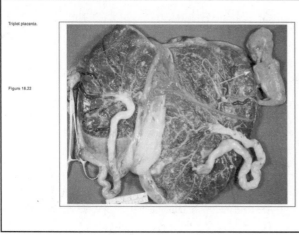

Conjoined twins exhibiting a large congenital defect in the abdominal wall (Case 18-3).

Figure 18.23a

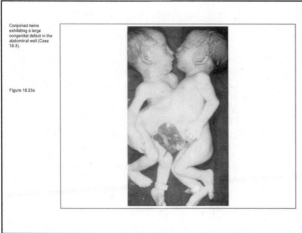

X-ray of conjoined twins demonstrating extreme curvature of fetal spine.

Figure 18.23b

Notes

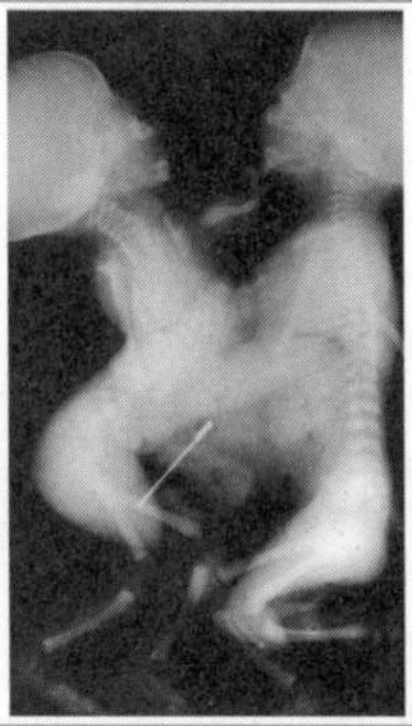

Gestational Trophoblast Disease (1 of 3)

- Trophoblastic cells covering villi continue to grow at excessive rate, producing higher HCG than in normal pregnancy
- Proliferating trophoblastic tissue may invade uterus, vagina, distant sites
- Hydatidiform mole ("hydatid": fluid-filled vesicle; "mole": shapeless structure)
  - Occurs in 80% of affected patients
  - Complete mole
  - Results from abnormal fertilization of an ovum lacking chromosomes and ovum fertilized by a single sperm bearing an X chromosome that is duplicated to form 46

Gestational Trophoblast Disease (2 of 3)

- Hydatidiform mole: complete mole
  - Both X chromosomes come from the father
  - No embryo develops
  - Chorionic villi become cystic structures resembling mass of grapes (complete mole)
- Hydatidiform mole: partial mole
  - Normal ovum fertilized by 2 sperm, resulting in a fertilized ovum with 3 sets of chromosomes (69 chromosomes)
  - Embryo forms but does not survive
  - Less likely to exhibit aggressive behavior

Gestational Trophoblast Disease (3 of 3)

- Invasive mole
  - Trophoblastic tissue invades deeply into uterine wall
  - Occurs in 15% of affected patients
  - Aggressive, destructive
- Choriocarcinoma
  - May arise following incomplete removal of invasive or incompletely removed mole
  - Masses of proliferating trophoblast may extend into vagina
  - Metastasizes to lungs and brain
- Treatment: curettage, periodic determination of HCG; hysterectomy; chemotherapy

Erythroblastosis Fetalis (1 of 2)

- Pathogenesis
  - 1. Sensitization of mother to a blood group antigen in fetal RBCs
  - 2. Mother forms antibodies that cross placenta
  - 3. Maternal antibodies damage fetal RBCs
  - 4. Fetus increases blood production to compensate for increased RBC destruction
- Variable severity
  - Hydrops fetalis
  - Less intense hemolytic process
  - Mild disease

Erythroblastosis Fetalis (2 of 2)

- Hydrops fetalis
  - Severe anemia causes heart failure and impaired hepatic plasma protein synthesis
  - Results in edema
  - Hemolytic process is extremely severe, causing death
  - Infant dies in uterus during last trimester
- Less intense hemolytic process
  - Infant is born alive but moderately or severely anemic
- Mild disease
  - Infant appears normal at birth then becomes anemic and jaundiced, develops edema

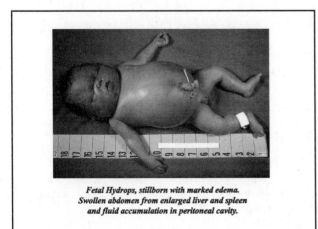

Fetal Hydrops, stillborn with marked edema.
Swollen abdomen from enlarged liver and spleen
and fluid accumulation in peritoneal cavity.

Rh Hemolytic Disease (1 of 3)

- Most cases: Rh-negative mother and Rh-positive infant
- Consists of a series of allelic genes that determine multiple Rh antigens on red cells
  - Rh-positive: red cells contain D (Rh_o) antigen
    - May be homozygous (genotype DD)
    - May be heterozygous (genotype Dd)
  - Rh-negative: red cells lack D (Rh_o) antigen
    - Genotype dd

Rh Hemolytic Disease (2 of 3)

- Mother sensitized to "foreign" antigen in infant's cells and forms anti-D antibodies that cross placenta into infant's blood
- Rarely occurs in first pregnancy
  - First Rh-positive infant born to Rh-negative mother is normal
  - Rh antibodies not yet formed
- Treatment
  - Exchange transfusion
  - Fluorescent light therapy for hyperbilirubinemia
  - Intrauterine fetal transfusion

Rh Hemolytic Disease (3 of 3)

- Prevention
  - Rh immune globulin administered to mother
    - Contains gamma globulin with Rh antibody
    - Given within 72 hours after delivery of Rh-positive infant
    - Rh antibody coats Rh antigen sites on surface of fetal red cells in maternal circulation to reduce sensitization
  - Not 100% effective: 1.5% still form antibodies
  - Some physicians recommend injections late in pregnancy and after delivery to reduce incidence of sensitization

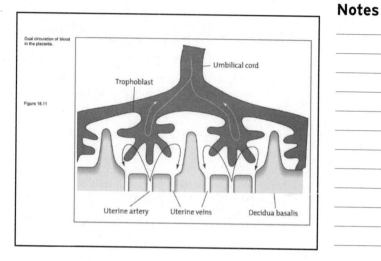

Dual circulation of blood in the placenta.

Figure 18.11

- Umbilical cord
- Trophoblast
- Uterine artery
- Uterine veins
- Decidua basalis

Discussion

- A 30-year old woman prematurely delivered normal, well-formed female twins at 36 weeks of gestation. However, on examination of the placenta following delivery, a third amnionic sac was noted with a degenerated fetus measuring 13 centimeters in length
  - A. Vanishing twin
  - B. Twin transfusion syndrome
  - C. Blighted twin
  - D. Conjoined twins
  - E. Placenta previa

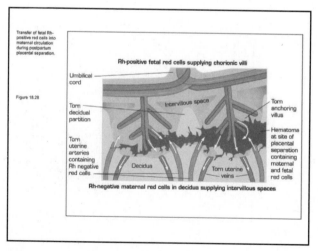

Transfer of fetal Rh-positive red cells into maternal circulation during postpartum placental separation.

Figure 18.28

Rh-positive fetal red cells supplying chorionic villi

- Umbilical cord
- Torn decidual partition
- Torn uterine arteries containing Rh negative red cells
- Intervillous space
- Decidua
- Torn uterine veins
- Torn anchoring villus
- Hematoma at site of placental separation containing maternal and fetal red cells

Rh-negative maternal red cells in decidua supplying intervillous spaces

ABO Hemolytic Disease (1 of 2)

- Pathogenesis
  - Mother is type 0 (has anti-A and anti-B antibodies in her serum) while infant is type A or type B
  - Maternal anti-A and anti-B antibodies attach to fetal red cells
  - Can occur in first ABO-incompatible pregnancy due to pre-existing anti-A and anti-B antibodies
- Manifestations
  - Milder disease than Rh hemolytic disease because fetal A and B antigens are not as well developed unlike in adult cells; antibodies do not attach as firmly to fetal cells

ABO Hemolytic Disease (2 of 2)

- Manifestations
  - A and B antigens also present in other fetal tissues, absorbing some of the antibodies that would otherwise attach to fetal cells
  - Complications: anemia; hyperbilirubinemia; kernicterus
  - Excess unconjugated bilirubin from red cell breakdown
- Treatment
  - Control hyperbilirubinemia by fluorescent light therapy
  - Exchange transfusion not usually required

Diagnosis of hemolytic disease.

Table 18.02

TABLE 18-2

Diagnosis of hemolytic disease

CHARACTERISTIC FEATURE	MEANS OF RECOGNITION
Production of antigenic fetal cells	Maternal-fetal blood group differences; mother lacks antigen present in fetal cells
Maternal sensitization	Mother's blood contains antibody against antigenic cells
Transplacental passage of maternal antibody	Positive direct Coombs test on cord blood
Increased blood destruction in newborn infant	Decreased hemoglobin in cord blood; elevated bilirubin

Discussion

- The following are true of hemolytic disease of the newborn EXCEPT:
    - A. Mother forms antibodies that cross the placenta and attack fetal red cells
    - B. Infant's red cells are protected by the mother's antibodies
    - C. Infant suffers edema from heart failure and impaired protein synthesis
    - D. Infant compensates by increasing red blood cell production
    - E. Infant may suffer severe hemolytic anemia and edema

Notes

Chapter Outline

The chapter outline provides you with an organizational guide to the topics and ideas presented in this chapter of the text.

Structure and Function of the Urinary System
   The Kidneys
   The Ureters
   The Bladder and Urethra
Function of the Kidneys
   The Nephron
   Renal Regulation of Blood Pressure and Blood Volume
   Requirements for Normal Renal Function
Developmental Disturbances
Glomerulonephritis
   Immune-Complex Glomerulonephritis
   Anti-GBM Glomerulonephritis
Nephrotic Syndrome
Arteriolar Nephrosclerosis
Diabetic Nephropathy
Infections of the Urinary Tract
   Cystitis
   Pyelonephritis
   Vesicoureteral Reflux and Infection
Calculi
Foreign Bodies
Obstruction
Renal Tubular Injury
Renal Cysts
   Solitary Cysts
   Multiple Cysts
Tumors of the Urinary Tract
   Renal Cortical Tumors
   Transitional Cell Tumors
   Nephroblastoma (Wilms' Tumor)
Diagnostic Evaluation of Kidney and Urinary Tract Disease
   Urinalysis
   Clearance Tests
   Additional Techniques
Renal Failure (Uremia)
   Hemodialysis
   Renal Transplantation

Study Questions

The following questions are provided as a test for comprehension and as a study guide for use with the text chapters. Additional study material is located at http://health.jbpub.com/humandisease/8e, which contains useful tools such as an A&P review, animated flashcards, an interactive online glossary, crossword puzzles, and web links.

Key Terms

Define the following terms:

1. Diabetic nephropathy _____

2. Urea _____

3. Uremia _____

4. Glomerulonephritis _____

5. Pyelonephritis _____

6. Nephritic syndrome _____

7. Nephrosclerosis _____

Fill-in-the-Blank

1. The enzyme released by juxtaglomerular cells is called _____ , which converts a protein called_____ into _____. The converted protein then is converted by ACE into _____, which is a powerful vasoconstrictor and also stimulates the adrenal cortex to release a hormone called _____.

2. Glomerulonephritis results from an immunologic reaction within the glomeruli and is divided into two main types, which are called _____ and _____.

3. An infection of the bladder is called _____, and an infection of the kidney is called _____.

4. Dilatation of the renal pelvis, calyces, and ureter resulting from obstruction to outflow of urine is called

   _____.

5. A kidney stone is called a _____.

6. The hereditary kidney disease characterized by formation of multiple progressively enlarging renal cysts that gradually destroy the function of the kidneys is called _____.

7. Two methods of renal dialysis are called _____ and _____.

8. Malignant tumors occur in the kidneys and bladder. The malignant kidney tumor occurring in older adults is called _____. The malignant kidney tumor occurring in infants and young children is called _____. The malignant bladder tumor is called _____.

9. The laboratory test that is likely to show abnormal results in a patient with acute glomerulonephritis is

   _____.

True/False

Tell whether each statement is true or false. If false, explain why the statement is incorrect.

1. Blood and urine clearance tests measure the ability of the kidneys to remove ("clear") waste products from the blood and excrete the products in the urine. _____

_____

2. Diabetic nephropathy is characterized by nodular and diffuse thickening of glomerular basement membranes as well as by marked thickening and narrowing of glomerular arterioles (arteriolonephrosclerosis). _____

_____

3. Tell whether each statement is true or false regarding acute poststreptococcal glomerulonephritis. If false, explain why the statement is incorrect.

   a. It is induced by antigen–antibody complexes filtered from the blood that accumulate within the walls of the glomerular capillaries. _____

   _____

   b. It results from bacterial infection of the glomeruli. _____

   _____

   c. It usually causes a nephrotic syndrome. _____

   _____

   d. It is caused by damage done by enzymes released from leukocytes that accumulate within the glomeruli.

   _____

4. Tell whether each statement is true or false regarding the nephrotic syndrome. If false, explain why the statement is incorrect.

   a. The liver fails to produce plasma protein. _____

   _____

   b. Protein is lost in the urine more rapidly than it can be produced by the body. _____

   _____

   c. The nephrotic syndrome is usually associated with normal concentration of plasma protein and normal plasma osmotic pressure. _____

   _____

   d. It may result from any type of glomerular disease that allows large amounts of protein to escape in the urine.

   _____

   e. It usually is caused by a bacterial infection of the kidney. _____

   _____

   f. It may result from renal tubular disease. _____

   _____

5. Tell whether each statement is true or false regarding the renin–angiotensin–aldosterone syndrome. If false, explain why the statement is incorrect.

   a. Renin is secreted by cells of the juxtaglomerular apparatus in response to high blood sodium concentration, higher than normal blood pressure, or higher than normal blood volume. _____

   _____

   b. Renin converts angiotensinogen to angiotensin I. _____

   _____

   c. Angiotensin-converting enzyme (ACE) converts angiotensin I to angiotensin II. _____

   _____

   d. Angiotensin II stimulates aldosterone release and arteriolar vasoconstriction. _____

   _____

6. Tell whether each statement is true or false regarding congenital polycystic kidney disease. If false, explain why the statement is incorrect.

   a. It is transmitted as mendelian dominant trait. _____

   _____

   b. Manifestations occur in late childhood or adolescence. _____

   _____

   c. Progressively enlarging cysts slowly destroy kidney function. _____

   _____

   d. Affected kidneys become greatly enlarged. _____

   _____

7. Tell whether each statement is true or false regarding bladder carcinoma. If false, explain why the statement is incorrect.

   a. The bladder tumor arises from transitional epithelium of the urinary bladder. _____

   _____

   b. Hematuria (blood in urine) may be the first manifestation of the bladder tumor. _____

   _____

   c. The tumor usually is poorly differentiated and rapidly growing and has a very poor prognosis. _____

   _____

   d. Diagnosis of a tumor is made by cystoscopy and biopsy. _____

   _____

Matching

Match the item in the left column with its characteristic or property in the right column.

1. _____ Polycystic kidney disease   A. Kidney infection

2. _____ Gout   B. Mendelian dominant trait

3. _____ Pyelonephritis   C. Nodular and diffuse basement membrane thickening

4. _____ IgA nephropathy   D. Urate crystals plug tubules

5. _____ Diabetes   E. Immune complexes in mesangial cells

Identify

1. Identify three conditions that predispose a person to urinary tract infection.

   a. _____

   b. _____

   c. _____

2. Identify three features characteristic of the nephrotic syndrome.

   a. _____

   b. _____

   c. _____

Discussion Questions

1. What is the relationship between glomerulonephritis and beta streptococcal infection? _____
   _____
   _____
   _____

2. What is the difference between the nephrotic syndrome and nephrosclerosis? _____
   _____
   _____
   _____

3. Why does edema occur in a patient with nephrosis? _____
   _____
   _____
   _____

4. What are the common causes of urinary tract obstruction? What are its effects on the kidneys and lower urinary tract? _____
   _____
   _____
   _____

5. What conditions predispose a person to kidney stones? _____

_____

_____

6. Describe the conditions that may lead to renal tubular necrosis. What are its clinical manifestations? _____

_____

_____

_____

7. What is the significance of an elevated level of urea in the blood? _____

_____

_____

_____

8. What are the manifestations of uremia? How is it treated by the physician? _____

_____

_____

_____

9. How is kidney failure treated? _____

_____

_____

_____

10. What methods does the physician use to establish a diagnosis of renal disease? _____

_____

_____

11. What condition(s) may eventually lead to renal failure? _____

_____

_____

12. What adverse effects are caused by a foreign body inserted into the bladder? _____

_____

_____

Notes

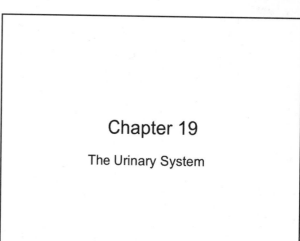

Chapter 19

The Urinary System

Learning Objectives (1 of 2)

- Describe normal structure and functions of the kidneys
- Explain pathogenesis and clinical manifestations of glomerulonephritis, nephrosis, nephrosclerosis, and glomerulosclerosis
- Describe clinical manifestations and complications of urinary tract infections
- Describe causes of renal tubular injury, manifestations, treatment

Learning Objectives (2 of 2)

- Explain mechanism of urinary tract calculi formation, complications, manifestations of urinary tract obstruction
- Differentiate major forms of cystic disease of the kidney and prognoses; common tumors affecting urinary tract
- Describe causes, clinical manifestations, treatment of renal failure
- Describe principles and techniques of hemodialysis

Notes

_____
_____
_____
_____
_____
_____
_____
_____
_____
_____
_____
_____
_____
_____
_____
_____
_____
_____
_____
_____
_____
_____
_____
_____
_____
_____
_____
_____
_____
_____
_____
_____
_____
_____
_____
_____

Urinary System

- Kidneys: produce urine
- Excretory duct system
  - Ureter: conveys urine into bladder by peristalsis
  - Renal pelvis: expanded upper portion of ureter
  - Major calyces: subdivisions of renal pelvis
  - Minor calyces: subdivisions of major calyces into which renal papillae discharge
- Bladder: stores urine
  - Discharges urine into urethra during voiding
  - Anatomic configuration of bladder and ureters normally prevents reflux of urine into ureters
- Urethra: conveys urine from the bladder for excretion

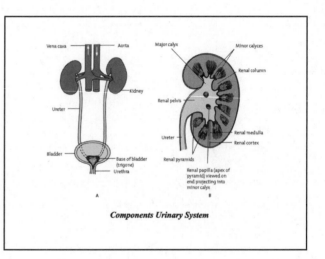

Components Urinary System

Kidneys (1 of 2)

- Paired, bean-shaped organs below diaphragm adjacent to vertebral column
- Divided into outer cortex and inner medulla (renal pyramids and columns)
- Excretory organs, functions along with lungs in excreting waste products of food metabolism
- Three basic functions
  - 1. Excrete waste products of food metabolism
    - CO_2 and H_2O: end-products of carbohydrate and fat metabolism
    - Urea and other acids: end-products of protein metabolism that only the kidneys can excrete

Kidneys (2 of 2)

– 2. Regulate mineral and H_2O balance
  - Excretes excess minerals and H_2O ingested and conserving them as required
  - Body's internal environment is determined not by what a person ingests but by what the kidneys retain

– 3. Produces erythropoietin and renin: specialized cells in the kidneys
  - Erythropoietin: regulates RBC production in marrow
  - Renin: helps regulate blood pressure

Nephron (1 of 2)

- Basic structural and functional unit of the kidney
- About 1 million nephrons in each kidney
- Consists of glomerulus and renal tubule
- Glomerulus
  – Tuft of capillaries supplied by an afferent glomerular arteriole that recombine into an efferent glomerular
  – Material is filtered by a 3-layered glomerular filter
    - Inner: fenestrated capillary endothelium
    - Middle: basement membrane
    - Outer: capillary endothelial cells (with foot processes and filtration slits)
  – Mesangial cells: contractile phagocytic cells that hold the capillary tuft together; regulate caliber of capillaries affecting filtration rate

Nephron (2 of 2)

- Renal tubule: reabsorbs most of filtrate; secretes unwanted components into tubular fluid; regulates H_2O balance
  – Proximal end: Bowman's capsule
  – Distal end: empties into collecting tubules
- Requirements for normal renal function
  – Free flow of blood through the glomerular capillaries
  – Normally functioning glomerular filter that restricts passage of blood cells and protein
  – Normal outflow of urine

Notes

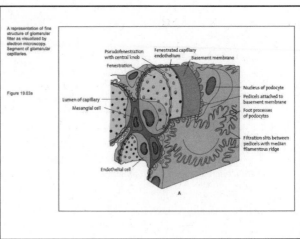

A representation of fine structure of glomerular filter as visualized by electron microscopy. Segment of glomerular capillaries.

Figure 19.03a

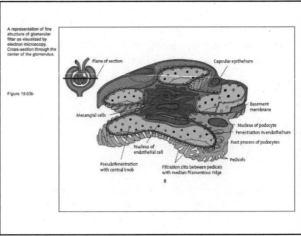

A representation of fine structure of glomerular filter as visualized by electron microscopy. Cross-section through the center of the glomerulus.

Figure 19.03b

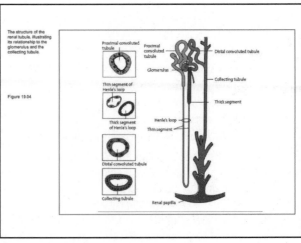

The structure of the renal tubule, illustrating its relationship to the glomerulus and the collecting tubule.

Figure 19.04

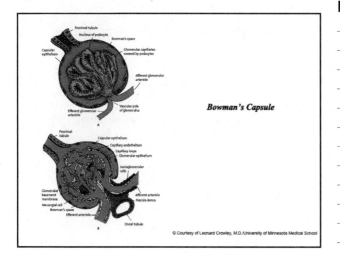

Bowman's Capsule

© Courtesy of Leonard Crowley, M.D./University of Minnesota Medical School

Renal Regulation of Blood Pressure

- Renin: released in response to decreased blood volume, low blood pressure, low sodium
- Angiotensin I → angiotensin II by angiotensin converting enzyme (ACE) as blood flows through the lungs
- Angiotensin II:
  - Powerful vasoconstrictor: raises blood pressure by causing peripheral arterioles to constrict
  - Stimulates aldosterone secretion from adrenal cortex: increases reabsorption of NaCl and H_2O by kidneys
  - Net effect: higher blood pressure, increased fluid in vascular system
- System is self-regulating

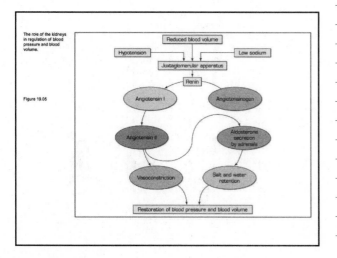

Figure 19.05

Developmental Abnormalities

- Developmental process is disturbed
- Normal development
  - Kidneys arise from mesoderm, develop in pelvis, ascend to final position
  - Bladder derived from lower end of intestinal tract
  - Excretory ducts (ureters, calyces, pelves) develop from ureteric buds that extend from bladder into the developing kidneys

Three congenital abnormalities result

- Renal agenesis: failure of one or both kidneys to develop
  - Bilateral: rare, associated with other congenital anomalies, incompatible with life
  - Unilateral: common, asymptomatic; other kidney enlarges to compensate
- Duplications of urinary tract
  - Complete duplication: formation of extra ureter and renal pelvis
  - Incomplete duplication: only upper part of excretory system is duplicated
- Malposition: one or both kidneys, associated with fusion of kidneys; horseshoe kidney; fusion of upper pole

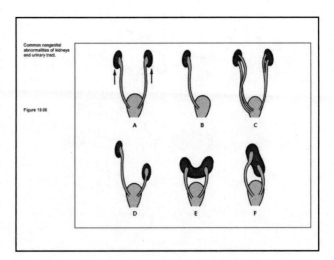

Common congenital abnormalities of kidneys and urinary tract.

Figure 19.06

Glomerulonephritis

- Inflammation of the glomeruli caused by antigen-antibody reaction within the glomeruli
- Immune-complex glomerulonephritis
  - Usually follows a beta-streptococcal infection
  - Circulating antigen and antibody complexes are filtered by glomeruli and incite inflammation
  - Leukocytes release lysosomal enzymes that cause injury to the glomeruli
  - Occurs in SLE; immune complexes trapped in glomeruli
  - Occurs in IgA nephropathy
- Anti-glomerular basement membrane (anti-GBM) glomerulonephritis: autoantibodies attack glomerular basement membrane

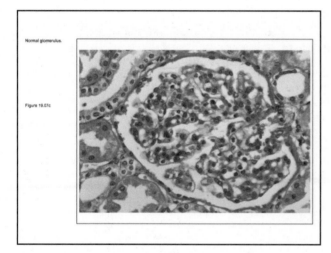

Normal glomerulus.

Figure 19.07c

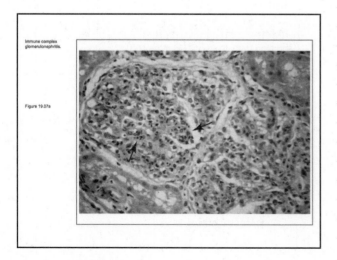

Immune complex glomerulonephritis.

Figure 19.07a

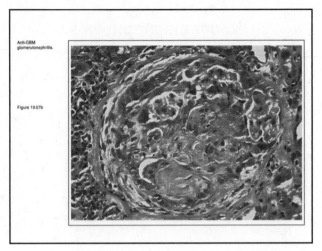

Anti-GBM
glomerulonephritis.

Figure 19.07b

Nephrotic Syndrome (1 of 2)

- Marked loss of protein in the urine
  - Urinary excretion of protein > protein production
  - Protein level in blood falls
  - Causes edema due to low plasma osmotic pressure
- Clinical manifestations
  - Marked leg edema
  - Ascites

Nephrotic Syndrome (2 of 2)

- Prognosis
  - In children: minimal glomerular change, complete recovery
  - In adults: a manifestation of severe progressive renal disease
- May result from
  - Glomerulonephritis
  - Diabetes (causing glomerular changes)
  - Systemic lupus erythematosus, SLE
  - Other kidney diseases

Arteriolar Nephrosclerosis

- Complication of severe hypertension
- Renal arterioles undergo thickening from carrying blood at a much higher pressure than normal
- Glomeruli and tubules undergo secondary degenerative changes causing narrowing of lumen and reduction in blood flow
  - Reduced glomerular filtration
  - Kidneys shrink
  - May die of renal insufficiency

Diabetic Nephropathy

- Complication of long-standing diabetes
- Nodular and diffuse thickening of glomerular basement membranes (glomerulosclerosis), usually with coexisting nephrosclerosis
- Manifestations
  - Progressive impairment of renal function
  - Protein loss may lead to nephrotic syndrome
  - No specific treatment can arrest progression of disease
  - Progressive impairment of renal function may lead to renal failure

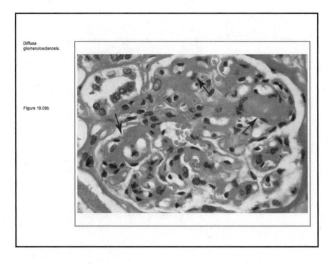

Diffuse glomerulosclerosis.

Figure 19.09b

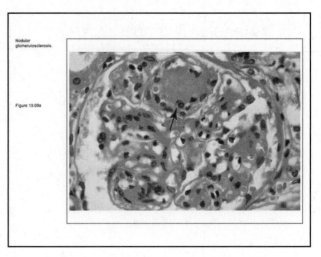

Nodular glomerulosclerosis.

Figure 19.09a

Gout Nephropathy

- Pathogenesis
  - Elevated blood uric acid levels lead to ↑ uric acid in tubular filtrate
  - Urate may precipitate in Henle's loops and collecting tubules
  - Tubular obstruction causes damage
- Manifestations
  - Impaired renal function
  - May lead to renal failure
  - Common in poorly-controlled gout

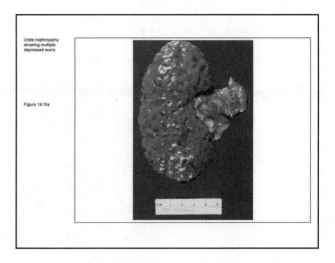

Urate nephropathy showing multiple depressed scars.

Figure 19.10a

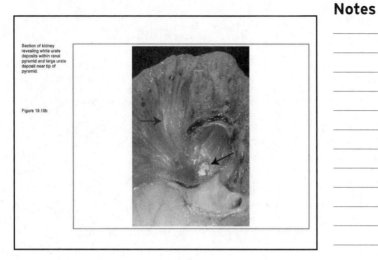

Section of kidney revealing white urate deposits within renal pyramid and large urate deposit near tip of pyramid.

Figure 19.10b

Urinary Tract Infections (1 of 2)

- Very common; maybe acute or chronic
- Most infections are caused by gram-negative bacteria
- Organisms contaminate perianal and genital areas and ascend urethra
- Conditions protective against infection
  - Free urine flow
  - Large urine volume
  - Complete bladder emptying
  - Acid urine: most bacteria grow poorly in an acidic environment

Urinary Tract Infections (2 of 2)

- Predisposing factors
  - Any condition that impairs free drainage of urine
  - Stagnation of urine favors bacterial growth
  - Injury to mucosa by kidney stone disrupts protective epithelium allowing bacteria to invade deeper tissue
  - Introduction of catheter or instruments into bladder may carry bacteria

Cystitis

- Affects only the bladder
  - More common in women than men; shorter female urethra, and, in young sexually active women, sexual intercourse promotes transfer of bacteria from urethra to bladder
  - Common in older men, because enlarged prostate interferes with complete bladder emptying
- Clinical manifestations
  - Burning pain on urination
  - Desire to urinate frequently
  - Urine contains many bacteria and leukocytes
  - Responds well to antibiotics
  - May spread upward into renal pelvis and kidneys

Pyelonephritis

- Involvement of upper urinary tract from
  - Ascending infection from the bladder (ascending pyelonephritis)
  - Carried to the kidneys from the bloodstream (hematogenous pyelonephritis)
- Clinical manifestations: similar with an acute infection
  - Localized pain and tenderness over affected kidney
  - Responds well to antibiotics
  - Cystitis and pyelonephritis are frequently associated
  - Some cases become chronic and lead to kidney failure

Vesicoureteral Reflux

- Urine normally prevented from flowing back into the ureters during urination
- Failure of mechanisms allows bladder urine to reflux into ureter during voiding
  - Predisposes to urinary tract infection
  - Predisposes to pyelonephritis

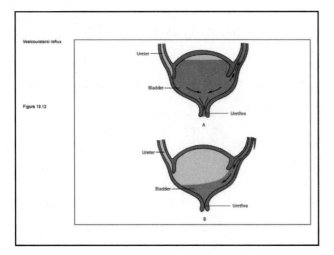

Vesicoureteral reflux.

Figure 19.12

Ureter
Bladder
Urethra
A

Ureter
Bladder
Urethra
B

Urinary Calculi (1 of 3)

- Stones may form anywhere in the urinary tract
- Predisposing factors
  - High concentration of salts in urine saturates urine causing salts to precipitate and form calculi
    - Uric acid in gout
    - Calcium salts in hyperparathyroidism
  - Urinary tract infections reduce solubility of salts in urine; clusters of bacteria are sites where urinary salts may crystallize to form stone
  - Urinary tract obstruction causes urine stagnation, promotes stasis and infection, further increasing stone formation

Urinary Calculi (2 of 3)

- Staghorn calculus: urinary stones that increase in size to form large branching structures that adopt to the contour of the pelvis and calyces
- Small stones may pass through ureters causing renal colic
- Some become impacted in the ureter and need to be removed
- Manifestations
  - Renal colic associated with passage of stone
  - Obstruction of urinary tract causes hydronephrosis-hydroureter proximal to obstruction

Urinary Calculi (3 of 3)

- Treatment
  - Cystoscopy: snares and removes stones lodged in distal ureter
  - Shock wave lithotripsy: stones lodged in proximal ureter are broken into fragments that are readily excreted

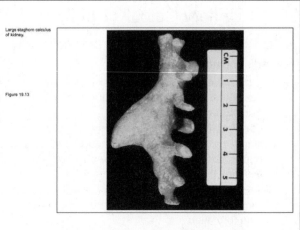

Large staghorn calculus of kidney.

Figure 19.13

Urinary Obstruction

- Blockage of urine outflow leads to progressive dilatation of urinary tract proximal to obstruction, eventually causes compression atrophy of kidneys
- Manifestations
  - Hydroureter: dilatation of ureter
  - Hydronephrosis: dilatation of pelvis and calyces
- Causes
  - Bilateral: obstruction of bladder neck by enlarged prostate or urethral stricture
  - Unilateral: ureteral stricture, calculus, tumor
- Complications: stone formation; infections
- Diagnosis and treatment: pyelogram, CT san

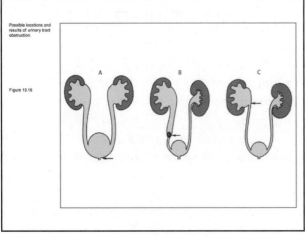

Possible locations and results of urinary tract obstruction.

Figure 19.16

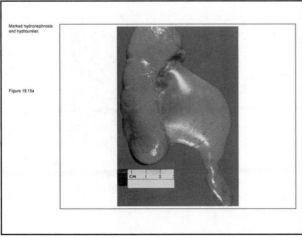

Marked hydronephrosis and hydroureter.

Figure 19.15a

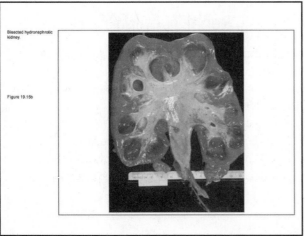

Bisected hydronephrotic kidney.

Figure 19.15b

Foreign Bodies in Urinary Tract

- Usually inserted by patient
- May injure bladder
- Predispose to infection
- Treatment
  - Usually removed by cystoscopy
  - Occasionally necessary to open bladder surgically

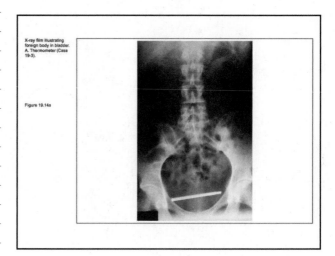

X-ray film illustrating foreign body in bladder. A. Thermometer (Case 19-3).

Figure 19.14a

Renal Tubular Injury

- Pathogenesis
  - Impaired renal blood flow
  - Tubular necrosis caused by toxic drugs or chemicals
- Clinical manifestation
  - Acute renal failure: oliguria, anuria
  - Tubular function gradually recovers
  - Treated by dialysis until function returns

Renal Cysts

- Solitary cysts common; not associated with impairment of renal function
- Multiple cysts
  - Congenital polycystic kidney disease
  - Most common cause of multiple cysts
  - Mendelian dominant transmission
  - Cysts enlarge and destroy renal tissue and function
  - Onset of renal failure by late middle age
  - Suspected by physical examination that reveals greatly enlarged kidneys
  - Some form cysts in liver or cerebral aneurysm

Renal Tumors

- Cortical tumors: arise from epithelium of renal tubules
  - Adenomas: usually small and asymptomatic
  - Carcinomas more common
  - Hematuria often first manifestation
  - Invades renal vein and metastasizes into bloodstream
  - Treated by nephrectomy
- Transitional cell tumor: Arise from transitional epithelium lining urinary tract
  - Most arise from bladder epithelium
  - Hematuria: common first manifestation
  - Low grade malignancy; good prognosis

Nephroblastoma (Wilms Tumor)

- Uncommon; highly malignant; affects infants and children
- Diagnosis
  - Urinalysis
  - Urine culture and sensitivity tests
  - Blood chemistry tests
  - Clearance tests
  - X-ray, ultrasound, cystoscopy
  - Renal biopsy
- Treatment: nephrectomy; radiotherapy; chemotherapy

Notes

Renal Failure (Uremia) (1 of 2)

- Retention of excessive byproducts of protein metabolism in the blood
- Acute renal failure
  - Causes: tubular necrosis from impaired blood flow to kidneys or effects of toxic drugs
  - Renal function usually returns
- Chronic renal failure
  - From progressive, chronic kidney disease; > 50% from chronic glomerulonephritis
  - Others include congenital polycystic kidney disease, nephrosclerosis, diabetic nephropathy

Renal Failure (Uremia) (2 of 2)

- Clinical manifestations
  - Weakness, loss of appetite, nausea, vomiting
  - Anemia
  - Toxic manifestations from retained waste products
  - Edema: retention of salt and water
  - Hypertension
- Treatment
  - Hemodialysis
  - Hypertension

Hemodialysis

- Substitutes for the functions of the kidneys by removing waste products from patient's blood
- Waste products in patient's blood diffuse across a semipermeable membrane into a solution (dialysate) into the other side of the membrane
- Two types
  - Extracorporeal dialysis (more common): patient's circulation connected to an artificial kidney machine
  - Peritoneal dialysis (less common): patient's own peritoneum is used as the dialyzing membrane

Renal Transplantation (1 of 2)

- Attempted when kidneys fail
- Kidney is from a close relative donor or cadaver
- Survival of transplant depends on similarity of HLA antigens between donor and recipient
  - Only identical twins have identical HLA antigens in their tissues; others invariably contain foreign HLA antigens
  - Consequently, patient's immunologic defenses will respond to the foreign antigens and attempt to destroy (reject) foreign kidney

Renal Transplantation (2 of 2)

- Patient's immune system must be suppressed by drugs
- Kidney is placed in the iliac area, outside the peritoneal cavity
- Prognosis
  - >90% of transplanted kidneys survive for 5 years when donor's HLA antigens resemble the patient's
  - Survival rate of cadaver transplants has improved in recent years

Discussion

- 6-year-old boy complained of abdominal discomfort. His mother noted that his face, abdomen, scrotum, and legs were edematous. His urine has large amounts of protein and a few casts. His serum albumin and serum protein were much lower than normal.
  - What is the boy most likely suffering from?
  - Explain the generalized edema in this boy.

Notes

_____
_____
_____
_____
_____
_____
_____
_____

Discussion

- How does diabetes affect the kidneys? What are the clinical manifestations in such case?
- What is the difference between acute and chronic renal failure in terms of causes, clinical manifestations, and treatment?
- What is the relationship between glomerulonephritis and beta-streptococcal infection?

_____
_____
_____
_____
_____
_____
_____
_____
_____
_____
_____
_____
_____
_____
_____
_____
_____
_____
_____
_____
_____
_____
_____
_____
_____
_____
_____
_____
_____
_____
_____
_____
_____

Chapter Outline

The chapter outline provides you with an organizational guide to the topics and ideas presented in this chapter of the text.

Study Questions

The following questions are provided as a test for comprehension and as a study guide for use with the text chapters. Additional study material is located at http://health.jbpub.com/humandisease/8e, which contains useful tools such as an A&P review, animated flashcards, an interactive online glossary, crossword puzzles, and web links.

Key Terms

Define the following terms:

1. Seminoma _____

2. Prostate-specific antigen _____

Fill-in-the-Blank

1. The infectious agents that are the two main causes of acute urethritis acquired by sexual contact are _____ and _____. These infections are treated by _____.

2. Benign prostatic hyperplasia (BPH) is a common problem in older men. It produces symptoms of _____, resulting from compression of the _____ by the nodules of enlarged prostatic tissue.

3. There are many ways to treat BPH. The surgical procedure is called _____.

4. Prostatic epithelial cells secrete a protein called _____, which also can be detected in the bloodstream. Higher than normal levels are detected in the bloodstream of man with a disease called _____.

5. Testicular carcinomas are uncommon tumors. Many of these tumors produce a hormone called _____ and a protein antigen called _____.

6. Testicular malignant tumors that are composed of many different types of immature tissues are called

   _____.

7. Carcinoma of the penis is an uncommon tumor that almost never occurs in circumcised men. The agent responsible for the carcinoma is _____.

8. The fibrous cord that guides the testis into the scrotum is called the _____.

9. Failure of the proximal end of the tunica vaginalis to close after the testis has entered the scrotum may be complicated by a condition called a/an _____.

True/False

Tell whether each statement is true or false. If false, explain why the statement is incorrect.

1. Most prostate carcinomas arise from the inner group of prostatic glands surrounding the prostatic urethra. _____

   _____

2. Prostate-specific antigen is secreted by prostatic epithelial cells. _____

   _____

3. Most prostate carcinomas are very poorly differentiated, grow rapidly, and have a very poor prognosis. _____

   _____

Matching

Match the disease or condition in the left column with its characteristic features in the right column.

1. _____ Cryptorchidism
2. _____ Hydrocele
3. _____ Varicocele
4. _____ Testicular torsion
5. _____ Prostate hyperplasia

A. Dilated spermatic cord veins
B. Twisted spermatic cord
C. Overgrowth of prostatic tissue
D. Undescended testis
E. Excess fluid in tunica vaginalis

Discussion Questions

1. What are the components of the male reproductive system? _____

_____

_____

_____

2. What methods are available to detect carcinoma of the prostate? _____

_____

_____

_____

3. How is carcinoma of the prostate treated? _____

_____

_____

_____

4. Why do many physicians recommend conservative treatment of prostatic carcinoma in older men with well-differentiated tumors? _____

_____

_____

_____

Notes

Chapter 20

The Male Reproductive System

Learning Objectives

- Differentiate benign prostatic hyperplasia and prostatic carcinoma as to clinical manifestations and methods of treatment
- Describe three most common types of testicular cancer, manifestations, and methods of treatment
- List anatomic structures, functions, and diseases of the male reproductive system

Anatomy

- Components of the male reproductive system
- Penis
- Prostate
- Accessory glands
- Testes
- Duct system to transport sperm from testes to urethra
  - Starts at epididymis
  - Continues on as vasa deferentia
  - Vasa deferentia extend upward in spermatic cords
  - Enter prostatic urethra as ejaculatory ducts
  - Urethra divided into long penile urethra and a short segment traversing the prostate (prostatic urethra)

Notes

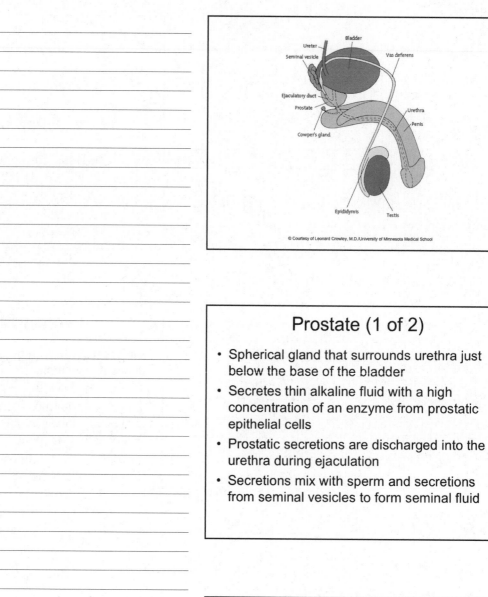

© Courtesy of Leonard Crowley, M.D./University of Minnesota Medical School

Prostate (1 of 2)

- Spherical gland that surrounds urethra just below the base of the bladder
- Secretes thin alkaline fluid with a high concentration of an enzyme from prostatic epithelial cells
- Prostatic secretions are discharged into the urethra during ejaculation
- Secretions mix with sperm and secretions from seminal vesicles to form seminal fluid

Prostate (2 of 2)

- Composed of numerous branched glands intermixed with masses of smooth muscle and fibrous tissue
- Inner group of glands
  - Surround urethra as it passes through the prostate
  - May give rise to benign hyperplasia
- Outer or main group of glands
  - Makes up bulk of prostatic glandular tissue
  - May give rise to prostatic carcinoma

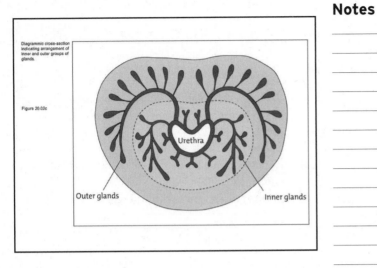

Diagrammic cross-section indicating arrangement of inner and outer groups of glands.

Figure 20.02c

Urethra

Outer glands

Inner glands

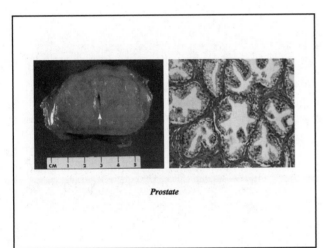

Prostate

Benign Prostatic Hyperplasia (1 of 2)

- Moderate enlargement of the prostate gland is relatively common in elderly men
- Usually **involves inner group of glands** surrounding the urethra
- Obstructs the outflow of urine
- Enlargement is significant if it obstructs neck of the bladder, leading to incomplete emptying, or causes complete urinary tract obstruction

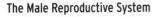

Benign Prostatic Hyperplasia (2 of 2)

- Complications
  - Cystitis: inflammation of urinary bladder
  - Pyelonephritis: inflammation of kidneys and pelvis
  - Calculi formation: stones
  - Hydronephrosis: distention of renal pelvis and calyces with urine due to obstruction
- Gold standard: transurethral resection

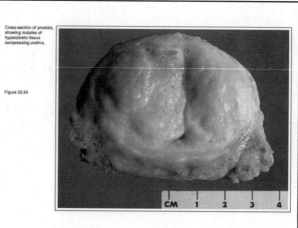

Cross-section of prostate, showing nodules of hyperplastic tissue compressing urethra.

Figure 20.04

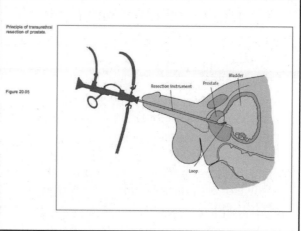

Principle of transurethral resection of prostate.

Figure 20.05

Prostatitis

- Acute
  - Acute inflammation of the prostate
    - Spread of infection from bladder or urethra
    - May be secondary to gonococcal infection of posterior urethra
- Chronic
  - Mild inflammation
  - Common
  - Causes few symptoms

Gonorrhea and Chlamydia

- A common sexually transmitted disease
  - Initially, acute inflammation of anterior urethra
  - Inflammation may spread to posterior urethra and transport ducts
  - May also cause an acute inflammation of the rectal mucosa
  - Obstruction of vasa may block sperm transport and cause sterility
- Nongonococcal urethritis
  - Caused by *Chlamydia*
  - Causes an acute urethritis
  - Clinically very similar to gonorrhea

Carcinoma of the Prostate (1 of 3)

- Usually originates in outer group of glands of the prostate
- Manifestations
  - Common in elderly men; early case may be asymptomatic
  - Urinary obstruction from encroachment of bladder neck
  - Infiltration of tissues surrounding prostate
- Metastasizes to bones of spine and pelvis
- Acid phosphatase: secreted by normal prostatic cells and tumor cells; leaks into bloodstream; high levels in prostate cancer

Notes

Carcinoma of the Prostate (2 of 3)

- Prostate-specific antigen, PSA
  - Secreted by prostatic epithelial cells
  - Not specific for prostate cancer
  - Also elevated in prostatic hyperplasia and other benign prostatic diseases
- Tumor grows slowly; may take ≥ 10 before it obstructs bladder or metastasizes to the bones
- Diagnosis
  - Digital rectal exam: irregularity or nodularity
  - PSA or acid phosphatase test
  - Biopsy
  - Ultrasound

Carcinoma of the Prostate (3 of 3)

- Surgery
- Radical prostatectomy and radiation: seems to improve survival; controversy on effectiveness in elderly men
- Radical prostatectomy
  - For small, localized tumor; may cause impotence due to disruption of nerve supply to penis
- If with metastasis:
  - Surgical removal of testes to eliminate source of testosterone that stimulates tumor growth
  - May administer estrogen
  - Drugs that suppress gonadotropic hormones to inhibit testicular testosterone secretion

Cryptorchidism (1 of 2)

- Testis does not descend normally into scrotum
  - Usually retained in abdominal cavity; sometimes in inguinal canal
  - Germ cells require a temperature lower than the normal body temperature
  - Interstitial cells function normally at body temperature
- Manifestations
  - Germ cells are destroyed at higher intra-abdominal temperature
  - Interstitial cells of Leydig function normally and produce testosterone
  - Undescended testis more prone to developing testicular cancer; treat by surgically replacing testis in scrotum

Cryptorchidism (2 of 2)

- In some newborns, testes may not have descended yet into scrotum but usually descend within 6 months after birth
- If descent has not occurred by 12 months, an ectopic testis that is not in the scrotum should be surgically brought into the scrotum

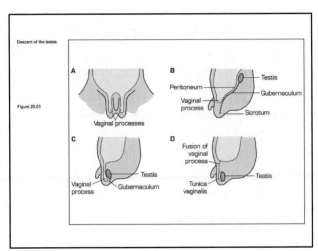

Descent of the testes.

Figure 20.03

A

Vaginal processes

B
Peritoneum — Testis
Vaginal process — Gubernaculum
— Scrotum

C
Vaginal process — Testis
— Gubernaculum

D
Fusion of vaginal process — Testis
Tunica vaginalis

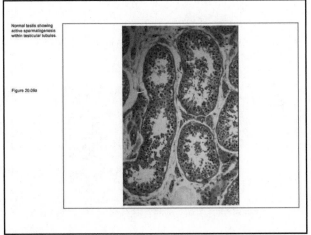

Normal testis showing active spermatogenesis within testicular tubules.

Figure 20.09a

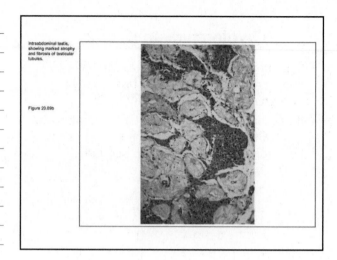

Intraabdominal testis, showing marked atrophy and fibrosis of testicular tubules.

Figure 20.09b

Testicular Torsion

- Abnormal attachment of testis in scrotum
  - Predisposes to rotary twisting of testis and spermatic cord within scrotum
  - Shuts blood supply to testes
- Manifestations and treatment
  - Acute onset of testicular pain and swelling
  - Leads to hemorrhagic infarction unless promptly untwisted
- Surgery
  - Untwist the torsion, firmly anchor affected testis within scrotum
  - Other testis also anchored in scrotum to prevent possible torsion

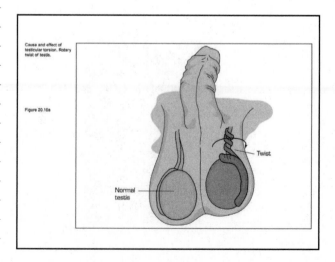

Cause and effect of testicular torsion. Rotary twist of testis.

Figure 20.10a

Twist

Normal testis

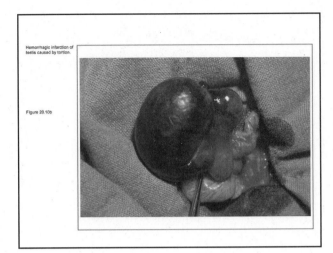

Hemorrhagic infarction of testis caused by tortion.

Figure 20.10b

Scrotal Abnormalities

- Hydrocele
  - Excess fluid accumulates in tunica vaginalis
  - Treated by aspiration or resection of tunica vaginalis
- Varicocele
  - Varicose veins in spermatic cord
  - Usually involves left side of scrotum
  - May impair fertility
  - Treatment required only if varicocele causes discomfort or impairs infertility

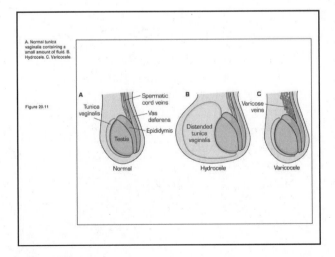

A. Normal tunica vaginalis containing a small amount of fluid. B. Hydrocele. C. Varicocele.

Figure 20.11

A — Spermatic cord veins / Tunica vaginalis / Vas deferens / Epididymis / Testis — Normal

B — Distended tunica vaginalis — Hydrocele

C — Varicose veins — Varicocele

Notes

Penis

- Consists of 3 cavernous bodies or cylinders of extremely vascular erectile tissue
  - Two lateral: corpora cavernosa
  - Midline: corpora spongiosum that surrounds penile urethra
  - Surrounded by thick fibrous connective tissue capsule (spongy meshwork of endothelium-lined blood sinuses)
  - Supported by connective tissue and smooth muscle

Erectile Dysfunction (1 of 2)

- Inability to achieve and maintain a penile erection
- Common problem and frequency increases with age
- Causes
  - Low testosterone level inhibits sexual desire and arousal
  - Damage to nerves supplying penis (prostate surgery; neurologic disease)
  - Impaired blood supply to penis: arteriosclerosis, diabetes
  - Certain anti-hypertensive drugs that target autonomic nervous system
  - Stress, emotional factors, chronic diseases

Erectile Dysfunction (2 of 2)

- Treatment: depends on cause of dysfunction
  - Use of drugs that inhibit phosphodiesterase to promote blood flow to penis
- Examples:
  - Sildenafil (Viagra)
  - Vardenafil (Levitra)
  - Tadenafil (Cialis)
- Differ in duration of action

Physiology of Penile Erection
(1 of 3)

- Complex process
- Factors
  - Sexual desire: initiates physiologic events that increase blood flow to penis
  - Arteries supplying cavernous bodies must dilate to deliver a large volume of blood to penis
  - Pressure of blood in cavernous bodies must be high to compress draining veins
  - Blood must flow into penis faster than it drains out or erection cannot be maintained

Physiology of Penile Erection
(2 of 3)

- Penile arteries are normally constricted
  - Little blood flows into cavernous bodies
  - Vascular sinuses are collapsed
- In sexual arousal
  - Parasympathetic nerve impulses from sacral part of spinal cord cause release nitric oxide
  - Nitric oxide causes relaxation of smooth muscle walls of penile arteries and trabeculae
  - Penile arteries dilate and sinuses in cavernous bodies expand

Physiology of Penile Erection
(3 of 3)

- In sexual arousal
  - Blood pours under high pressure into the sinuses
  - Increased blood pressure compresses veins retarding outflow of blood from penis
  - Engorgement of sinuses with results in rigidity and erection

Carcinoma of the Testis

- Seminoma: malignant neoplasm of semen-producing epithelium
- Malignant teratoma: composed of several types of malignant tissues
- Choriocarcinoma: arises from trophoblastic tissues in the uterus
- Treatment:
  - Resection of testicle and associated structures
  - Chemotherapy
- Methods for monitoring response to therapy
  - Chorionic gonadotropin (HCG) test
  - Alpha fetoprotein (AFP) test

Carcinoma of the Penis

- Rare in circumcised males
- Secretions accumulating under foreskin may be carcinogenic
- Papilloma virus may play role
- Treatment: partial or complete amputation of penis; removal of inguinal lymph nodes

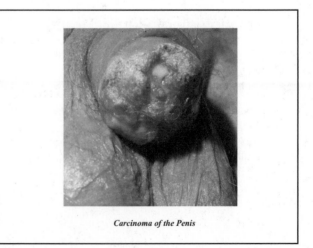

Carcinoma of the Penis

Discussion

- A young man has undescended testis within the abdomen. How does this affect testicular function? What are the likely complications?
- The following statements are true of benign prostatic hyperplasia EXCEPT:
  - A. A precancerous condition
  - B. Causes incomplete emptying of the bladder
  - C. Involves the inner group of glands of the prostate
  - D. Hyperplasia is secondary to the response to dihydrotestosterone
  - D. Obstructing prostatic tissue may be surgically removed

Notes

Chapter Outline

The chapter outline provides you with an organizational guide to the topics and ideas presented in this chapter of the text.

Structure and Function of the Liver
Bile
    Formation and Excretion
    Composition and Properties
Causes and Effects of Liver Injury
Viral Hepatitis
    Clinical Manifestations and Course
    Hepatitis A
    Hepatitis B
    Hepatitis C
    Hepatitis D (Delta Hepatitis)
    Hepatitis E
    Other Hepatitis Viruses
    Hepatitis Among Male Homosexuals
Fatty Liver
Alcoholic Liver Disease
Cirrhosis of the Liver
    Derangements of Liver Structure and Function
    Procedures to Treat Manifestations of Cirrhosis
    Biliary Cirrhosis
Reye's Syndrome
Cholelithiasis
    Factors Affecting the Solubility of Cholesterol in Bile
    Complications of Gallstones
    Treatment of Gallstones
Cholecystitis
Tumors of the Liver and Gallbladder
Jaundice
    Hemolytic Jaundice
    Hepatocellular Jaundice
    Obstructive Jaundice
Biopsy of the Liver

Study Questions

The following questions are provided as a test for comprehension and as a study guide for use with the text chapters. Additional study material is located at http://health.jbpub.com/humandisease/8e, which contains useful tools such as an A&P review, animated flashcards, an interactive online glossary, crossword puzzles, and web links.

Key Terms

Define the following terms:

1. Hepatitis _____

2. Bilirubin _____

3. Bile _____

4. Jaundice _____

Fill-in-the-Blank

1. The iron-free pigment derived from breakdown of hemoglobin is called _____.

2. The substance present in bile that may precipitate within the bile to form gallstones is _____.

3. Some persons may have chronic hepatitis but show no symptoms of infection. This condition is called

   _____.

4. The antigen present in the blood of persons infected with hepatitis B is _____.

5. The most frequent cause of chronic hepatitis in the United States is _____.

6. Approximately _____ percent of persons infected with HCV are unable to eliminate the virus and become chronic carriers of the virus.

7. Persons with chronic hepatitis are at risk of two major complications, which are _____

   _____ and _____.

8. The two most common causes of cirrhosis are _____ and _____.

9. Two common causes of obstructive biliary cirrhosis are _____ and _____.

10. A child with a viral infection and a fever is given acetaminophen (Tylenol) rather than aspirin to control the fever to avoid the risk of a liver and central nervous system disease called _____.

11. Most gallstones are composed of _____.

True/False

Tell whether each statement is true or false. If false, explain why the statement is incorrect.

1. The infectious particle in the blood of persons with HBV infection is hepatitis B surface antigen. _____

   _____

2. Most HCV-infected persons are unable to eradicate the virus and become chronic carriers of the virus. _____

   _____

3. Many HCV-infected persons are asymptomatic. _____

_____

4. Chronic HCV infection is caused by ingestion of virus-contaminated food or water. _____

_____

5. Primary biliary cirrhosis is caused by chronic HCV infection. _____

_____

6. Primary biliary cirrhosis is an autoimmune disease in which the autoantibody is directed against bile duct epithelial cells. _____

_____

7. Secondary biliary cirrhosis is caused by longstanding obstruction of large extrahepatic bile ducts. _____

_____

Identify

1. Construct a table comparing the major features of the three main types of hepatitis. (*Hint:* see Table 21-1.)

Characteristic	*Hepatitis A*	*Hepatitis B*	*Hepatitis C*

2. Alcoholic liver disease can be divided into three states of progressively increasing severity:

a. _____

b. _____

c. _____

Discussion Questions

1. What are some of the main functions of the liver? _____

_____

_____

_____

2. How does the blood supply to the liver differ from the blood supply to other organs? _____

_____

_____

_____

3. Why does severe liver disease cause disturbances in blood clotting? _____

_____

_____

_____

4. What is the difference between hemoglobin and bilirubin? How does conjugated bilirubin differ from unconjugated bilirubin? _____

_____

_____

_____

5. What is the difference between bilirubin and bile? What role does bile play in digestion? _____

_____

_____

_____

6. Describe the major structural changes and physiological derangements in patients with cirrhosis. What conditions are associated with cirrhosis? _____

_____

_____

_____

7. Why is the pressure in the portal vein elevated in patients with cirrhosis? _____

_____

_____

_____

8. Why do patients with cirrhosis often accumulate a fluid within their peritoneal cavity that is called ascites?

_____

_____

_____

9. Why do patients with cirrhosis often develop varicose veins in their esophagus? _____

_____

_____

_____

10. In patients with cirrhosis, laboratory tests that measure the amounts of proteins concerned with the coagulation of the blood are frequently abnormal. Why? _____

_____

_____

_____

11. What is jaundice? How is jaundice classified? Under what circumstances do gallstones cause jaundice? _____

_____

_____

_____

12. What is hepatitis B virus (HBV) infection? How is it transmitted? What populations are at risk? How can it be prevented? _____

_____

_____

_____

13. What is fatty liver? With what other conditions is it associated? _____

_____

_____

_____

14. What is cholelithiasis? With what other conditions is it associated? _____

_____

_____

_____

15. What conditions may lead to hepatic cirrhosis? _____

_____

_____

_____

Notes

_____

_____

_____

_____

_____

_____

_____

_____

_____

_____

_____

_____

_____

_____

_____

_____

_____

_____

_____

_____

_____

_____

_____

_____

_____

_____

_____

_____

_____

_____

_____

_____

_____

_____

_____

_____

_____

Chapter 21

The Liver and the Biliary System

Learning Objectives

- Describe normal structure and functions of the liver in relation to the major diseases of the liver
- Describe causes of liver injury and the effects on hepatic function
- Differentiate three major types of viral hepatitis (pathogenesis, incubation period, incidence of complications, frequency of carriers, diagnostic tests)
- Explain adverse effects of alcohol intake on liver structure, function
- Explain formation of gallstones, causes and effects
- Compare three major causes of jaundice

The Liver (1 of 2)

- Largest organ in body, right upper abdominal area, beneath the diaphragm
- Main functions
  - 1. Metabolism: carbohydrates, protein, and fat delivered through the portal circulation
  - 2. Synthesis: plasma proteins, clotting factors
  - 3. Storage: vitamin B12 and other materials
  - 4. Detoxification and excretion: various substances

Notes

_____
_____
_____
_____
_____
_____
_____
_____
_____
_____
_____
_____
_____
_____
_____
_____
_____
_____
_____
_____
_____
_____
_____
_____
_____
_____
_____
_____
_____
_____
_____
_____
_____
_____
_____

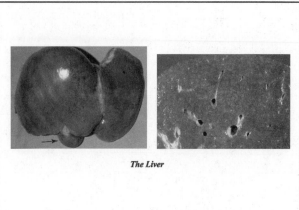

The Liver

The Liver (2 of 2)

- Has a double blood supply
  - Portal vein: 75% of blood, drains spleen and GI tract, rich in nutrients absorbed from intestines, low in oxygen
  - Hepatic artery: rest of blood, high in oxygen, low in nutrients
  - Both blood mix in the liver eventually collecting into right and left hepatic veins that drain into inferior vena cava
- Portal triad, portal tracts travel together
  - Hepatic artery branches
  - Portal vein
  - Bile ducts
  - Lymphatic vessels

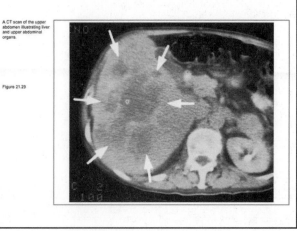

A CT scan of the upper abdomen illustrating liver and upper abdominal organs.

Figure 21.29

Bile (1 of 2)

- From the breakdown of red blood cells
- When red blood cells break down, iron is reused and iron-free heme pigment or bilirubin is excreted in the bile
- Small quantities of bile are continually present in blood
- When blood passes through liver, bilirubin is removed by conjugation or by combining bilirubin with glucuronic acid
- Bile: aqueous solution with various dissolved substances
  - 1. Conjugated bilirubin
  - 2. Bile salts: major constituent of bile; derivatives of cholesterol and amino acids; emulsify fat; function as detergents

Bile (2 of 2)

- Other substances present in bile
  - Lecithin: lipid that also functions as a detergent
  - Cholesterol
  - Water
  - Minerals
- Bile is secreted continually
  - Concentrated and stored in gallbladder
  - During digestion, gallbladder contracts, releasing bile into the duodenum
  - Bile does not contain digestive enzymes, but acts as a biologic detergent

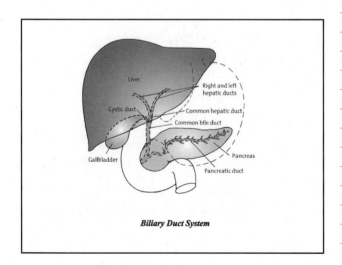

Biliary Duct System

Notes

Types of Liver Injury

- Manifestations
  - Cell necrosis
  - Fatty change
  - Mixed necrosis and fatty change
- Common types of liver injury
  - Viral hepatitis
  - Fatty liver
  - Alcoholic liver disease or alcoholic hepatitis
  - Cirrhosis

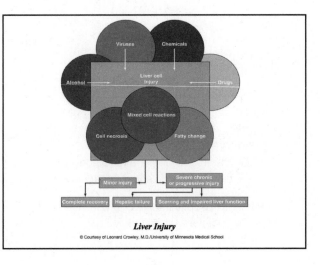

Liver Injury

© Courtesy of Leonard Crowley, M.D./University of Minnesota Medical School

Hepatitis A

- RNA-containing virus
- Incubation period: 2 to 6 weeks
- Excreted through nose, throat, stools
- Transmission
  - Person-to-person contact
  - Fecal contamination of food or water
- Self-limited; no carriers; no chronic liver disease
- Prevention
  - Hepatitis A vaccine
  - Hepatitis A immune globulin: given after exposure

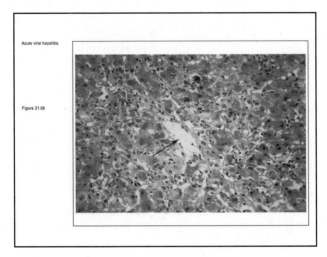

Acute viral hepatitis.

Figure 21.06

Hepatitis B

- DNA-containing virus
- Incubation period: 6 weeks to 4 months
- Transmission: blood or body fluids
- Diagnosis: antigen-antibody test results
  - Infected persons: HBsAg positive; lack anti-HBs
  - Immune persons: presence of anti-HBs
  - 10% become carriers and may develop chronic liver disease
- Prevention
  - Hepatitis B vaccine
  - Hepatitis B immune globulin: given after exposure

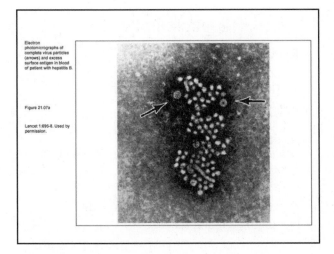

Electron photomicrographs of complete virus particles (arrows) and excess surface antigen in blood of patient with hepatitis B.

Figure 21.07a

Lancet 1:695-8. Used by permission.

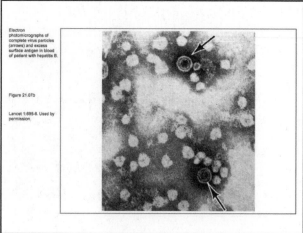

Electron photomicrographs of complete virus particles (arrows) and excess surface antigen in blood of patient with hepatitis B.

Figure 21.07b

Lancet 1:695-8. Used by permission.

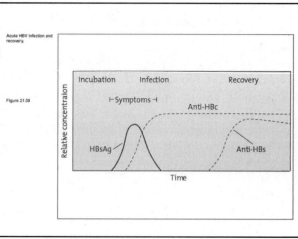

Acute HBV infection and recovery.

Figure 21.08

Hepatitis C (1 of 2)

- RNA virus
- Incubation period: 3 to 12 weeks
- Transmission: blood and body fluids
- Antigen-antibody test results
  - HCV RNA: presence of virus in blood and active infection
  - Anti-HCV: infection but does not confer immunity
- 75% become carriers and many develop chronic liver disease
- No prevention of disease after exposure
- No immunization available

Hepatitis C (2 of 2)

- Testing for asymptomatic HCV infection
- Recommendations
  - 1. Persons who have injected illegal drugs
  - 2. Persons who received antihemophilic globulin or other clotting factor concentrates before 1987
  - 3. Persons who received blood transfusions before 1992
  - 4. Health care personnel who have been exposed to blood or body fluids

Hepatitis D: Delta Hepatitis

- Small, defective RNA virus
- **Only infects persons with acute or chronic HBV infection**
- Delta virus is unable to produce its own virus coat and uses HBsAg produced by HBV
- Most U.S. cases from sharing needles

Hepatitis E

- RNA-containing virus
- Transmission
  - Oral-fecal
  - Contaminated water
- No prevention of disease after exposure
- No immunization available

Notes

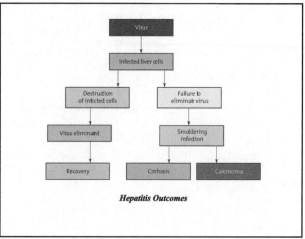

Hepatitis Outcomes

Fatty Liver

- Fat accumulates in liver secondary to injury
- Common in heavy drinkers and alcoholics
- May be caused by chemicals and solvents
- Impaired liver function but injury is still reversible

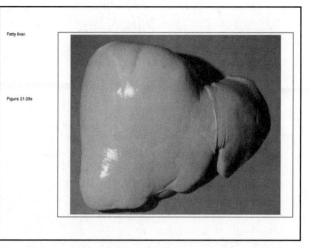

Fatty liver.

Figure 21.09a

Alcoholic Liver Disease

- Refers to a group of structural and functional changes in the liver resulting from excessive alcohol consumption
- Severity depends on amount and duration of alcohol consumption
- 3 stages of progression
  - 1. Alcoholic fatty liver: mildest form
  - 2. Alcoholic hepatitis: causes degenerative changes and necrosis of liver cells
  - 3. Alcoholic cirrhosis: most advanced, diffuse scarring, disturbed liver function

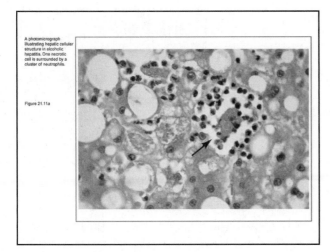

A photomicrograph illustrating hepatic cellular structure in alcoholic hepatitis. One necrotic cell is surrounded by a cluster of neutrophils.

Figure 21.11a

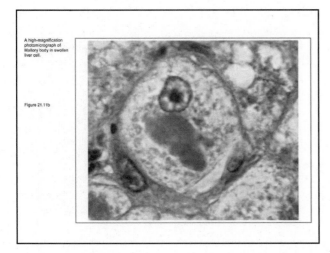

A high-magnification photomicrograph of Mallory body in swollen liver cell.

Figure 21.11b

Cirrhosis (1 of 3)

- Diffuse scarring of the liver from any cause with derangement of liver function and regeneration
  - Alcoholic liver disease
  - Chronic hepatitis
  - Severe liver necrosis
  - Repeated liver injury: drugs and chemicals
  - Longstanding bile duct obstruction
- Manifestations
  - Liver failure
  - Portal hypertension
  - Ascites, collateral circulation formation

Cirrhosis (2 of 3)

- Manifestations
  - Bypass routes connect systemic-portal venous systems
  - Anastomoses develop between branches of portal and system veins
  - Blood shunted away from high pressure portal system into low pressure veins of systemic circulation
    - Esophageal veins become distended
    - Risk of fatal hemorrhage from esophageal varices
  - Inability to inactivate estrogen in males
    - Testicular atrophy, loss of sex drive, breast hypertrophy

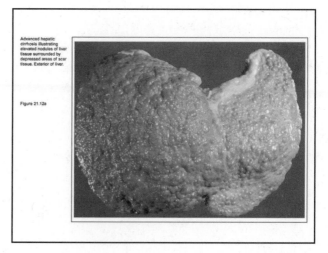

Advanced hepatic cirrhosis illustrating elevated nodules of liver tissue surrounded by depressed areas of scar tissue. Exterior of liver.

Figure 21.12a

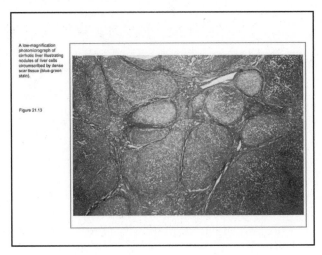

A low-magnification photomicrograph of cirrhotic liver illustrating nodules of liver cells circumscribed by dense scar tissue (blue-green stain).

Figure 21.13

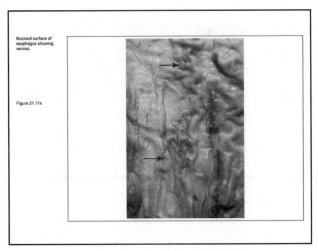

Mucosal surface of esophagus showing varices.

Figure 21.17a

Cirrhosis (3 of 3)

- Surgical procedures
  - Portal-systemic anastomoses to control varices
    - Splenorenal shunt
    - Portacaval shunt
    - Intrahepatic portosystemic shunt
  - Transjugular intrahepatic portosystemic shunt (TIPS)
    - An alternative to an open operative procedure
    - Intrahepatic shunt between hepatic and portal vein branches
- Materials in ascitic fluid may cause intravascular coagulation syndrome, other complications

Notes

Notes

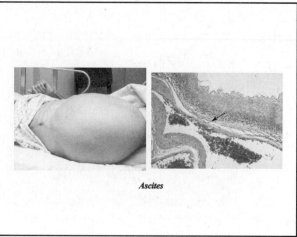

Ascites

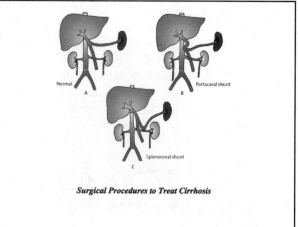

Surgical Procedures to Treat Cirrhosis

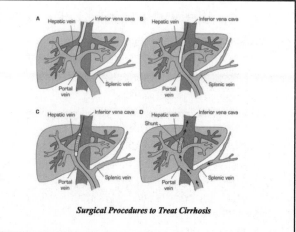

Surgical Procedures to Treat Cirrhosis

Chapter 21

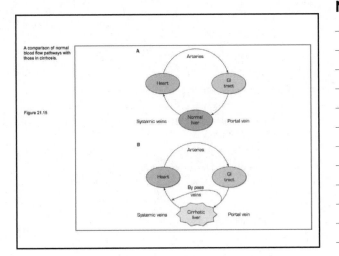

A comparison of normal blood flow pathways with those in cirrhosis.

Figure 21.15

Hepatic Encephalopathy

- Deterioration of brain function characterized by impaired consciousness, confusion, disorientation, and eventually coma
  - From accumulation of toxic substances in the blood that are normally detoxified and excreted by the liver
  - Toxic products include ammonia from deamination of amino acids and bacterial decomposition products of colonic fecal material
- Precipitating events
  - Conditions that reduce hepatic blood flow or liver cell functions

Biliary Cirrhosis

- Primary biliary cirrhosis
  - Autoimmune disease attacking small intrahepatic bile ducts
  - No specific treatment, may lead to liver failure
  - Require liver transplant
- Secondary biliary cirrhosis
  - Obstruction of large extrahepatic bile ducts
    - Gallstone, carcinoma in pancreas, cancer from common bile duct
  - Treatment: relieve or bypass duct obstruction

Notes

Cholelithiasis (1 of 2)

- Formation of stones in the gallbladder
- Incidence
  - Higher in women than men
  - Higher in women who have borne several children
  - Twice as high in women who use contraceptive pills
  - Higher in obese women
- Factors influencing solubility of cholesterol in bile
  - Cholesterol is insoluble in aqueous solution
  - Dissolved in micelles composed of bile salts and lecithin
  - Solubility of cholesterol depends on ratio of cholesterol to bile salts and lecithin

Cholelithiasis (2 of 2)

- Complications
  - Asymptomatic
  - Biliary colic if stone is extruded into ducts
    - Common duct obstruction: obstructive jaundice
    - Cystic duct obstruction: no jaundice, acute cholecystitis may occur if with preexisting infection in gallbladder
- Treatment
  - Cholecystectomy
  - Chenodeoxycholic acid dissolves gallstones

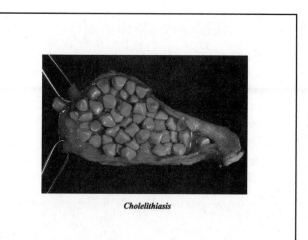

Cholelithiasis

Cholecystitis

- Inflammation of gallbladder
  - Chronic infection is common
  - Gallstones may predispose to cholecystitis
  - Impaction of a stone in neck of gallbladder may cause acute cholecystitis

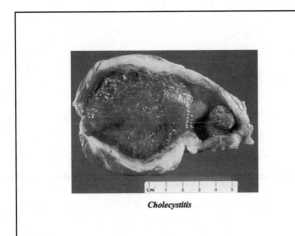

Cholecystitis

Reye Syndrome

- Pathogenesis
  - Evidence suggests the combined effect of viral illness and use of acetylsalicylic acid (aspirin)
  - Aspirin may increase injurious effects of virus
  - Liver damage
  - Brain damage
- Characteristics
  - Affects infants and children
  - Fatty liver with liver dysfunction
  - Cerebral edema with neurologic dysfunction
  - No specific treatment

Liver Tumors

- Benign adenomas: uncommon, occur in women taking contraceptive pills
- Primary carcinoma
  - Uncommon in U.S. and Canada but common in Asia and Africa due to high incidence HBV carriers
  - HBV carriers have a high risk for develop liver disease and primary liver carcinoma
- Metastatic carcinoma
  - Common in developed countries
  - Spread from primary sites such as GI tract, lung, breast
  - Tumor cells carried in the blood and delivered to the liver via hepatic artery

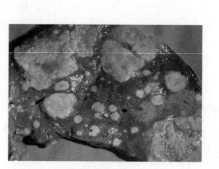

Metastatic Carcinoma

Jaundice

- Yellow discoloration of skin and sclera from accumulation of bile pigment in tissues and body fluids
- Causes of accumulation
  - Hemolytic jaundice: increased breakdown of red cells
  - Hepatocellular jaundice: liver injury impairing conjugation of bilirubin
  - Obstructive jaundice: bile duct obstructed by tumor or stone impairing delivery of bile into duodenum

Liver Biopsy

- Indications
  - To determine cause of liver disease
  - To evaluate extent of liver cell damage in persons with chronic hepatitis
- Needle inserted through abdominal skin directly into liver
- Biopsy specimen examined histologically by pathologist
  - Provides specific diagnosis
  - Provides basis for treatment

Discussion (1 of 2)

- Individuals at risk for developing Hepatitis C include the following EXCEPT:
  - A. Intranasal cocaine users
  - B. Health care personnel exposed to blood and body fluids
  - C. Intravenous drug users
  - D. Children born to mothers who tested positive for Hepatitis C
  - E. Children's day care personnel

Discussion (2 of 2)

- What groups of people are considered at risk for hepatitis C?
- What is anicteric hepatitis?
- What is subclinical hepatitis?
- Chronic liver disease is a complication of which types of viral hepatitis?
- What is the clinical significance of Mallory bodies?

Notes

Chapter Outline

The chapter outline provides you with an organizational guide to the topics and ideas presented in this chapter of the text.

Study Questions

The following questions are provided as a test for comprehension and as a study guide for use with the text chapters. Additional study material is located at http://health.jbpub.com/humandisease/8e, which contains useful tools such as an A&P review, animated flashcards, an interactive online glossary, crossword puzzles, and web links.

Key Terms

Define the following terms:

1. Ketone bodies _____

2. Ketosis _____

3. Diabetes _____

Fill-in-the-Blanks

1. After each of these diabetes-related conditions, mark *type 1* if the condition affects only persons with type 1 diabetes; mark *type 2* if the condition affects only persons with type 2 diabetes; mark *both* if the condition affects both type 1 and type 2 diabetics.

   a. Insulin essential to control the diabetes _____

   b. An autoimmune disease _____

   c. Responds to oral drugs that lower blood glucose _____

   d. May lead to blindness _____

   e. May lead to hyperosmolar hyperglycemic nonketotic coma _____

   f. Proper diet and weight reduction may control disease _____

   g. May lead to ketoacidosis _____

   h. May damage kidneys if poorly controlled _____

   i. Poor control associated with higher than normal glycosylated hemoglobin test _____

Identify

1. Identify two factors that predispose a person to pancreatitis.

   a. _____

   b. _____

2. Construct a table comparing the major characteristics of the two major types of diabetes with respect to age of onset, body build, major complications, response to insulin, and response to oral antidiabetic drugs.

Characteristic Features	*Type 1 Diabetes*	*Type 2 Diabetes*

3. Identify six complications of poorly controlled diabetes.

a. _____

b. _____

c. _____

d. _____

e. _____

f. _____

Discussion Questions

1. Describe the major abnormalities in the pancreas of persons with cystic fibrosis of the pancreas. _____

_____

_____

_____

2. Describe the major abnormalities in the lungs of persons with cystic fibrosis of the pancreas. _____

_____

_____

_____

3. What are ketone bodies, and why are they elevated in persons with poorly controlled type 1 diabetes? _____

_____

_____

_____

4. Why do some persons with type 2 diabetes develop diabetic coma even though they do not have ketosis? _____

_____

_____

_____

5. Which of the following descriptors applies to cystic fibrosis of the pancreas.

a. Transmitted as mendelian dominant trait _____

_____

b. Red cells sickle under low oxygen tension _____

_____

c. Characterized by secretion of thin, watery mucus _____

_____

d. Pancreas secretes excessive digestive enzymes that may digest the pancreas _____

_____

e. Frequently complicated by symptoms of chronic pulmonary disease _____

_____

6. A 27-year-old woman has insulin-dependent diabetes. What abnormalities would be expected in this condition?

_____

_____

_____

7. List the 4 characteristic features of the metabolic syndrome. _____

_____

_____

8. A woman had pregnancy-related diabetes and her blood glucose returned to normal after delivery. What steps should she take to reduce her risk of developing permanent diabetes when she grows older? _____

_____

_____

Notes

Chapter 22

The Pancreas and Diabetes Mellitus

Learning Objectives

- Describe pathogenesis and treatment of acute and chronic pancreatitis
- Describe pathogenesis, manifestations, complications, prognosis of cystic fibrosis
- Differentiate type 1 and type 2 diabetes mellitus
  - Pathogenesis
  - Incidence
  - Manifestations
  - Complications
  - Treatment

Pancreas (1 of 2)

- Two glands in one
  - Digestive gland
  - Endocrine gland
- Exocrine function: exocrine tissue of the pancreas
  - Concerned solely with digestion
  - Secretes alkaline pancreatic juice rich in digestive enzymes into the duodenum through the pancreatic duct to aid digestion

Notes

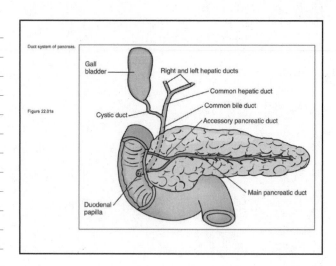

Figure 22.01a

Duct system of pancreas.

Gall bladder
Right and left hepatic ducts
Common hepatic duct
Common bile duct
Accessory pancreatic duct
Cystic duct
Main pancreatic duct
Duodenal papilla

Pancreas (2 of 2)

- Endocrine function: endocrine tissue of the pancreas
- Consists of multiple small clusters of cells scattered throughout the gland as pancreatic islets or Islets of Langerhans
  - Discharge secretions directly into the bloodstream
  - Each islet is composed of different types of cells
    - Alpha cells: secrete glucagon; raise blood glucose
    - Beta cells: secrete insulin; lower blood glucose
    - Delta cells: secrete somatostatin; inhibit secretion of glucagon and insulin

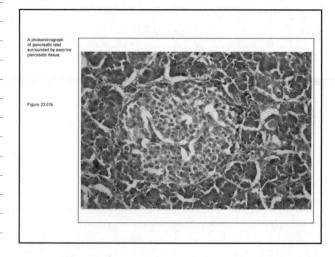

A photomicrograph of pancreatic islet surrounded by exocrine pancreatic tissue.

Figure 22.01b

Acute Pancreatitis (1 of 3)

- Pathogenesis
  - Escape of pancreatic juice from the ducts into the pancreatic tissue
  - Pancreatic digestive enzymes cause destruction and severe hemorrhage
  - Involves active secretion of pancreatic juice despite an obstructed pancreatic duct at its entrance into the duodenum
  - Resulting build-up of pancreatic juice increases pressure within the duct system, causing ducts to rupture

Acute Pancreatitis (2 of 3)

- Predisposing factors
  - Gallbladder disease/gallbladder stones
    - Common bile duct and common pancreatic duct enter the duodenum via the ampulla of Vater
    - Impacted stone in ampulla obstructs pancreatic duct
  - Excessive alcohol consumption
    - Potent stimulus for pancreatic secretions
    - Induces edema, spasm of pancreatic sphincter, in ampulla of Vater
    - Result in high intraductal pressure, duct necrosis, and escape of pancreatic juice

Acute Pancreatitis (3 of 3)

- Clinical manifestations
  - Severe abdominal pain
  - Seriously ill
  - High mortality rate

Notes

_____
_____
_____
_____
_____
_____
_____
_____
_____
_____
_____
_____
_____
_____
_____
_____
_____
_____
_____
_____
_____
_____
_____
_____
_____
_____
_____
_____
_____
_____
_____
_____
_____
_____
_____
_____

Chronic Pancreatitis

- Repeated episodes of mild inflammation of pancreas
- Each bout destroys some pancreatic tissue
- Inflammation subsides and damaged pancreatic tissue is replaced by scar tissue, leading to progressive destruction of pancreatic tissue
- Manifestations
  - Difficulty digesting and absorbing nutrients
  - Not enough surviving pancreatic tissue to produce adequate enzymes
  - Destruction of pancreatic islets may lead to diabetes

Cystic Fibrosis (1 of 3)

- Serious hereditary disease, autosomal recessive trait
- Mutation of a normal gene, CF gene, on long arm of chromosome 7
- Manifests in infancy and childhood
- Incidence in whites: 1 in 3,000
- Incidence in blacks and other races: rare
- Mortality, more than 50% die before age 32
- Pathogenesis
  - Defective transport of chloride, sodium, and H_2O across cell membrane
  - Deficient electrolyte and H_2O in the mucus secreted by the pancreas, bile ducts, respiratory tract, and other secretory cells

Cystic Fibrosis (2 of 3)

- Pathogenesis
  - Mucus becomes abnormally thick, precipitates, and forms dense plugs that obstruct the pancreatic ducts, bronchi, bronchioles, and bile ducts
  - Obstruction of pancreatic ducts: causes atrophy and fibrosis
  - Obstruction of bronchi: causes lung injury
  - Obstruction of biliary ducts: causes liver scarring
  - Abnormal function of sweat glands: unable to conserve sodium and chloride with excessively high salt concentration in sweat; basis of diagnostic test

Cystic Fibrosis (3 of 3)

- Treatment
  - Oral capsules containing pancreatic enzymes to compensate for lack of pancreatic digestive enzymes
  - Various treatments to preserve as much pulmonary function as possible
  - Vigorous treatment of pulmonary bacterial infections
  - Lung transplant may eventually be required if lungs are severely damaged

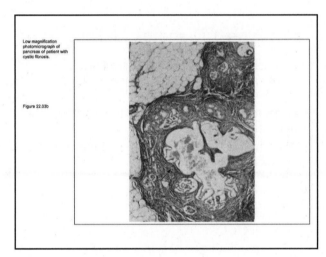

Low magnification photomicrograph of pancreas of patient with cystic fibrosis.

Figure 22.03b

Diabetes Mellitus

- Very common and important metabolic disease
- Two major groups depending on cause
  - Type 1 diabetes
    - Insulin deficiency
    - Occurs primarily in children and young adults
  - Type 2 diabetes
    - Inadequate response to insulin
    - Typically an adult-onset diabetes
    - More common than Type 1
    - Becoming more common in children
- Manifestation: Increased glucose levels in blood or hyperglycemia

Notes

TABLE 22-1

Comparison of two major types of diabetes mellitus

	TYPE 1	TYPE 2
Usual age of onset	Childhood Young adulthood	Middle age or later
Body build	Normal	Overweight
Plasma insulin	Absent or low	Normal or high
Complications	Ketoacidosis	Hyperosmolar coma
Response to insulin	Normal	Reduced
Response to oral antidiabetic drugs	Unresponsive	Responsive

Type 1 Diabetes Mellitus

- Results from damage to pancreatic islets leading to reduction or absence of insulin secretion
- Often follows a viral infection that destroys the pancreatic islets
- Abnormal immune response may play part: production of autoantibodies directed against islet cells
- With a hereditary predisposition
- Complication
  - Diabetic ketosis

Type 2 Diabetes Mellitus (1 of 2)

- Complex metabolic disease
- Occurs in older, overweight, or obese adults
- Increasingly seen among younger people who are overweight or obese
- **Insulin secretion is normal or increased**
- **Reduced response of tissues to insulin**
- Cause is not completely understood but weight reduction restores insulin responsiveness
- Islet function is not completely normal as pancreas is not able to increase insulin output to compensate for the insulin resistance

Type 2 Diabetes Mellitus (2 of 2)

- Hereditary disease
- Children of parents with diabetes are at a significant risk
- Incidence in some populations as high as 40% (Pima Indians of Arizona)
- Complication
- Hyperosmolar nonketotic coma due to marked hyperglycemia

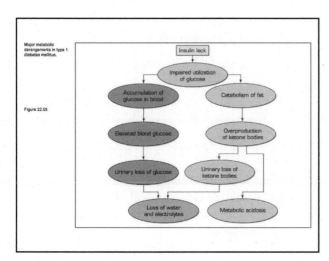

Major metabolic derangements in type 1 diabetes mellitus.

Figure 22.05

Complications of Diabetes

- Increased susceptibility to infection
- Diabetic coma
- Ketoacidosis
- Hyperosmolar coma
- Arteriosclerosis
- Blindness
- Renal failure
- Peripheral neuritis

Notes

Ketone Bodies (1 of 2)

- Glucose is absorbed normally but is not used properly for energy due to insulin deficiency or insensitivity
- Body turns to fat as a source of energy
- Fat is broken down into a fatty acid and glycerol
- Fatty acid broken down further into 2 carbon fragments combined with carrier molecule, acetyl coenzyme A
- Some acetyl-CoA are converted by the liver into ketone bodies
- More acetyl-CoA molecules are produced than can be oxidized as a source of energy
- Ketosis: accumulation of ketone bodies in blood and excreted in the urine together with H_2O and electrolytes

Ketone Bodies (2 of 2)

- Acetoacetic acid: from condensation of 2 acteyl-CoA molecules
- Beta-hydroxybutyric acid: from addition of a hydrogen atom to an oxygen atom and converted into a –OH group
- Acetone: from removal of a carboxyl group of acetoacetic
- Type 1 diabetes complication
- Ketoacidosis: overproduction of ketone bodies
  - Buffer systems cannot maintain normal pH
  - May lead to coma

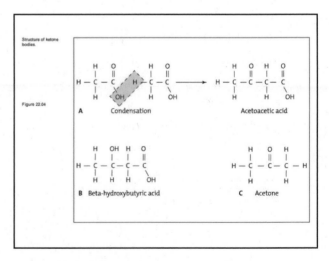

Structure of ketone bodies.

Figure 22.04

A Condensation Acetoacetic acid

B Beta-hydroxybutyric acid

C Acetone

Hyperosmolar Hyperglycemic Nonketotic Coma

- Type 2 diabetes complication
- Severe hyperglycemia
  - Blood glucose increases 10 to 20 x normal value
- Absence of ketosis
  - Less insulin is required to inhibit fat mobilization than is needed to promote entry of glucose into cells
  - Patients have enough insulin to prevent ketosis, not enough to prevent hyperglycemia
- Results in coma due to extreme hyperosmolarity of blood
  - H_2O moves out of the cells into the extracellular fluid
  - Cells become dehydrated disturbing functions of neurons leading to coma

Insulin

- Influences carbohydrate, protein, and fat metabolism on liver cells, muscle, and adipose tissues
- Main stimulus for release: high glucose in blood
- Promotes
  - Entry of glucose into cells
  - Utilization of glucose as source of energy
  - Storage of glucose as glycogen
  - Conversion of glucose into triglycerides
  - Storage of newly formed triglyceride in fat cells
  - Entry of amino acids into cells and stimulates protein synthesis

Hyperglycemia

- Elevated blood glucose levels
- Also from other conditions that impair glucose utilization but are less common than diabetes
  - Chronic pancreatic disease: damage or destruction of pancreatic islets
  - Endocrine diseases: overproduction of pituitary or adrenal hormones that raise blood glucose
  - Drugs that impair glucose utilization as a side effect
  - Hereditary diseases characterized by disturbed carbohydrate metabolism

Notes

Hypoglycemia in Diabetes (1 of 2)

- Pancreas regulates the glucose in blood by adjusting its output of insulin
  - Hypoglycemia: low blood sugar
  - Adrenal medulla: responds by discharging epinephrine that raises blood glucose
- Neurologic manifestations appear if blood glucose continues to fall
- Other causes of hypoglycemia
  - Oral hypoglycemic drugs in type 2 diabetics
  - Self-administration of oral hypoglycemic drugs or insulin by emotionally disturbed person
  - Islet cell tumor

Hypoglycemia in Diabetes (2 of 2)

- Must adjust dose of insulin to match the amount of ingested carbohydrate
  - Insufficient insulin, glucose levels increase
  - Too much insulin, glucose levels decrease
- Conditions predisposing to hypoglycemia in a diabetic patient taking insulin
  - Skipping a meal: carbohydrate intake is insufficient in relation to amount insulin and blood glucose falls
  - Vigorous exercise: with high physical activity there is high glucose utilization; excess insulin
- Too much insulin causes a precipitous drop in glucose leading to insulin reaction or insulin shock

Treatment of Diabetes

- Diet
- Type 1 diabetes: requires insulin; dosage adjusted to control level of blood glucose
- Type 2 diabetes
  - Management: weight reduction and diet
  - Oral hypoglycemic drugs if patient does not respond adequately to diet and exercise regimen

Monitoring Control of Diabetes

- Goal: achieve control of blood glucose as close as possible to normal
  - 1. Frequent periodic measurements of blood glucose
  - 2. Urine test: detects glucose spilling into the urine when blood glucose is too high
  - 3. Measurement of glycosylated hemoglobin: serves as an index of long-term control of hyperglycemia

Glycosylated Hemoglobin, HgA1c

- Glycosylated hemoglobin monitors how well blood glucose is being controlled by treatment
  - Excess glucose molecules attach permanently to red blood cells that circulate in body for about 3 months before they die
  - Concentration of glycosylated hemoglobin is directly proportional to average blood glucose for the preceding 6-12 weeks
- Normal persons: 6% of hemoglobin is glycosylated
- Well-controlled diabetes: 7% or less
- Poorly controlled diabetes: 8% and above

Tumors of the Pancreas

- Carcinoma of the pancreas
  - Usually develops in the head of the pancreas
    - Blocks common bile duct
    - Causes obstructive jaundice
  - Tumors elsewhere in pancreas: no specific symptoms, usually far advanced when first detected
- Islet cell tumors
  - Benign
  - Beta cell tumors produce hyperinsulinism and hypoglycemia

Notes

Notes

_____
_____
_____
_____
_____
_____
_____
_____
_____
_____
_____
_____
_____
_____
_____
_____
_____
_____
_____
_____
_____
_____
_____
_____
_____
_____
_____
_____
_____
_____
_____
_____
_____
_____
_____
_____
_____
_____

Discussion

- Insulin performs all of the following functions EXCEPT
  - A. It promotes entry of amino acids into the cells
  - B. It promotes storage of glucose in muscle and liver cells
  - C. It promotes entry and absorption of glucose into cells for use as energy
  - D. It promotes the breakdown of fat
  - E. It lowers blood glucose

Chapter Outline

The chapter outline provides you with an organizational guide to the topics and ideas presented in this chapter of the text.

Chapter 23

Study Questions

The following questions are provided as a test for comprehension and as a study guide for use with the text chapters. Additional study material is located at http://health.jbpub.com/humandisease/8e, which contains useful tools such as an A&P review, animated flashcards, an interactive online glossary, crossword puzzles, and web links.

Key Terms

Define the following terms:

1. Reflux esophagitis _____

2. Barrett's esophagus _____

Fill-in-the-Blank

1. The inheritance of cleft lip and palate, which is related to interaction of multiple genes and environmental factors, is called a _____ inheritance pattern.

2. Each tooth is formed from a separate tooth bud, and _____ is deposited in the dentine and enamel as the tooth is formed.

3. To prevent staining of the teeth, the antibiotic _____ is not given to pregnant women or to children during the time when the teeth are forming.

4. Masses of bacteria intermixed with bacterial products and proteins from saliva form aggregates called_____ _____ that adhere to the teeth and predispose a person to tooth decay.

5. The substance _____, when added to water supplies and toothpaste, helps prevent tooth decay.

6. Chronic gingivitis complicated by spread of the infection into the space between the teeth and gums to form pockets of pus is called _____.

7. A small superficial ulcer in the oral cavity is called _____.

8. Failure of the lower esophageal sphincter to open properly is called _____.

9. Inability of the lower esophageal sphincter to close properly is called _____. It leads to a condition called _____, which eventually may be complicated by a condition called _____.

10. The metaplastic change in the epithelium of the distal esophagus is called _____. It may predispose a person to the development of _____ in the distal esophagus.

11. An enzyme called _____ is required for the synthesis of prostaglandins, which have many functions. There are _____ forms of the enzyme.

12. Many cases of chronic gastritis appear to be caused by an organism called _____. This organism may also slightly increase the risk of developing two different types of gastric tumors, which are called _____ and _____.

13. If a person has a gastric or duodenal ulcer and is also colonized by an organism called _____, the person is treated not only with antacids but also with _____ to eradicate the organism.

True/False

Tell whether each statement is true or false. If false, explain why the statement is incorrect.

1. Many cases of acute gastritis are caused by nonsteroidal anti-inflammatory drugs (NSAIDs), which act by inhibiting an enzyme (cyclooxygenase) that is required to synthesize prostaglandins. _____

_____

2. There are two forms of cyclooxygenase (COX). One form (COX-1) promotes the synthesis of prostaglandins that protect the gastric mucosa from the harmful effects of gastric acid. The other form (COX-2) promotes the synthesis of prostaglandins that function as mediators of inflammation. _____

_____

Matching 1

Match the abnormalities in the right column with the diseases in the left column.

Disease or Condition

1. ____ Regional enteritis (Crohn's disease)
2. ____ Meckel's diverticulitis
3. ____ Mesenteric artery thrombosis
4. ____ Chronic ulcerative colitis
5. ____ Antibiotic-associated colitis
6. ____ Nontropical sprue
7. ____ Lactose intolerance
8. ____ Irritable bowel syndrome
9. ____ Colon diverticulosis
10. ____ Colon diverticulitis
11. ____ Intussusception
12. ____ Colon volvulus

Abnormality

A. Protrusion of mucosa through weak area in bowel wall
B. Hypersensitivity to wheat protein (gluten)
C. Inflammation of colon diverticula
D. Inflammation and ulceration of colon mucosa
E. Chronic inflammation and scarring of distal ileum
F. Deficiency of lactase enzyme
G. Overgrowth of *Clostridium difficile*
H. Inflammation of congenital small bowel diverticulum
I. Disturbed bowel function without structural changes
J. Rotary twist of sigmoid colon on its mesentery
K. Telescoping of proximal colon into distal colon
L. Extensive necrosis of small bowel and proximal colon

Matching 2

Match the eating disturbance with its manifestations:

1. ____ obesity
2. ____ bulimia nervosa
3. ____ anorexia nervosa
4. ____ binge-eating disorder

a. Excessive weight loss by restricting food intake and other means because the person believes that she or he is too fat.

b. Excessive weight gain because of chronic overeating despite knowledge of the harmful effects of obesity.

c. Frequent bouts of compulsive overeating in older adults without self-induced vomiting or other methods to prevent weight gain.

d. Bouts of compulsive overeating followed by self-induced vomiting and other means to prevent weight gain.

Discussion Questions

1. What are some of the major causes of esophageal obstruction? What symptoms does esophageal obstruction produce?

   _____

   _____

   _____

2. How does acute appendicitis usually develop? What is the pathogenesis of acute appendicitis? _____

   _____

   _____

   _____

3. What is intestinal obstruction? What symptoms does it produce? What are some of the common causes of intestinal obstruction? _____

   _____

   _____

   _____

4. What symptoms and physical findings are likely to be encountered in a patient with a carcinoma of the colon? Why?

   _____

   _____

   _____

5. What conditions predispose a person to chronic diverticulosis of colon? _____

   _____

   _____

   _____

6. As a result of the tumor, what conditions might be encountered in a patient with a small ulcerated carcinoma of the cecum? _____

   _____

   _____

   _____

7. What condition usually results from a complete thrombosis or embolic occlusion of the superior mesenteric artery?

   _____

   _____

   _____

Notes

Chapter 23

The Gastrointestinal Tract

Learning Objectives (1 of 2)

- Identify major types of cleft lip and cleft palate deformity
- Explain pathogenesis and prevention of dental caries and periodontal disease
- Describe common congenital anomalies of the GIT, clinical manifestations, diagnosis, treatment
- Describe three most common lesions of the esophagus that lead to esophageal obstruction
- Explain pathogenesis, complications, and treatment of peptic ulcer
- Describe types and clinical manifestations of acute and chronic enteritis

Learning Objectives (2 of 2)

- Differentiate acute appendicitis and Meckel's diverticulitis in terms of pathogenesis, clinical manifestations, and treatment
- Describe pathogenesis of diverticulitis and the role of diet in its development
- Discuss causes, clinical manifestations, complications
  - Intestinal obstruction
  - Colon cancer
  - Diverticulosis

Gastrointestinal Tract

- Digestion and absorption of food
- Oral cavity
- Esophagus, stomach, small and large intestines, anus

Cleft Lip and Cleft Palate

- Embryologically, face and palate formed by coalescence of cell masses that merge to form facial structures
- Palate formed by two masses of tissues that grow medially and fuse at midline to separate as nose and mouth
- Maldevelopment leads to defects
  - 1 per 1000 births
  - Multifactorial inheritance pattern
- Surgical correction (cheiloplasty)
  - Cleft lip: soon after birth
  - Cleft palate: 1 to 2 years of age followed by speech therapy to correct nasal speech

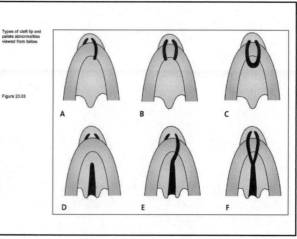

Types of cleft lip and palate abnormalities viewed from below.

Figure 23.03

A B C
D E F

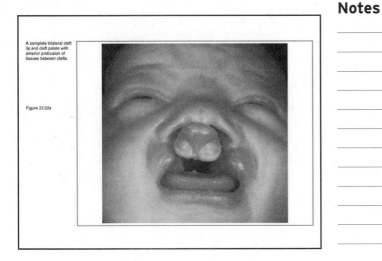
A complete bilateral cleft lip and cleft palate with anterior protrusion of tissues between clefts.

Figure 23.02a

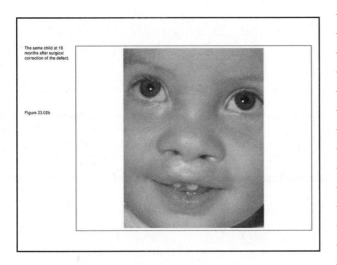
The same child at 18 months after surgical correction of the defect.

Figure 23.02b

Abnormalities of Tooth Development

- Teeth: specialized structures that develop in tissues of the jaws
- Two sets
  - Temporary or deciduous teeth (20 teeth)
  - Permanent teeth (32 teeth)
- Missing teeth or extra teeth: common abnormality
- Enamel forms at specific times during embryologic period
- Tetracycline: administered during enamel formation causes permanent yellow-gray to brown discoloration of the crown

Notes

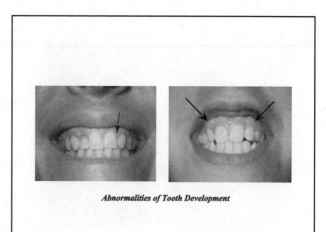

Abnormalities of Tooth Development

Dental Caries and Periodontal Disease

- Oral cavity: diverse collection of aerobic and anaerobic bacteria that mix with saliva, forming sticky film on teeth (dental plaque)
- Plaque + action of bacteria result in tooth decay (caries)
- Dental cavity: loss of tooth structure from bacterial action
- Gingivitis: inflammation of the gums due to masses of bacteria and debris accumulating around base of teeth
- Periodontal disease: inflammation extends to tissues that support teeth; forms small pockets of infection between teeth and gums
    - Two types: gingivitis and periodontitis

Stomatitis

- Inflammation of the oral cavity
- Causes
    - Irritants: alcohol, tobacco, hot or spicy foods
    - Infectious agents: *Herpes* virus, *Candida albicans* fungus, bacteria that cause trench mouth

Carcinoma of the Oral Cavity

- Arises from squamous epithelium
  - Lips
  - Cheek
  - Tongue
  - Palate
  - Back of throat

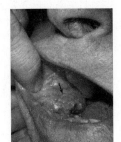

Esophagus (1 of 3)

- Muscular tube that extends from pharynx to stomach with sphincters at both upper and lower ends
  - Upper sphincter relaxes to allow passage of swallowed food
  - Lower (gastroesophageal or cardiac) sphincter relaxes to allow passage of food to the stomach
- Diseases
  - Failure of cardiac sphincter to function properly
  - Tears in lining of esophagus from retching and vomiting
  - At gastroesophageal junction from repetitive, intermittent, vigorous contractions that increase intraabdominal pressure
  - Esophageal obstruction from carcinoma, food impaction, or stricture

Esophagus (2 of 3)

- Symptoms
  - Difficulty swallowing (dysphagia)
  - Substernal discomfort or pain
  - Inability to swallow (complete obstruction)
  - Regurgitation of food into trachea
  - Choking and coughing
- Two major disturbances of cardiac sphincter
  - 1. Cardiospasm: sphincter fails to open properly due to malfunction of nerve plexus; esophagus becomes dilated proximal to constricted sphincter from food retention
    - Treatment: periodic stretching of sphincter; surgery
  - 2. Incompetent cardiac sphincter: sphincter remains open; gastric juices leak back into esophagus

Esophagus (3 of 3)

- Complications of incompetent cardiac sphincter
  - Reflux esophagitis: inflammation
  - Ulceration and scarring of squamous mucosal lining
  - Barrett's esophagus: glandular metaplasia; change from squamous to columnar epithelium; ↑ risk for cancer
- Esophageal obstruction
  - Carcinoma: can arise anywhere in esophagus
  - Tumor narrows lumen of esophagus, infiltrates surrounding tissue, invades trachea (tracheoesophageal fistula)
  - Food impaction: distal part
  - Stricture: from scar tissue due to necrosis and inflammation from corrosive chemicals such as lye

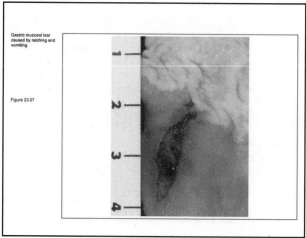

Gastric mucosal tear caused by retching and vomiting.

Figure 23.07

Acute Gastritis

- Inflammation of the gastric lining
- Self-limited inflammation of short duration
- May be associated with mucosal ulceration or bleeding
- From nonsteroidal anti-inflammatory drugs (NSAID) that inhibit cyclooxygenase (COX) enzyme: aspirin, ibuprofen, naproxen
  - COX-1: promotes synthesis of prostaglandin that protects gastric mucosa
  - COX-2: promotes synthesis of prostaglandin that mediate inflammation
    - Drugs that selectively inhibit COX-2 increase risk for heart attack and stroke
- Alcohol: a gastric irritant; stimulates gastric acid secretion

H. Pylori Gastritis (1 of 2)

- Small, curved, gram-negative organisms that colonize surface of gastric mucosa
- Grow within layer of mucus covering epithelial cells
- Produce urease that decomposes urea, a product of protein metabolism, into ammonia
- Ammonia neutralizes gastric acid allowing organisms to flourish; organisms also produce enzymes that break down mucus layer

H. Pylori Gastritis (2 of 2)

- Common infection that increases with age (50% by age 50)
- Spreads via person-to-person through close contact and fecal-oral route
- Increased risk of gastric carcinoma: intestinal metaplasia
- Increased risk of malignant lymphoma (mucosa-associated lymphoid tissue, MALT)

Peptic Ulcer

- Pathogenesis
  - Digestion of mucosa due to increased acid secretions and digestive enzymes (gastric acid and pepsin)
  - *Helicobacter pylori* injures mucosa directly or through increased acid secretion by gastric mucosa
  - **Common sites: distal stomach or proximal duodenum**
- Complications: hemorrhage, perforation, peritonitis, obstruction from scarring
- Treatment
  - Antacids: block acid secretion by gastric epithelial cells
  - Antibiotic therapy: against *H. pylori*
  - Surgery if medical therapy fails

Notes

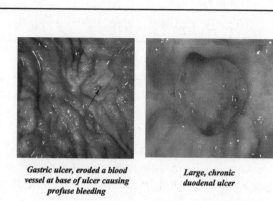

Gastric ulcer, eroded a blood vessel at base of ulcer causing profuse bleeding

Large, chronic duodenal ulcer

Carcinoma of the Stomach

- Manifestations
  - Vague upper abdominal discomfort
  - Iron-deficiency anemia (chronic blood loss from ulcerated surface of tumor)
- Diagnosis: biopsy by means of gastroscopy
- Treatment: surgical resection of affected part, surrounding tissue and lymph nodes
- Long-term survival: relatively poor; often far-advanced at time of diagnosis

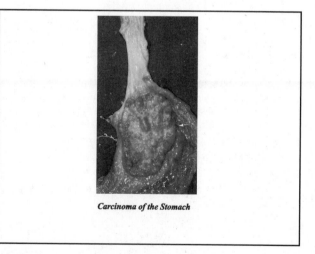

Carcinoma of the Stomach

Inflammatory Diseases of the Intestines

- Acute enteritis
  - Intestinal infections; common; of short duration
  - Nausea, vomiting, abdominal discomfort, loose stools
- Chronic enteritis: less common, more difficult to treat
- Regional enteritis or Crohn's disease: distal ileum
  - Chronic inflammation and ulceration of mucosa with thickening and scarring of bowel wall
  - Inflammation may be scattered with normal intervening areas or "skip areas"
  - Treatment: drugs and possible surgical resection of affected part of bowel

Ulcerative Colitis (1 of 2)

- Ulcerative colitis: large intestines and rectum
  - Inflammation is limited to mucosa, bowel not thickened unlike in Crohn's
  - Frequently begins in rectal mucosa and spreads until entire colon is involved
- Complications
  - Bleeding; bloody diarrhea
  - Perforation: from extensive inflammation with leakage of intestinal contents into peritoneal cavity
  - Long-standing disease may develop cancer of colon and/or rectum

Ulcerative Colitis (2 of 2)

- Treatment
  - Symptomatic and supportive measures
  - Antibiotics, corticosteroids to control flare-ups
  - Immunosuppressive drugs
  - Surgical resection

Notes

Inflammatory Diseases of the Intestines (1 of 3)

- Antibiotic-associated colitis: broad-spectrum antibiotics destroy normal intestinal flora
  - Allows growth of anaerobic spore-forming bacteria, *Clostridium difficile* not inhibited by antibiotic taken
  - Organisms produce toxins causing inflammation and necrosis of colonic mucosa
  - Diarrhea, abdominal pain, fever
- Diagnosis: stool culture, toxin in stool
- Treatment: stop antibiotic treatment; give vancomycin or metronidazole
  - Drugs that decrease intestinal motility will prolong illness

Inflammatory Diseases of the Intestines (2 of 3)

- Appendicitis: most common inflammatory lesion of the bowel
  - Narrow caliber of appendix may be plugged with fecal material
  - Secretions of appendix drain poorly, create pressure in appendiceal lumen, compressing blood supply
  - Bacteria invade appendiceal wall causing inflammation
- Manifestations
  - Generalized abdominal pain localizing in right lower quadrant; rebound tenderness; rigidity
- Treatment: surgery

Inflammatory Diseases of the Intestines (3 of 3)

- Meckel's diverticulum
  - Outpouching at distal ileum, 12-18 inches proximal to cecum
  - From persistence of a remnant of the vitelline duct, narrow tubular channel connecting small intestine with yolk sac embryologically
  - Found in 2% of population; usually asymptomatic
- May become infected causing features and complications similar to acute appendicitis
- Lining may consist of ectopic acid-secreting gastric mucosa and may cause peptic ulcer

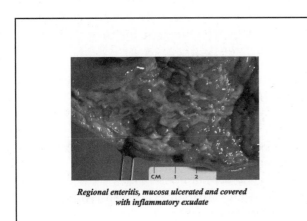

Regional enteritis, mucosa ulcerated and covered with inflammatory exudate

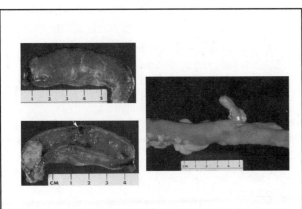

Inflammatory Disease Intestines

Disturbances in Bowel Function (1 of 2)

- Food intolerance: Crampy abdominal pain, distention, flatulence, loose stools
- Lactose intolerance
  - Unable to digest lactose into glucose and galactose for absorption due to lactase deficiency
  - Enzyme abundant in infants and young children
  - Unabsorbed lactose remains in intestinal lumen and raises osmotic pressure of bowel contents
  - Fermented by bacteria in colon, yielding lactic acid that further increases intraluminal pressure
  - Common in Asians; 90% in Native Americans; 70% Blacks

Disturbances Bowel Function (2 of 2)

- Gluten intolerance (Celiac disease; Gluten enteropathy or Nontropical sprue)
  - Gluten: protein in wheat, rye, barley; imparts elasticity to bread dough
  - Chronic diarrhea impairing absorption of fats and nutrients; weight loss, vitamin deficiencies
  - Leads to atrophy of intestinal villi
  - Diagnosis: clinical features and biopsy of intestinal mucosa
  - Treatment: gluten-free diet

Irritable Bowel Syndrome

- Also known as spastic colitis or mucous colitis
- Episodes of crampy abdominal discomfort, loud gurgling bowel sounds, and disturbed bowel function without structural or biochemical abnormalities
- Alternating diarrhea and constipation
- Excessive mucus secreted by colonic mucosal glands
- Diagnosis: by exclusion
  - Rule out pathogenic infections, food intolerance, and inflammatory conditions
- Treatment
  - Reduce emotional tension
  - Improve intestinal motility

Intestinal Infections in Homosexual Men

- *Shigella*
- *Salmonella*
- *Entamoeba Histolytica*
- *Giardia*
- Transmission: anal-oral sexual practices
- Treatment: treat underlying cause

Colon Diverticulosis and Diverticulitis

- Diverticulosis: outpouchings or diverticula of colonic mucosa through weak areas in the muscular wall of large intestine
  - Low-residue diet predisposes to condition as increased intraluminal pressure must be generated to propel stools through colon
  - Acquired, usually asymptomatic, seen in older people
  - Common site: sigmoid colon
- Diverticulitis: inflammation incited by bits of fecal material trapped within outpouchings
- Complications: inflammation, perforation, bleeding, scarring, abscess

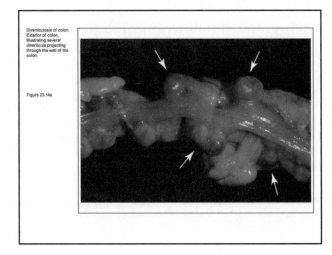

Diverticulosis of colon. Exterior of colon, illustrating several diverticula projecting through the wall of the colon.

Figure 23.14a

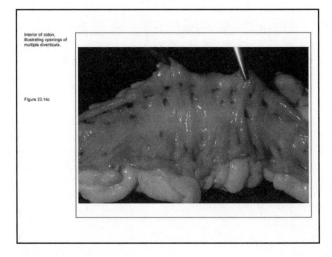

Interior of colon, illustrating openings of multiple diverticula.

Figure 23.14c

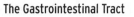

Diverticula of colon demonstrated by injection of barium contrast material into colon (barium enema).

Figure 23.15

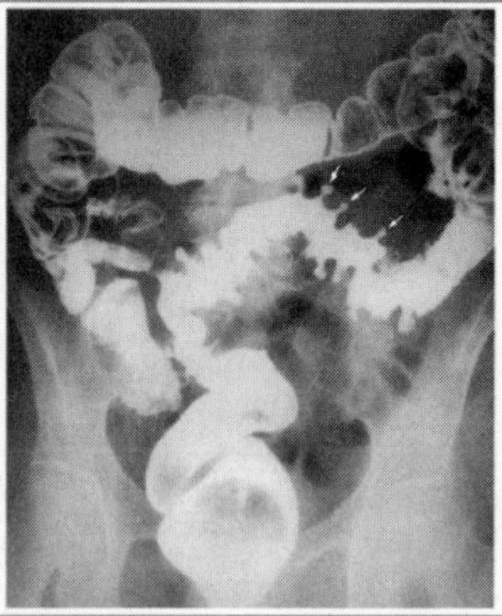

Intestinal Obstructions (1 of 5)

- Conditions blocking normal passage of intestinal contents
- Always considered as a serious condition
- Severity depends on location of obstruction, completeness, interference with blood supply
- High intestinal obstruction
  - Severe, crampy abdominal pain from vigorous peristalsis
  - Vomiting with loss of H_2O and electrolytes, may result in dehydration

Intestinal Obstructions (2 of 5)

- Low intestinal obstruction
  - Symptoms less acute
  - Mild, crampy abdominal pain
  - Moderate distention of abdomen
- Common causes of intestinal obstruction
  - Adhesions
  - Hernia
  - Tumor
  - Volvulus
  - Intussusception

Intestinal Obstructions (3 of 5)

- Adhesions
  - Adhesive bands of connective tissue
  - May cause loop of bowel to become kinked, compressed, twisted
  - Causes obstruction proximal to site of adhesion
- Hernia
  - Protrusion of loop of bowel through a small opening, usually in abdominal wall
  - Herniated loop pushes through peritoneum to form hernial sac

Intestinal Obstructions (4 of 5)

- Hernia
  - Inguinal hernia: common in men; loop of small bowel protrudes through a weak area in inguinal ring and descends downward into scrotum
  - Umbilical and femoral hernia: common in both sexes
    - Umbilical hernia: loop of bowel protrudes into umbilicus through defect in the abdominal wall
    - Femoral hernia: loop of intestine extends under inguinal ligament along course of femoral vessels into the groin

Intestinal Obstructions (5 of 5)

- Reducible hernia: herniated loop of bowel can be pushed back into abdominal cavity
- Incarcerated hernia: cannot be pushed back
- Strangulated hernia: loop of bowel is tightly constricted obstructing the blood supply to the herniated bowel; requires prompt surgical intervention
- Volvulus: rotary twisting of bowel impairing blood supply; common site: sigmoid colon
- Intussusception: telescoping of a segment of bowel into adjacent segment; from vigorous peristalsis or tumor
  - Common site: terminal ileum

Notes

Notes

_____
_____
_____
_____
_____
_____
_____
_____
_____
_____
_____
_____
_____
_____
_____
_____
_____
_____
_____
_____
_____
_____
_____
_____
_____
_____
_____
_____
_____
_____
_____
_____

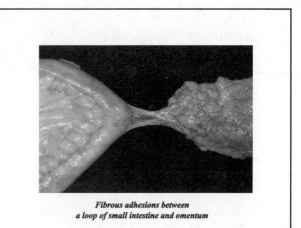

Fibrous adhesions between
a loop of small intestine and omentum

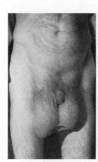

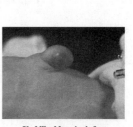

Umbilical hernia, infant

Inguinal hernia,
bilateral, extending
into scrotum

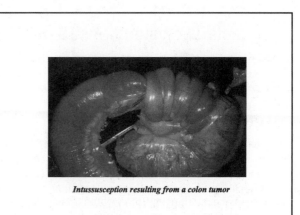

Intussusception resulting from a colon tumor

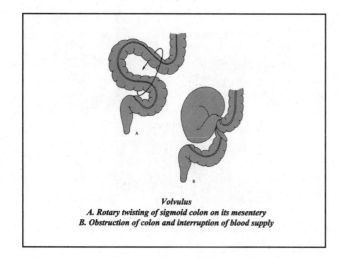

Volvulus
A. Rotary twisting of sigmoid colon on its mesentery
B. Obstruction of colon and interruption of blood supply

Mesenteric Thrombosis

- Thrombosis of superior mesenteric artery
  - Artery supplies blood to small bowel and proximal half of colon
  - May develop arteriosclerosis
  - Become occluded by thrombus, embolus, or atheroma
  - Obstruction causes extensive bowel infarction

Tumors of the Colon

- Benign pedunculated polyps
  - Frequent
  - Tip may erode causing bleeding
  - Removed by colonoscopy
- Carcinoma
  - Cecum and right half of colon
    - Does not cause obstruction as caliber is large and bowel contents are relatively soft
    - Tumor can ulcerate, bleed; leads to chronic iron-deficiency anemia
    - Symptoms of anemia: weakness and fatigue
  - Left half of colon
    - Causes obstruction and symptoms of lower intestinal obstruction

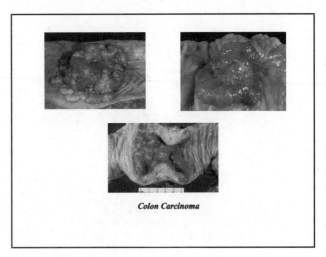

Colon Carcinoma

Imperforate Anus

- Congenital anomaly, colon fails to acquire a normal anal opening
- Two types
- 1. Rectum and anus normally formed and extends to level of skin but no anal orifice
  - Easily treated by incising tissue covering anal opening
- 2. Entire distal rectum fails to develop, with associated abnormalities of urogenital and skeletal system
  - Corrected surgically but technically more difficult
  - Less satisfactory results

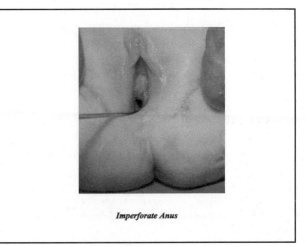

Imperforate Anus

Hemorrhoids

- Varicose veins of hemorrhoidal venous plexus that drains rectum and anus
- Constipation and straining predispose to development
- Relieved by high-fiber diet rich in fruits and vegetables, stool softeners, rectal ointment, or surgery
  - Internal hemorrhoids
    - Veins of the lower rectum
    - May erode and bleed, become thrombosed, or prolapse
  - External hemorrhoids
    - Veins of anal canal and perianal skin
    - May become thrombosed, causing discomfort

Diagnosis of GI Disease

- Endoscopic procedures
  - To directly visualize and biopsy abnormal areas such as esophagus, stomach, intestines
- Radiologic examination
  - To examine areas that cannot be readily visualized
  - To evaluate motility problems
  - To visualize contours of GIT mucosa
  - To identify location and extent of disease
    - Examples: Upper gastrointestinal tract – UGI
    - Colon – BE (barium enema)

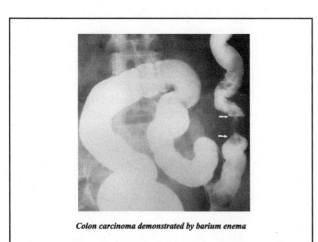

Colon carcinoma demonstrated by barium enema

Notes

Discussion

- A 45-year-old patient has a large right-sided colon carcinoma with iron deficiency anemia. The anemia is most likely due to:
  - A. Impaired absorption of nutrients due to the tumor
  - B. Chronic blood loss from ulcerated surface of the tumor
  - C. Poor appetite
  - D. Metastases to the liver
  - E. Obstruction of the colon by the tumor

Chapter 24 Water, Electrolyte, and Acid-Base Balance

Chapter Outline

The chapter outline provides you with an organizational guide to the topics and ideas presented in this chapter of the text.

Body Water and Electrolytes
Interrelations of Intracellular and Extracellular Fluid
Units of Concentration of Electrolytes
Regulation of Body Fluid and Electrolyte Concentration
Disturbances of Water Balance
    Dehydration
    Overhydration
Disturbances of Electrolyte Balance
Acid–Base Balance
    Buffers
    Respiratory Control of Carbonic Acid
    Control of Bicarbonate Concentration
    Relation between pH and Ratio of Buffer Components
Disturbances of Acid–Base Balance
    Compensatory Mechanisms Responding to Disturbances in pH
    Metabolic Acidosis
    Respiratory Acidosis
    Metabolic Alkalosis
    Respiratory Alkalosis
    Diagnostic Evaluation of Acid–Base Balance

Study Questions

The following questions are provided as a test for comprehension and as a study guide for use with the text chapters. Additional study material is located at http://health.jbpub.com/humandisease/8e, which contains useful tools such as an A&P review, animated flashcards, an interactive online glossary, crossword puzzles, and web links.

Key Terms

Define the following terms:

1. Acidosis _____

2. Alkalosis _____

3. Electrolyte _____

4. pH _____

Fill-in-the-Blank

1. Positively charged ions are called _____, and negatively charged ions are called _____.

2. The units of concentration of electrolytes are expressed as _____.

3. The principal ions in intracellular fluids are _____.

Matching

The numbered column lists several clinical conditions associated with acid–base balance disturbances. The lettered column lists the four types of acid–base disturbances. Match the letter with the clinical condition. There are six conditions but only four acid–base disturbances; thus, some letters are used more than once, and some may not be used at all.

1. _____ Diabetes. Excessive ketone bodies formed.

2. _____ Hyperventilation. Fall in alveolar PCO_2 and blood carbonic acid.

3. _____ Impaired lung function caused by chronic pulmonary disease.

4. _____ Kidney failure. Retention of nonvolatile acids.

5. _____ Excess loss of gastric juice resulting from vomiting.

6. _____ Adrenal corticosteroid excess.

A. Metabolic acidosis

B. Respiratory acidosis

C. Metabolic alkalosis

D. Respiratory alkalosis

Discussion Questions

1. Body fluids are distributed within "compartments" as intracellular fluids and extracellular fluids. The extracellular fluids, in turn, are distributed between the fluid surrounding the cells (interstitial fluid) and that within the blood and lymph vessels (intravascular fluid). Which of these fluid compartments most closely resemble each other in electrolyte composition? _____

_____

_____

_____

2. What percentage of body weight consists of water? _____

_____

_____

_____

3. What factors lead to overhydration of patients? _____

_____

_____

_____

4. What is the effect of prolonged use of diuretics on fluid and electrolyte balance? _____

_____

_____

_____

5. What is the source of the carbonic acid produced by the body? _____

_____

_____

_____

6. What is the source of the ketone bodies produced by the body? _____

_____

_____

_____

7. What is the source of the lactic acid produced by the body? _____

_____

_____

_____

8. What is the normal pH of blood and body fluids? _____

_____

_____

_____

9. What regulatory mechanisms does the body use to maintain the normal body fluid pH? _____

_____

_____

_____

10. How do blood buffers function to maintain normal body fluid pH? _____

_____

_____

11. How do the lungs control the concentration of carbonic acid in the blood? _____

_____

_____

12. How do the kidneys regulate the concentration of bicarbonate in the blood? _____

_____

_____

13. What is the normal ratio of bicarbonate to carbonic acid at the normal pH of blood and body fluids? _____

_____

_____

14. How does the body respond to a disease or condition characterized by an increase in carbonic acid in blood and body fluids? _____

_____

_____

15. How does the body respond when bicarbonate levels fall as a result of buffering of excess acids produced within the body? _____

_____

_____

16. What is metabolic acidosis? _____

_____

_____

17. What are the principal causes of metabolic acidosis? _____

_____

_____

18. What is respiratory alkalosis? _____

_____

_____

_____

19. What are the principal causes of respiratory alkalosis? _____

_____

_____

_____

20. What compensatory mechanisms does the body employ in an attempt to correct the pH change resulting from the respiratory alkalosis? _____

_____

_____

_____

21. Why does excessive use of antacids disturb body pH? _____

_____

_____

_____

22. What effect do excess adrenal corticosteroids have on body pH? What mechanism is responsible for the pH disturbance? What effect do the corticosteroids have on blood electrolytes? _____

_____

_____

_____

Notes

Chapter 24

Water, Electrolyte, and Acid–Base Balance

Learning Objectives

- Explain regulation of electrolytes in the body; major ions in the intracellular and extracellular fluid and units of concentration
- Describe common disturbances of water balance and pathogenesis
- Explain physiologic mechanisms in the control of pH
- Describe pathogenesis of 4 common disturbances of acid-base balance and body's compensatory mechanisms
- Define role of kidneys and lungs in regulating acid–base balance

---

Body Water and Electrolytes

- Body water contains dissolved mineral salts or electrolytes that dissociate in solution, yielding
  - Cations: positively charged ions
  - Anions: negatively charged ions
- Body fluids: electrically neutral
- Sum of cations balanced by sum of anions
- In disease, ion concentrations may vary but the electrical neutrality is always maintained

Notes

Intracellular and Extracellular Fluid (1 of 5)

- Disturbances of body water are associated with corresponding change in electrolytes
- If electrolyte concentration changes, there is a corresponding change in body water and vice versa
- Body consists of 70% water
  - Intracellular water (inside cells)
  - Extracellular water (within interstitial tissues surrounding cells, blood plasma, and lymph)
- "Rule of thirds"
  - 2/3 of body weight is H_2O
  - 2/3 of H_2O is within cells
  - 1/3 of H_2O is extracellular in tissues surrounding cells (interstitial fluid)

Intracellular and Extracellular Fluid (2 of 5)

- Adult female: water content is 10% lower than adult male due to higher body fat than water
- Fluids and electrolytes diffuse freely between the intravascular and interstitial fluids
- Because capillaries are impermeable to protein, the interstitial fluid contains very little protein
- Cell membrane: separates intracellular fluid from interstitial fluid by a cell membrane
  - Freely permeable to water
  - Impermeable to Na^+ and K^+ ions

Intracellular and Extracellular Fluid (3 of 5)

- Chief intracellular ions
  - K^+ (potassium)
  - PO_4^{2-} (phosphate)
- Chief extracellular ions
  - Na^+ (sodium)
  - Cl^- (chloride)
- Differences in concentration of ions on different sides of the cell membrane result from metabolic activity of the cell
- Amount of sodium in the body determines the volume of extracellular fluid as the chief extracellular cation

Intracellular and Extracellular Fluid (4 of 5)

- Amount of potassium in the body determines the volume of intracellular fluid as the chief intracellular cation
- In electrolyte disturbances: primary concern is the concentration of various ions and the interrelation of positively and negatively charged ions with one another than the actual number

Intracellular and Extracellular Fluid (5 of 5)

- Units of concentration of electrolytes
- Expressed in units that define ability to combine with other ions
- Equivalent weight: molecular weight of substance in grams divided by valence
  - 1 equivalent weight dissolved in a liter equals one equivalent per liter (1Eq/L)
  - Units expressed in milliequivalents per liter (1000 mEq = 1Eq)

Regulation of Body Fluid and Electrolyte Concentration (1 of 3)

- Amount of H_2O and electrolytes in body: represents the balance between amounts ingested in food and fluids and amounts excreted via urine, GI tract, perspiration, and as H_2O vapor excreted by lungs
- Disturbances of H_2O balance
  - Dehydration: most common
    - Inadequate intake: diarrhea or vomiting
    - Excess H_2O loss: comatose or debilitated patients
  - Overhydration: less common
    - Excessive fluid intake when renal function is impaired: renal disease; excessive intake of fluids; excessive administration of IV fluids

Notes

Regulation of Body Fluid and Electrolyte Concentration (2 of 3)

- Disturbances of electrolyte balance
  - Conditions that produce H_2O imbalance also disturb electrolyte composition
  - Most result from depletion of body electrolytes
- Depletion of electrolytes
  - Vomiting or diarrhea: sodium and potassium depletion
  - Excessive use of diuretics
  - Excessive diuresis in diabetic acidosis
  - Renal tubular disease

Regulation of Body Fluid and Electrolyte Concentration (3 of 3)

- Diuretics promote excretion of salt and H_2O by the kidneys while impairing reabsorption of these substances
  - Patients with heart failure, liver cirrhosis, kidney disease
- Uncontrolled diabetes: excessive loss of H_2O in urine from the diuretic effect of glucose
- Renal tubular disease: regenerating renal tubules unable to conserve electrolytes and water

Acid–Base Balance

- Body produces large amounts of acid from normal metabolic processes, such as breakdown of proteins and glucose or oxidation of fat
- Body fluids remain slightly alkaline
- pH is maintained within a narrow range: 7.38 to 7.42
- Regulatory mechanisms maintain pH
- Neutralize and eliminate the acids as soon as they are produced to maintain normal pH
  - Blood buffers: resist pH change
  - Lungs: control carbonic acid (H_2CO_3)concentration
  - Kidneys: control bicarbonate concentration

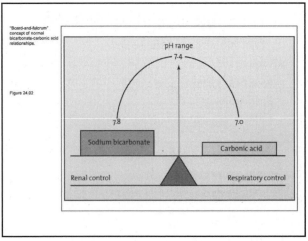

"Board-and-fulcrum" concept of normal bicarbonate-carbonic acid relationships.

Figure 24.02

Blood Buffer System (1 of 2)

- Minimize change in hydrogen ion by converting strong acids and bases into weaker ones chemically
  - Weak acid and its salt
  - Weak base and its salt
- Respiratory control of carbonic acid
  - Carbonic acid (H_2CO_3): dissolved as CO_2 in plasma
  - Hyperventilation: lowers CO_2 and H_2CO_3 in plasma
  - Decreased or inadequate ventilation: raises CO_2 and H_2CO_3 in plasma

Blood Buffer System (2 of 2)

- Renal control of bicarbonate concentration
  - Kidneys selectively reabsorb filtered bicarbonate
  - Kidneys can manufacture bicarbonate to replace amounts lost in buffering acids from metabolic processes
- In any buffer system
  - pH depends on ratio of bicarbonate to H_2CO_3
  - Normal ratio: 20 parts Na bicarbonate: 1 part H_2CO_3

Disturbances in Acid–Base Balance

- Acidosis
  - Blood pH shifts to acidic side
  - From an excess of H_2CO_3
  - From a reduced amount of bicarbonate
- Alkalosis
  - Blood pH shifts to basic side
  - From a decrease in H_2CO_3
  - From an excess of bicarbonate

TABLE 24-1

Comparison of common acid–base disturbances

DISTURBANCE	PRIMARY ABNORMALITY	COMPENSATION	USUAL CAUSES
Metabolic acidosis	Excess endogenous acid depletes bicarbonate	Hyperventilation lowers PCO_2; kidney excretes more hydrogen ions and forms more bicarbonate	Renal failure; ketosis; overproduction of lactic acid
Respiratory acidosis	Inefficient excretion of carbon dioxide by lungs	Formation of additional bicarbonate by kidneys	Chronic pulmonary disease
Metabolic alkalosis	Excess plasma bicarbonate	None	Loss of gastric juice; chloride depletion; excess corticosteroid hormones; ingestion of excessive bicarbonate or other antacids
Respiratory alkalosis	Hyperventilation lowers PCO_2	Increased excretion of bicarbonate by kidneys	Severe anxiety with hyperventilation; stimulation of respiratory center by drugs; central nervous system disease

Classification of Acid–Base Disturbances (1 of 3)

- Metabolic: disturbance lies in bicarbonate member of the buffer pair
- Respiratory: disturbance lies in carbonic acid member of the buffer pair
- Metabolic acidosis: increased endogenous acid generated
  - Amount of acid generated exceeds body's buffering capacity
  - Excess acid is neutralized by bicarbonate
  - Bicarbonate in plasma falls from being consumed in neutralizing excess acid
  - Uremia, ketosis, lactic acidosis
- Compensation: by hyperventilation to lower PCO_2 and increased bicarbonate production in kidneys

Notes

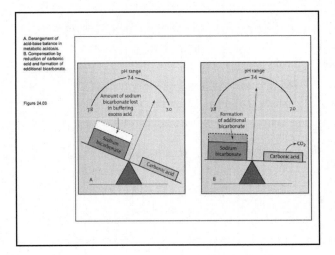

A. Derangement of acid-base balance in metabolic acidosis. B. Compensation by reduction of carbonic acid and formation of additional bicarbonate.

Figure 24.03

Classification of Acid–Base Disturbances (2 of 3)

- Respiratory acidosis: increased H_2CO_3 concentration
  - Inefficient excretion of CO_2 by lungs
  - Leads to retention of CO_2 and rise in H_2CO_3
  - Compensation: increased bicarbonate production in kidneys
- Metabolic alkalosis: increased plasma bicarbonate
  - From loss of gastric juice, chloride depletion, excess corticosteroids, excess antacids
  - With coexisting potassium deficiency
  - Compensation: inefficient, requires simultaneous correction of potassium deficiency

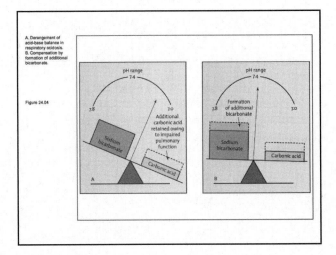

A. Derangement of acid-base balance in respiratory acidosis. B. Compensation by formation of additional bicarbonate.

Figure 24.04

Classification of Acid–Base Disturbances (3 of 3)

- Respiratory alkalosis: Reduced H_2CO_3 concentration
  - Hyperventilation lowers PCO_2 and H_2CO_3 level falls
  - Relative excess of bicarbonate
  - Compensation: excretion of bicarbonate by kidneys

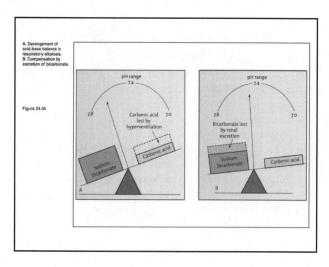

A. Derangement of acid-base balance in respiratory alkalosis. B. Compensation by excretion of bicarbonate.

Figure 24.06

Diagnostic Evaluation of Acid–Base Balance

- Clinical evaluation: determination of concentration of bicarbonate in plasma as an index of patient's overall status
- Laboratory studies
  - Blood pH
  - PCO_2
  - Bicarbonate

Discussion

- What is the difference between intracellular and extracellular fluid?
- What are the differences between metabolic acidosis and respiratory acidosis as to causes and compensatory mechanisms of the body?
- What are the differences between metabolic alkalosis and respiratory alkalosis as to causes and compensatory mechanisms of the body?

Notes

Chapter Outline

The chapter outline provides you with an organizational guide to the topics and ideas presented in this chapter of the text.

Study Questions

The following questions are provided as a test for comprehension and as a study guide for use with the text chapters. Additional study material is located at http://health.jbpub.com/humandisease/8e, which contains useful tools such as an A&P review, animated flashcards, an interactive online glossary, crossword puzzles, and web links.

Key Terms

Define the following terms:

1. Acromegaly _____

2. Amenorrhea _____

3. Goiter _____

4. Cretinism _____

5. Thyroiditis _____

6. Pheochromocytoma _____

7. Myxedema _____

Matching 1

Match the abnormalities in the right column with the diseases in the left column.

1. _____ Acromegaly
2. _____ Amenorrhea–galactorrhea syndrome
3. _____ Exophthalmic goiter
4. _____ Addison disease
5. _____ Cushing disease
6. _____ Cushing syndrome
7. _____ Cretinism
8. _____ Chronic thyroiditis
9. _____ Hyperparathyroidism
10. _____ Hyperaldosteronism
11. _____ Pheochromocytoma

A. Neonatal hypothyroidism
B. ACTH-producing pituitary tumor
C. Growth hormone-secreting pituitary tumor
D. Administration of excess adrenal corticosteroids
E. Autoantibody-induced thyroid hyperfunction
F. Autoantibody-induced destruction of adrenal cortex
G. Autoantibody-induced destruction of thyroid gland
H. Prolactin-secreting pituitary tumor
I. Hormone-secreting parathyroid tumor
J. Catecholamine-secreting adrenal tumor
K. Aldosterone-secreting adrenal cortical tumor

Matching 2

Match the disease or condition in the left column with the features of the disease in the right column.

1. _____ Addison disease
2. _____ Cushing syndrome
3. _____ Hypertension with high aldosterone
4. _____ Hypertension with high catecholamines
5. _____ Amenorrhea–galactorrhea syndrome

A. Corticosteroid-producing adrenal tumor
B. Pituitary tumor
C. Adrenal medullary tumor
D. Aldosterone-producing adrenal tumor
E. Atrophy or destruction of adrenal glands

Discussion Questions

1. What are the major hormones produced by the anterior lobe of the pituitary gland? What factors regulate secretion of anterior lobe pituitary hormones? _____

_____

_____

_____

2. What is the effect of overproduction of growth hormone? _____

_____

_____

3. What factors regulate the rate of production of thyroid hormone? What are the major effects of an abnormal output of thyroid hormone? _____

_____

_____

_____

4. What is the difference between cretinism and myxedema? _____

_____

_____

_____

5. Why does the thyroid gland become enlarged in persons with a nontoxic goiter? _____

_____

_____

_____

6. What is the difference between chronic thyroiditis (Hashimoto disease) and thyrotoxicosis (Graves disease)? What are the roles played by autoantibodies in thepathogenesis of these diseases? _____

_____

_____

7. What are the main classes of adrenal cortical hormones, and what are their functions? _____

_____

_____

_____

8. What diseases result from adrenal cortical dysfunction? _____

_____

_____

9. How is parathyroid hormone output regulated? What are the possible effects of parathyroid dysfunction?

_____

_____

_____

10. A 27-year-old woman has small, diffuse toxic goiter. What manifestations would you expect in this patient?

_____

_____

_____

11. A 25-year-old woman has acromegaly. What manifestations would you expect in this patient? _____

_____

_____

_____

12. A 35-year-old woman has hypothyroidism caused by chronic thyroiditis. What manifestations would you expect in this condition?

_____

_____

_____

13. A 64-year-old man has Addison disease caused by atrophy of both adrenal glands. What clinical manifestations would you expect in this condition? _____

_____

_____

_____

14. A 46-year-old woman has Cushing disease associated with hyperplasia of both adrenal glands. What are the manifestations that are often encountered in this condition?

_____

_____

_____

_____

Notes

_____
_____
_____
_____
_____
_____
_____
_____
_____
_____
_____
_____
_____
_____
_____
_____
_____
_____
_____
_____
_____
_____
_____
_____
_____
_____
_____
_____
_____
_____
_____
_____
_____
_____
_____
_____
_____
_____
_____

Chapter 25

The Endocrine Glands

Learning Objectives (1 of 2)

- Explain normal physiologic functions of pituitary hormones, common endocrine disturbances, and treatment
- Describe major thyroid abnormalities, clinical manifestations, and treatment
- Explain normal physiologic functions of adrenal cortex and medulla, common disturbances, and treatment
- Define causes and effects of parathyroid dysfunction and treatment

Learning Objectives (2 of 2)

- Discuss concept of ectopic hormone production by nonendocrine tumors
- Explain adverse health effects of obesity, surgical procedures for obesity and their rationale
- Explain stress and its effects on the endocrine system

Endocrine Glands (1 of 2)

- Major endocrine glands
  - Pituitary
  - Thyroid
  - Parathyroid
  - Adrenal cortex and medulla
  - Pancreatic islets
  - Ovaries and testes

Endocrine Glands (2 of 2)

- Level of hormone in circulation: controls amount of hormone synthesized and released by an endocrine gland
- Disorders: hypersecretion or hyposecretion
- Determination of clinical effects
  - Degree of dysfunction
  - Age and sex of affected individual

Pituitary Gland (1 of 6)

- Suspended by stalk from hypothalamus at base of brain
  - Anterior lobe
  - Intermediate lobe: rudimentary structure
  - Posterior lobe
- Tropic hormones (regulate other endocrine glands)
  - Regulated by level of hormone produced by the target gland
  - Self-regulating mechanism maintains uniform hormone output
  - Prolactin secretion controlled by prolactin inhibitory factor
  - Thyroid stimulating hormone stimulates release of prolactin and thyroid hormones

Pituitary Gland (2 of 6)

- Anterior lobe hormones
  - Growth hormone: stimulates growth of tissues
  - Prolactin: stimulates milk production
  - Thyroid-stimulating hormone (TSH)
  - Adrenocorticotrophic hormone (ACTH)
  - Follicle-stimulating hormone (FSH)
  - Luteinizing hormone (LH)
- Posterior lobe hormones
  - Antidiuretic hormone (ADH): causes more concentrated urine
  - Oxytocin: stimulates uterine contractions and milk secretion

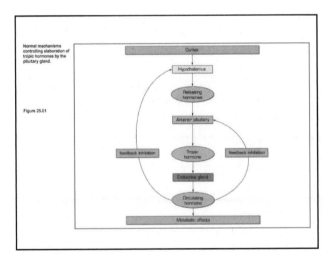

Normal mechanisms controlling elaboration of tropic hormones by the pituitary gland.

Figure 25.01

Pituitary Gland (3 of 6)

- Panhypopituitarism
  - Anterior lobe fails to secrete all hormones
- Pituitary dwarfism
  - Deficiency of growth hormone
  - Causes retarded growth and development
- Diabetes insipidus
  - Failure of posterior lobe to secrete ADH or failure of kidney to respond to ADH (nephrogenic diabetes insipidus)
  - Unable to absorb H_2O
  - Causes excretion of large amounts of diluted urine
  - From a pituitary tumor

Notes

Pituitary Gland (4 of 6)

- Growth hormone overproduction
  - Caused by pituitary adenoma
  - Causes **gigantism** in children
  - Causes **acromegaly** in adults
  - May cause visual disturbances from tumor encroachment in optic chiasm
- Prolactin overproduction
  - Result of small pituitary adenoma
  - Also from conditions affecting function of hypothalamus
  - Causes **amenorrhea and galactorrhea** (milk secretion from non-pregnant breasts)

Pituitary Gland (5 of 6)

- Pituitary tumors
  - Many pituitary endocrine disturbances caused by anterior lobe pituitary tumors
  - Clinical manifestations depend on size of tumor and the hormone produced
    - Functional tumors: produce hormones that cause clinical manifestations
    - Nonfunctional tumors: do not produce hormones but exert other effects
    - May encroach on important structures adjacent to optic chiasm; disrupt hormone-producing functions of anterior lobe cells

Pituitary Gland (6 of 6)

- Pituitary tumors
  - Treatment determined by type, size, and hormone produced by tumor
    - Drugs to suppress tumor growth
    - Surgical resection: usual surgical approach is through the nasal cavity (transsphenoidal resection)

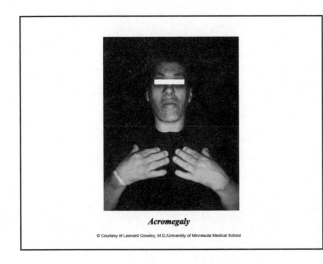

Acromegaly

© Courtesy of Leonard Crowley, M.D./University of Minnesota Medical School

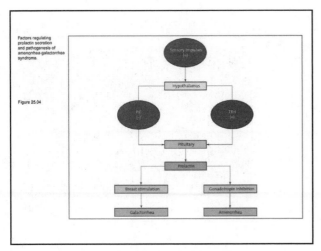

Factors regulating prolactin secretion and pathogenesis of amenorrhea-galactorrhea syndrome.

Figure 25.04

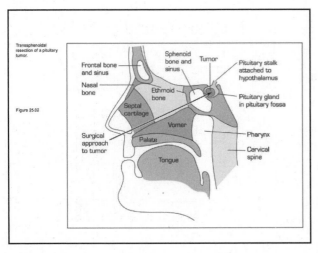

Transsphenoidal resection of a pituitary tumor.

Figure 25.02

The Endocrine Glands

Thyroid Gland

- Structure
- Two lateral lobes connected by isthmus
- Composed of thyroid follicles that produce and store hormones
- Hormone production regulated by TSH (thyroid stimulating hormone)
- Parafollicular cells: secrete calcitonin

- Actions
- Controls rate of metabolic processes
- Required for normal growth and development

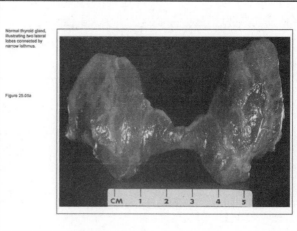

Normal thyroid gland, illustrating two lateral lobes connected by narrow isthmus.

Figure 25.05a

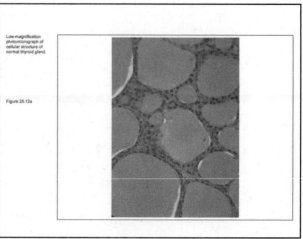

Low-magnification photomicrograph of cellular structure of normal thyroid gland.

Figure 25.12a

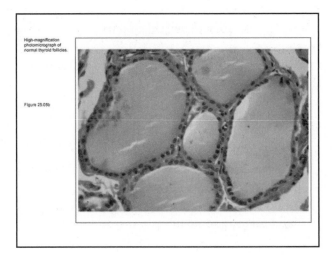

High-magnification photomicrograph of normal thyroid follicles.

Figure 25.05b

Thyroid Gland

Hyperthyroidism	Hypothyroidism
Rapid pulse	Slow pulse
Increased metabolism	Decreased metabolism
Hyperactive reflexes	Sluggish reflexes
Emotional lability	Placid and phlegmatic
GI effect: diarrhea	GI effect: constipation
Warm, moist skin	Cold, dry skin

Comparison of major effects of hyperthyroidism and hypothyroidism.

Table 25.01

TABLE 25-1

Comparison of major effects of hyperthyroidism and hypothyroidism		
	HYPERTHYROIDISM	HYPOTHYROIDISM
Cardiovascular effects	Rapid pulse, increased cardiac output.	Slow pulse, reduced cardiac output.
Metabolic effects	Increased metabolism, skin hot and flushed, weight loss	Decreased metabolism, cold skin, weight gain
Neuromuscular effects	Tremor, hyperactive reflexes	Weakness, lassitude, sluggish reflexes
Mental, emotional effects	Restlessness, irritability, emotional lability	Mental processes sluggish and retarded, personality placid and phlegmatic
Gastrointestinal effects	Diarrhea	Constipation
General somatic effects	Warm, moist skin	Cold, dry skin

Nontoxic Goiter

- Thyroid gland enlarges to increase hormone secretion
- Causes
  - Inadequate hormone output
  - Iodine deficiency
  - Enzyme deficiency
  - Inefficient enzyme function
  - Increased hormone requirements
- Treatment: administer thyroid hormone; may need surgical removal

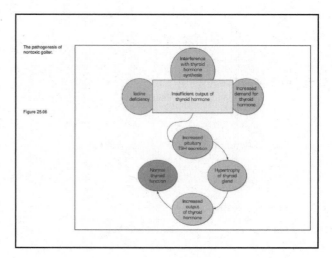

The pathogenesis of nontoxic goiter.

Figure 25.06

Hyperthyroidism

- Toxic goiter or Graves disease
- Caused by antithyroid antibody that stimulates gland
- Mimics effects of TSH but not subject to normal control mechanisms
- Treatment
  - Antithyroid drugs, thyroidectomy, large doses of radioactive iodine

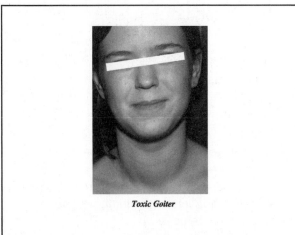

Toxic Goiter

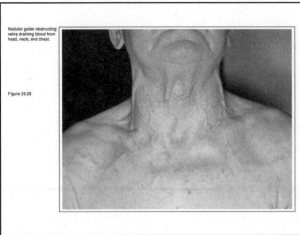

Nodular goiter obstructing veins draining blood from head, neck, and chest.

Figure 25.08

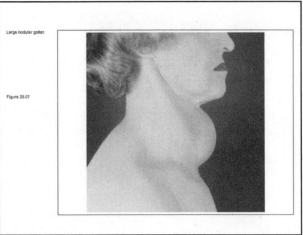

Large nodular goiter.

Figure 25.07

Hypothyroidism

- In adult
  - Myxedema
  - Causes metabolic slowing
  - Treatment: administration of thyroid hormone
- In an infant
  - Cretinism
  - Causes impaired growth and CNS development
  - Causes hypometabolism
  - Early diagnosis and treatment required for normal development

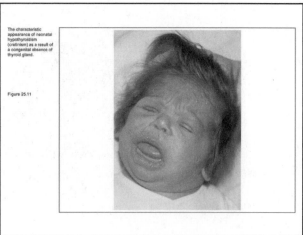

The characteristic appearance of neonatal hypothyroidism (cretinism) as a result of a congenital absence of thyroid gland.

Figure 25.11

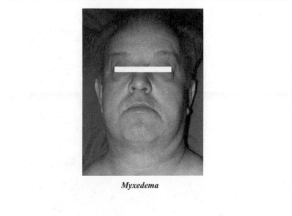

Myxedema

Chronic Thyroiditis or Hashimoto Thyroiditis

- Autoantibody destroys thyroid tissue
- Results in hypothyroidism
- An immunologic reaction, not from an infection
- Cellular infiltration from an immunologic reaction between antigen and antibody

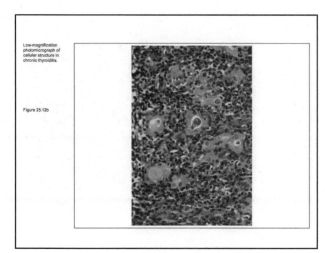

Low-magnification photomicrograph of cellular structure in chronic thyroiditis.

Figure 25.12b

Thyroid Tumors

- Benign adenoma
- Carcinoma
  - Well-differentiated follicular and papillary carcinoma
    - Good prognosis; treatment by surgical resection
  - Poorly-differentiated carcinoma
    - Poor prognosis; rapidly growing
    - Treatment: surgery, radiation, chemotherapy
  - Medullary carcinoma
    - Rare, secretes calcitonin

Radiation and Thyroid Tumors

- Radiation: increases incidence of benign and malignant thyroid tumors after latent period of 5-10 years
- Most tumors are well-differentiated and easily treated
- Persons who received head or neck radiation should have periodic follow-up examinations

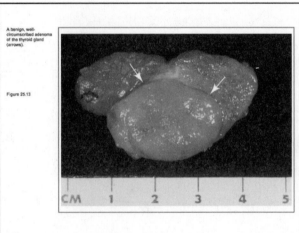

A benign, well-circumscribed adenoma of the thyroid gland (arrows).

Figure 25.13

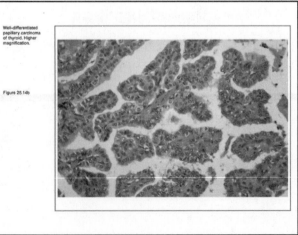

Well-differentiated papillary carcinoma of thyroid. Higher magnification.

Figure 25.14b

Parathyroid Glands

- Blood calcium level is in equilibrium with calcium in the bone
- Actions: Calcium level: regulated by parathyroid glands
  - Low calcium in blood: causes tetany (increased neuromuscular excitability causing spasm of skeletal muscle)
  - High calcium in blood: causes lowered neuromuscular excitability

Hyperparathyroidism

- Usually from a hormone-secreting parathyroid adenoma
- Effects
  - Hypercalcemia: blood calcium rises
  - Renal calculi: from excessive calcium excreted in urine
  - Calcium deposition in tissues
  - Decalcification of bone: from excessive calcium withdrawn from bone
- Treatment: Removal of tumor

Hypoparathyroidism

- Usually from accidental removal of parathyroid glands during thyroid surgery
- Effects
  - Hypocalcemia: blood calcium falls precipitously
  - Leads to neuromuscular excitability and tetany
- Treatment: raise calcium levels
  - High-calcium diet
  - Supplementary vitamin D

Notes

Adrenal Cortex (1 of 2)

- Adrenals: paired glands above kidneys
- Hormones secreted by adrenal cortex
  - Glucocorticoids
  - Mineralocorticoids
  - Aldosterone: major hormone
  - Renin-angiotensin system is main stimulus
  - Sex hormones
- Overproduction of aldosterone
  - From aldosterone-producing tumor of adrenal cortex
  - High sodium, blood volume, blood pressure
  - Low potassium level leading to neuromuscular manifestations

Adrenal Cortex (2 of 2)

- Overproduction of adrenal sex hormones
  - Congenital adrenal hyperplasia
  - Sex-hormone-producing tumors

Adrenal Medulla

- Produces catecholamines that stimulate the sympathetic nervous system
  - Norepinephrine (noradrenaline)
  - Epinephrine (adrenaline)
- Pheochromocytoma: increased secretion of catecholamines
  - Produces pronounced CV effects
  - May cause cerebral hemorrhage from hypertension
  - Any emotional stress causes release of hormones
  - Treatment: tumor resection

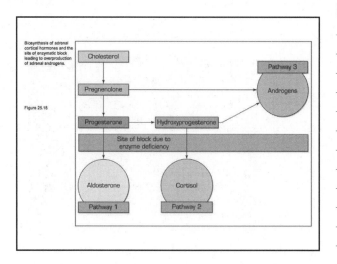

Biosynthesis of adrenal cortical hormones and the site of enzymatic block leading to overproduction of adrenal androgens.

Figure 25.18

Addison Disease

- An adrenal cortical hypofunction
- Deficiency of all steroid hormones
  - Glucocorticoid deficiency: hypoglycemia
  - Mineralocorticoid deficiency: lowblood volume and low blood pressure
  - Hyperpigmentation: from increased ACTH due to loss of feedback inhibition
- Autoimmune disorder
  - Treatment: administration of corticosteroids

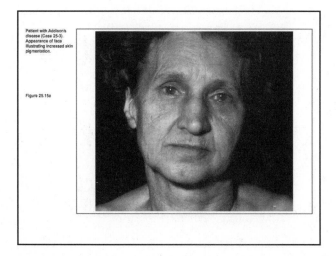

Patient with Addison's disease (Case 25-3). Appearance of face illustrating increased skin pigmentation.

Figure 25.15a

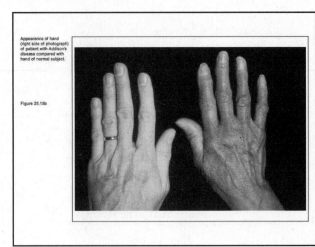

Appearance of hand (right side of photograph) of patient with Addison's disease compared with hand of normal subject.

Figure 25.15b

Cushing Disease

- Excessive production of adrenal corticosteroids
  - Glucocorticoid excess: disturbed carbohydrate, fat, and protein metabolism
  - Mineralocorticoid excess: high blood volume and high blood pressure
  - Treatment: tumor removal
- Causes
  - Hormone-producing pituitary microadenoma
  - Hormone-producing adrenal cortex adenoma
  - Hyperplastic adrenal glands
  - Administration of large amounts of corticosteroid
  - Other tumors

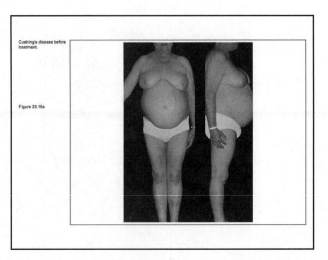

Cushing's disease before treatment.

Figure 25.16a

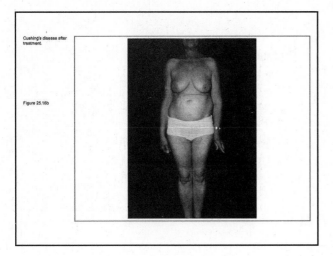

Cushing's disease after treatment.

Figure 25.16b

Overproduction of Other Adrenal Cortex Hormones

- Overproduction of aldosterone
  - Aldosterone secreting adenoma
- Overproduction of adrenal sex hormones
  - Congenital adrenal hyperplasia
  - Adrenal sex-hormone–producing tumor

Pancreatic Islets

- Pancreatic tissue that functions as an endocrine gland
- Produce hormones
  - Beta cells: insulin production
  - Alpha cells: glucagon
  - Delta cells: somatostatin

Gonads

- Function
  - Production of germ cells
  - Production of sex hormones: controlled by gonadotropic hormones of pituitary gland FSH and LH
- Tumors may secrete hormones
- Treatment: surgical excision

Nonendocrine Tumors

- Ectopic hormones: hormones secreted by nonendocrine tumors that are identical with or mimic action of true hormones
- Usual origin: produced by malignant tumors
- Lung, pancreas, kidneys, connective tissue

Stress and Endocrine System

- Stress: any event that disturbs homeostasis
- Causes: injury, surgery, prolonged exposure to cold, vigorous exercise, pain, or strong emotional stimulus such as anxiety or fear
- Acute response to stress
  - Fear-fight-flight reaction
  - Mediated by sympathetic nervous system and adrenal medulla
- Chronic response to stress: alters metabolism, taxes CV system, impairs inflammatory and immune responses
  - Involves adrenal cortex; predisposes to illness

Obesity (1 of 2)

- Occurs when caloric intake > requirements
- Usually NOT result of endocrine or metabolic disturbance
- Health consequences
  - Cardiovascular disease
  - Diabetes
  - Cancer
  - Musculoskeletal problems
  - Impaired pulmonary function

Obesity (2 of 2)

- Treatment
- Medical: diet
- Drugs: suppress appetite
  - Combination of fenfluramine and phentermine (fen-phen) causes heart valve damage
- Surgery
  - Ileal bypass: several complications, infrequently performed
  - Gastric bypass
  - Vertical-banded gastroplasty

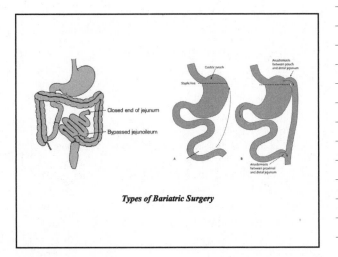

Types of Bariatric Surgery

Notes

_____

_____

_____

_____

_____

_____

_____

_____

_____

_____

_____

_____

_____

_____

_____

_____

_____

_____

_____

_____

_____

_____

_____

_____

_____

_____

_____

_____

_____

_____

_____

_____

_____

_____

_____

_____

_____

_____

_____

_____

_____

_____

_____

Discussion
• What are the major hormones produced by the pituitary gland?
• What are the major effects of abnormal output of thyroid hormone?
• What is the usual cause of obesity and its complications?

Chapter Outline

The chapter outline provides you with an organizational guide to the topics and ideas presented in this chapter of the text.

Study Questions

The following questions are provided as a test for comprehension and as a study guide for use with the text chapters. Additional study material is located at http://health.jbpub.com/humandisease/8e, which contains useful tools such as an A&P review, animated flashcards, an interactive online glossary, crossword puzzles, and web links.

Key Terms

Define the following terms:

1. Upper motor neuron lesion _____

2. Lower motor neuron lesion _____

3. Parkinson disease _____

4. Meningitis _____

5. Stroke _____

6. Anencephaly _____

Fill-in-the-Blank

1. The frequency of neural tube defects can be reduced significantly by ingestion of the vitamin _____ before conception and during pregnancy.

2. Failure of the cephalic end of the neural tube to close leads to a condition called _____, and failure of the caudal end to close properly leads to a condition called _____.

3. A stroke is a vascular injury to the brain that is classified as either an _____ or a _____.

4. A sac-like protrusion of the lining of a cerebral artery through a defect or weak area in the arterial wall is called a _____. The major complication of this condition is _____, and the treatment of this complication is _____.

5. A brief, temporary episode of neurologic dysfunction, followed by return of normal cerebral functions, is called a _____.

6. Recent onset of marked atrophy and weakness of skeletal muscles that were previously affected by poliomyelitis many years previously but were followed by complete recovery is called _____.

7. Creutzfeldt-Jakob disease is caused by an abnormal form of a protein called a _____. The disease may result either from a spontaneous mutation of a normal gene that codes for a normal protein or from _____.

8. This type of abnormal protein causes a disease in cows called _____, which can be transmitted to humans by _____.

9. A hereditary disease characterized by formation of multiple tumors arising from peripheral nerves is called _____.

10. Multiple sclerosis plaques within the brain can be demonstrated by a procedure called _____.

11. A poorly differentiated astrocytic tumor arising in older adults is called a _____.

12. A malignant brain tumor arising from the cerebellum in children is called a _____.

13. A brain tumor arising from the cerebral meninges is called a _____, and a brain tumor arising from the ependymal lining of the ventricular system is called an _____.

14. Persons with an immunodeficiency disease called _____ are prone to develop lymphomas of the nervous system that respond poorly to treatment.

True/False

Tell whether each statement is true or false. If false, explain why the statement is incorrect.

1. Postpolio syndrome is characterized by late onset of muscle atrophy, weakness, and fatigue many years after recovery from poliomyelitis. _____

_____

2. The abnormal form of the prion protein is identical to the normal form except for the configuration of the abnormal protein (the way the protein is folded). _____

_____

3. Mad cow disease is a type of rabies that causes cows to become aggressive and hostile. _____

_____

4. New-variant Creutzfeldt-Jakob disease is acquired by eating meat from cows infected with abnormal prions.

_____

Identify

1. What are the two principal types of neural tube defects?

a. _____

b. _____

2. Identify three neurologic manifestations of HIV infection.

a. _____

b. _____

c. _____

Discussion Questions

1. Briefly describe the organization of the central nervous system. Describe the function and circulation of cerebrospinal fluid. _____

_____

_____

_____

2. Describe how flaccid paralysis differs from spastic paralysis. _____

_____

_____

_____

_____

3. List or describe possible harmful effects of a severe blow to the head. _____

_____

_____

_____

4. Explain how atherosclerosis of a carotid artery can cause a stroke. _____

_____

_____

_____

5. What are the common causes of hydrocephalus? How does a brain tumor cause hydrocephalus? _____

_____

_____

_____

6. List and describe briefly the methods available to detect a neural tube defect in a fetus. _____

_____

_____

_____

7. Describe the two types of shunt procedures used to treat hydrocephalus, distinguishing between them with respect to the site of drainage from the shunt. _____

_____

_____

_____

8. What is a brief episode of neurologic dysfunction that subsides spontaneously in a short time? _____

_____

_____

_____

9. What are the effects of hydrocephalus in a middle-aged adult? _____

_____

_____

_____

10. What is a congenital aneurysm of the circle of Willis? _____

_____

_____

_____

Chapter 26   The Nervous System

Notes

_____
_____
_____
_____
_____
_____
_____
_____
_____
_____
_____
_____
_____
_____
_____
_____
_____
_____
_____
_____
_____
_____
_____
_____
_____
_____
_____
_____
_____
_____
_____
_____
_____
_____
_____
_____
_____
_____

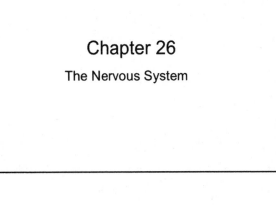

Chapter 26
The Nervous System

Learning Objectives (1 of 2)

- Describe normal structure and function of the brain, meninges, CSF in relation to neurologic disease
- Define muscle tone, voluntary motor activity and relate to two forms of muscle paralysis
- Explain pathogenesis, prenatal diagnosis, clinical manifestations of closure defects of the CNS
- Describe pathogenesis, clinical manifestations of hydrocephalus and relate to treatment measures
- Describe causes, manifestations, treatment of transient ischemic attack, TIA

Learning Objectives (2 of 2)

- Differentiate types of stroke as to pathogenesis, prognosis, and treatment
- Describe pathogenesis, manifestations, treatment of congenital cerebral aneurysms
- Explain pathogenesis, origin, clinical manifestations, and treatment of CNS tumors
- Explain pathogenesis, clinical manifestations, and treatment of Parkinson's disease, meningitis, multiple sclerosis, and Guillian Barre syndrome

Nervous System

- Central nervous system, CNS
  - Brain
  - Spinal cord
- Meninges: surrounding membranes
  - Neurons (nerve cells) and neuroglia (supporting cells)
  - Sensory or afferent nerve: transmits impulses to the nervous system
  - Motor or efferent nerve: transmits impulses from brain or spinal cord to muscle
  - Transmission of a nerve impulse via neurotransmitters
    - Acetylcholine, norepinephrine, dopamine

Meninges

- Dura: firm, outer covering
- Arachnoid: middle
  - Subarachnoid space: space between arachnoid and pia contains
    - CSF (cerebrospinal fluid)
    - Strands of arachnoid connective tissue
- **Pia**: thin, inner membrane
  - Adheres to brain and spinal cord

Brain

- Cerebrum
- Cerebellum
- Brain stem
- Brain: four cavities called ventricles
  - Tissues of brain and spinal cord
    - Nerve cells = neurons
    - Supporting cells = neuroglia
  - Arterial blood supply
    - Large vessels enter base of skull
    - Vessels join to form arterial circle at base of brain
  - Venous blood
    - From brain into large venous sinuses in dura
    - Sinuses eventually drain into jugular veins

Development of Nervous System

- Neural plate becomes neural tube
- Forebrain forms cerebral hemispheres and diencephalon
- Midbrain and hindbrain form remainder of adult brain
- Mesoderm surrounding neural tube forms cranial cavity, vertebral bodies, and surrounding structures

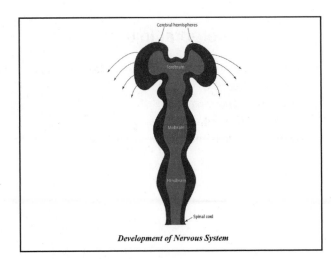

Development of Nervous System

Voluntary Motor Activity

- Controlled by nerve impulses originating in motor neurons of the cerebral cortex (cortical neurons)
- Muscle tone caused by reflex arcs
- Pyramidal system controls voluntary motor functions
- Extrapyramidal system regulates muscle groups concerned with automatic functions such as walking

Muscle Paralysis

- Flaccid paralysis
  - Destruction of motor neurons by disease
  - Interruption of reflex arc responsible for muscle tone
  - Muscle deprived of innervation
  - Low muscle tone
  - Peripheral nerve destruction
- Spastic paralysis
  - Reflex arc not disturbed
  - Injury to cortical neurons stops voluntary control
  - Muscle retains innervation
  - Increased muscle tone

Cerebral Injury

- Large blood vessels over surface of brain may be torn by force of injury
  - Epidural hemorrhage
  - Subdural hemorrhage
  - Subarachnoid hemorrhage

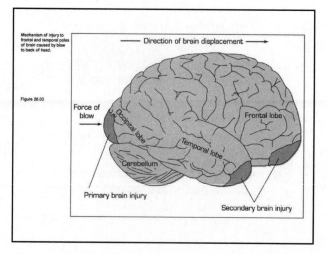

Mechanism of injury to frontal and temporal poles of brain caused by blow to back of head.

Figure 26.03

Direction of brain displacement

Force of blow

Occipital lobe

Frontal lobe

Temporal lobe

Cerebellum

Primary brain injury

Secondary brain injury

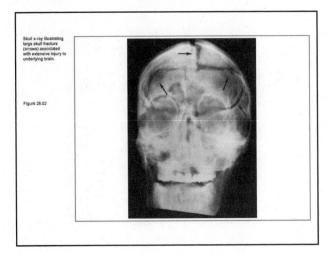

Skull x-ray illustrating large skull fracture (arrows) associated with extensive injury to underlying brain.

Figure 26.02

Neural Tube Defects

- Anencephaly
  - Failure of normal development of brain and cranial cavity
  - Multifactorial inheritance
- Spina bifida
  - Diagnosis: amniocentesis and alpha-fetoprotein levels
  - Alpha-fetoprotein leaks from fetal blood into amnionic fluid through open neural tube defect; high levels found in amnionic fluid
    - Occult
    - Meningocele
    - Meningomyelocele

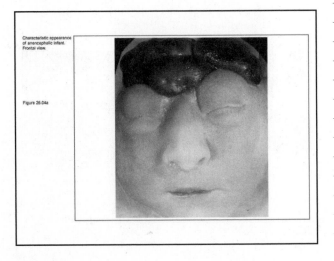

Characteristic appearance of anencephalic infant. Frontal view.

Figure 26.04a

Notes

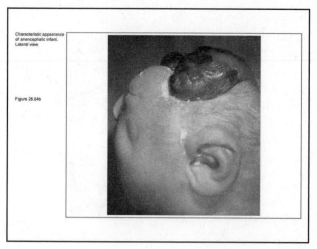

Characteristic appearance of anencephalic infant. Lateral view.

Figure 26.04b

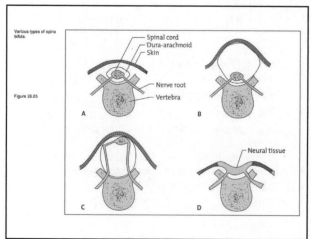

Various types of spina bifida.

Figure 26.05

Spinal cord
Dura-arachnoid
Skin

Nerve root
Vertebra

A

B

C

D

Neural tissue

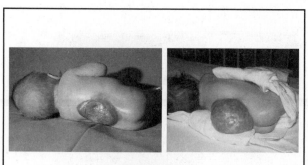

Neural Tube Defects
A. Thoracic meningomyelocele covered by thin membrane
B. Large meningomyelocele associated with neurologic deficit

Hydrocephalus

- Congenital hydrocephalus
  - From congenital obstruction of aqueduct or absence of openings in roof of 4th ventricle
  - Head enlarges as ventricles dilate because cranial structures have not fused
- Acquired hydrocephalus
  - Obstruction of CSF by tumor or adhesions blocking opening in 4th ventricle
  - Ventricles dilate but head does not enlarge because cranial structures are fused

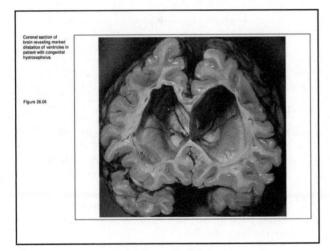

Coronal section of brain revealing marked dilatation of ventricles in patient with congenital hydrocephalus.

Figure 26.08

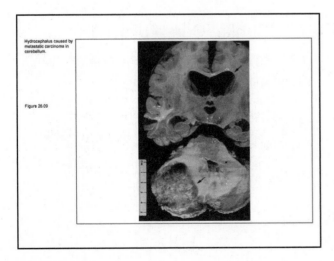

Hydrocephalus caused by metastatic carcinoma in cerebellum.

Figure 26.09

Notes

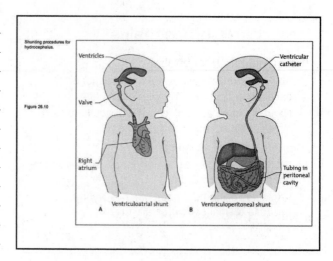

Shunting procedures for hydrocephalus.

Figure 26.10

Ventricles
Ventricular catheter
Valve
Right atrium
Tubing in peritoneal cavity
A Ventriculoatrial shunt
B Ventriculoperitoneal shunt

Stroke: Cerebrovascular Accident (1 of 5)

- Any injury to brain tissue from disturbance of blood supply to brain
- Types of stroke
  - Cerebral thrombosis: most common; thrombosis of cerebral artery narrowed by arteriosclerosis
  - Cerebral embolus: occurs less frequently; blockage of cerebral artery by fragment of blood clot from an arteriosclerotic plaque or from heart
  - Cerebral hemorrhage: most serious type of stroke; usually from rupture of a cerebral artery in person with hypertension

---

Stroke: Cerebrovascular Accident (2 of 5)

- Predisposing Factors
  - 1. Mural thrombus formed on wall of left ventricle adjacent to a healing myocardial infarction
  - 2. Thrombus formed on rough surface of diseased mitral or aortic valve
  - 3. Small thrombus in left atrium of person with atrial fibrillation

Stroke: Cerebrovascular Accident (3 of 5)

- Ischemic infarct: no blood leaks into brain
- Hemorrhagic infarct: blood leaks into damaged brain tissue
- Arteriosclerosis of extracranial arteries
  - Sclerosis of a major artery from aorta that supply brain
  - Common affected site: carotid artery in neck; arteriosclerotic plaque may narrow lumen and reduce cerebral blood flow

Stroke: Cerebrovascular Accident (4 of 5)

- Diagnosis
  - Cerebral angiogram
  - Carotid endarterectomy
  - Less invasive methods: similar to balloon angioplasty and stent insertion procedures used to treat coronary artery plaques

Stroke: Cerebrovascular Accident (5 of 5)

- CT scan: can distinguish a cerebral infarct from cerebral hemorrhage
- Magnetic resonance imaging (MRI): provides similar information and is equally effective

Notes

An angiogram revealing narrowing of the carotid artery in the neck (arrows).

Figure 26.15

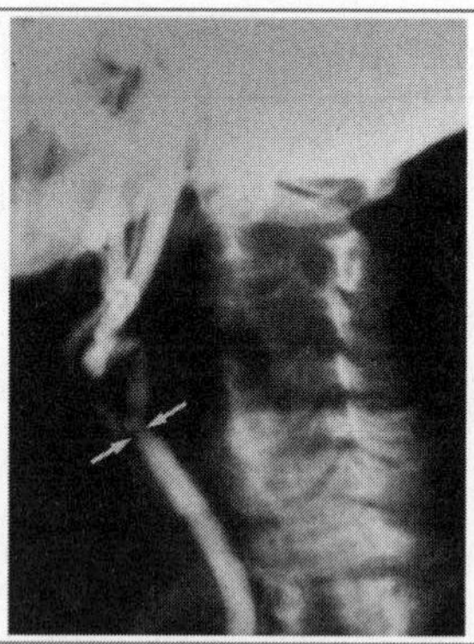

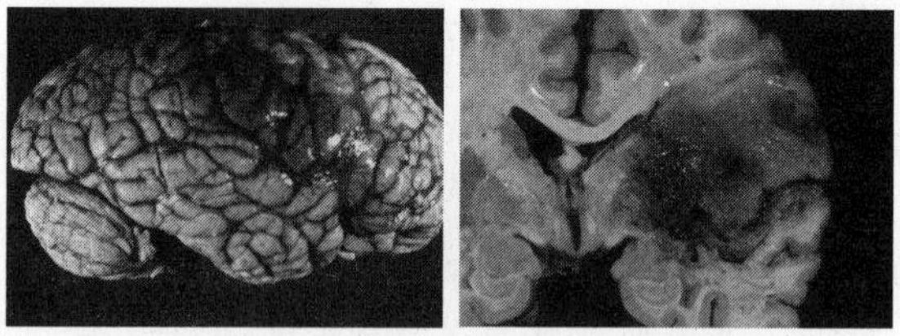

Infarct, right cerebral hemisphere from thrombosis of middle cerebral artery

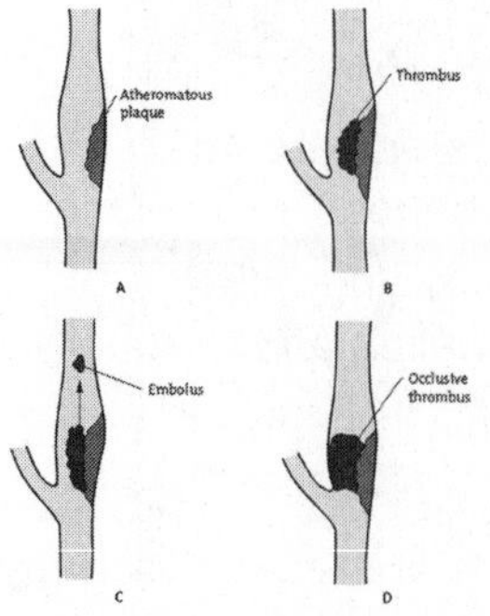

Effects of atherosclerosis of carotid artery

A. Narrowing of lumen
B. Thrombus formation
C. Thrombus dislodged & forms emboli
D. Complete occlusion of artery by thrombus

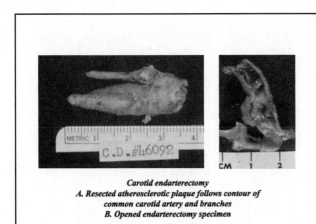

Carotid endarterectomy
A. Resected atherosclerotic plaque follows contour of
common carotid artery and branches
B. Opened endarterectomy specimen

Coronal section of
brain illustrating large
cerebral hemorrhage that
has compressed and
displaced the cerebral
ventricles.

Figure 26.17

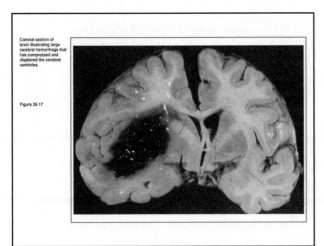

A computed tomographic
(CT) scan of a patient
with cerebral hemorrhage
(arrow), which appears
white because blood is
denser than brain tissue.

Figure 26.18

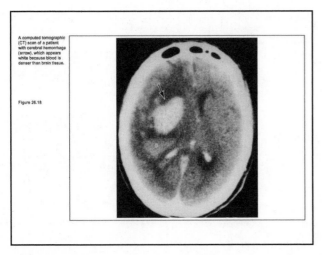

The Nervous System

Transient Ischemic Attack, TIA

- Brief episodes of neurologic disfunction
  - From embolization of material from plaque in carotid artery
  - One-third of patients eventually suffer major stroke
- Treatment: endarterectomy or medical therapy

Cerebral Aneurysm

- Congenital aneurysm of circle of Willis
  - Congenital weakness in arterial wall allows lining to protrude
  - Weakness is congenital but aneurysm develops in adult life
  - Rupture causes subarachnoid hemorrhage
  - Hypertension predisposes
  - Treatment: aneurysm occluded surgically
- Arteriosclerotic aneurysm
  - Cerebral artery dilates and compresses adjacent tissue
  - Rupture uncommon

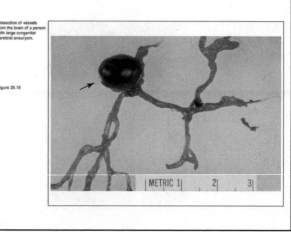

Dissection of vessels from the brain of a person with large congenital cerebral aneurysm.

Figure 26.19

METRIC 1   2   3

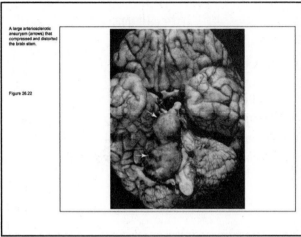

A large arteriosclerotic aneurysm (arrows) that compressed and distorted the brain stem.

Figure 26.22

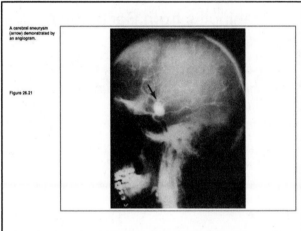

A cerebral aneurysm (arrow) demonstrated by an angiogram.

Figure 26.21

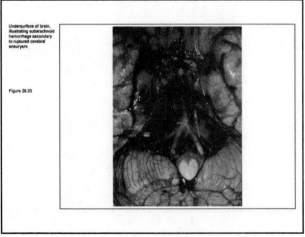

Undersurface of brain, illustrating subarachnoid hemorrhage secondary to ruptured cerebral aneurysm.

Figure 26.20

Notes

Infections

- Three types
  - Bacterial
  - Fungal
  - Viral
- Meningitis: infection affecting meninges
- Encephalitis: infection of brain tissue
- Meningoencephalitis: affects both meninges and brain tissue

Meningitis from Bacteria and Fungi

- Meningococcus (*Neisseria meningiditis*)
- Pneumococcus (*Streptococcus pneumoniae*)
- *Hemophilus influenzae*

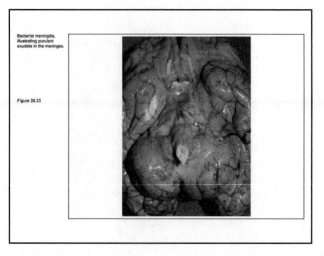

Bacterial meningitis, illustrating purulent exudate in the meninges.

Figure 26.23

Viral Infections That Affect the CNS (1 of 2)

- Measles, mumps, herpes simplex virus, intestinal and respiratory viruses, cytomegalovirus, poliomyelitis virus, and arboviruses
  - Manifestations
    - Systemic symptoms
    - Aseptic meningitis: caused by a virus
    - Suppurative meningitis: pus-producing; caused by bacteria
    - Encephalitis: brain tissue involvement
    - Spinal fluid abnormalities

Viral Infections That Affect the CNS (2 of 2)

- Arboviruses: responsible for cases of meningitis and encephalitis
  - Viruses infect birds, animals, humans; transmitted by mosquitoes
- Types of encephalitis
  - Western equine encephalitis
  - Eastern equine encephalitis
  - St. Louis encephalitis
  - California encephalitis
  - West Nile virus: "foreign" virus from Africa, first case identified in 1999 in New York City area

Creutzfeldt-Jakob Disease

- Caused by small protein particle produced as a result of gene **mutation**
  - Normal form of protein: "good prion" designated as PrPc
  - Abnormal form: "bad prion" designated as PrPsc
- Mad cow disease
  - Prion disease affecting cows
  - Cows become infected from animal feed mixed with protein-rich tissue from sheep infected with scrapie
  - Eating infected beef causes variant Creutzfeldt-Jakob disease in humans

Notes

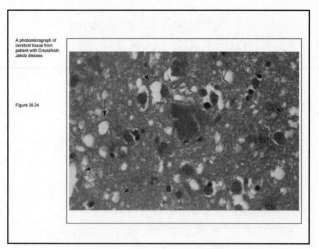

A photomicrograph of cerebral tissue from patient with Creutzfeldt-Jakob disease.

Figure 26.24

Alzheimer Disease

- Characteristics
  - Progressive mental deterioration
  - Emotional disturbances
- Anatomic and biochemical features
  - Neurofibrillary tangles: thickening of neurofilaments
  - Neurotic plaques: clusters of thick, broken neurofilaments
  - Biochemical abnormalities and brain enzyme deficiencies: acetylcholine and acetylcholine synthesizing enzyme
- No specific treatment; some drugs may temporarily improve cerebral function

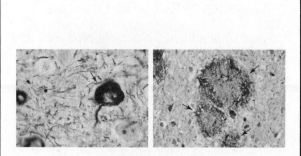

Alzheimer Disease
Thickened neurofilaments forming neurofibrillary tangles

Multiple Sclerosis

- Probably an autoimmune disease in generally predisposed individual
- Random foci of demyelination followed by glial scarring
- Neurologic symptoms depend on location of plaques
- Probably initiated by a viral infection in a genetically predisposed person
- Manifestations
  - Activated T lymphocytes, monocytes target myelin proteins, destroy myelin
- Treatment
  - MRI demonstrates plaques in CNS

Notes

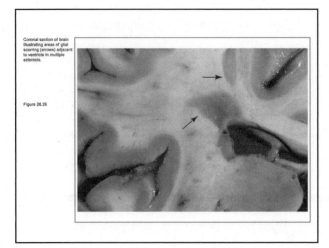

Coronal section of brain illustrating areas of glial scarring (arrows) adjacent to ventricle in multiple sclerosis.

Figure 26.26

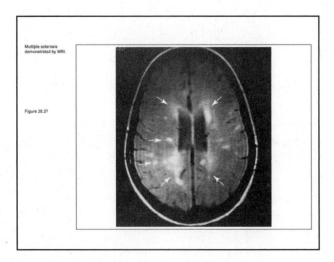

Multiple sclerosis demonstrated by MRI.

Figure 26.27

Parkinson Disease

- Most cases unknown etiology
- Some develop subsequent to viral infection of nervous system or toxic drugs
- Manifestations
  - Progressive loss of neurons in substantia nigra of midbrain
  - Rigidity of voluntary muscles
  - Tremors of fingers and extremities
  - Decreased dopamine in CNS
- Treatment: relieved by L-dopa
  - Embryonic stem cells may be key to successful treatment; possible to induce stem cells to differentiate into dopamine-producing neurons to treat disease

Huntington Disease

- Progressive hereditary autosomal dominant disease
- Abnormal gene contains too many CAG triplet repeats
- Greater number of repeats, the earlier the onset
- Uncommon but well-known hereditary disease
- Manifestations
  - Progressive mental deterioration; abnormal jerky and writhing movements
  - First manifestations occur between age 30 to 50
  - Progresses and usually fatal within 15 to 20 years
  - No way to arrest progression of disease
  - Drugs may help control some of its manifestations

Degenerative Disease of Motor Neurons

- Affects both upper and lower motor neurons
- From degeneration of neurons
- Causes: weakness, paralysis, respiratory problems
- No specific treatment
- Amyotrophic lateral sclerosis, ALS
  - Affects upper and lower motor neurons
  - Flaccid paralysis of muscles
  - Respiratory problems

Tumors of Peripheral Nerves

- Usually solitary; from Schwann cells
- Neuromas of cranial nerves: usually involves acoustic nerve; difficult to remove surgically
- Multiple nerve tumors occur in multiple neurofibromatosis
  - Transmitted as Mendelian dominant trait
  - Disfiguring skin nodules, thickened patches of skin, focal hyperpigmentation of skin
  - Sarcoma arises from preexisting tumors in 10-15% of cases

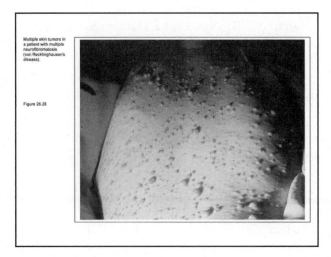

Multiple skin tumors in a patient with multiple neurofibromatosis (von Recklinghausen's disease).

Figure 26.28

Brain Tumors

- Metastatic tumors more common than primary tumors
- Primary tumors
  - Glioma: mostly poor prognosis with deep location in brain; surgery, radiation, chemotherapy; includes ependymoma and medulloblastoma
  - Astrocytoma
  - Glioblastoma multiforme
  - Oligodendroglioma
  - Lymphoma
  - Meningioma

Spinal Cord Tumors

- Same types of tumors that arise in brain
- Tumors in spinal vertebrae may extend from vertebrae to compress or invade spinal cord
  - Bone metastasis
  - Multiple myeloma

Peripheral Nerve Disorders (1 of 2)

- Peripheral nerve injury
  - Traumatic injury: lacerations, fractures, crush injury
  - Nerve entrapment neuropathy
    - External compression by fibrous band
    - Median nerve commonly involved
    - May require surgical release if unresponsive to conservative treatment
- Polyneuritis (Peripheral neuritis)
  - Sensory and motor dysfunction in "glove and stocking" distribution
  - Proximal sensation and motor function preserved
  - From systemic disease, toxins, alcoholism
  - Treat underling cause

Peripheral Nerve Disorders (2 of 2)

- Guillain Barré syndrome (Idiopathic polyneuritis)
  - **Patchy demyelination of nerves and nerve roots** with mild inflammation and sometimes, axon degeneration
  - Autoimmune reaction to myelin triggered by preceding viral infection
  - Progressive weakness followed by complete recovery
  - No specific treatment

HIV: Neurologic Manifestations

- Nervous system infections directly caused by AIDS virus
  - Acute viral meningitis
  - AIDS encephalopathy: chronic and progressive
  - Polyneuritis
- Nervous system infections caused by opportunistic pathogens
- Manifestations depend on location and extent of damage
  - Herpes
  - Cytomegalovirus
  - *Cryptococcus neoformans*
  - *Toxoplasma gondii*

AIDS-Related Tumors

- Primary tumor metastasizing to nervous system
  - Kaposi's sarcoma
  - Lymphoma
  - Other malignant tumors
- Primary lymphoma of brain may occur
- Tumors respond poorly to treatment

Discussion

- Which statement is TRUE regarding stroke?
  - A. Paralysis on right side of the body results from a stroke in the right cerebral hemisphere.
  - B. Flaccid paralysis occurs from a brain injury that damages the lower motor neurons.
  - C. Spastic paralysis occurs from a brain injury that damages lower motor neurons.
  - D. Smoking and use of oral contraceptives in women have no impact on their risk for stroke.
  - E. Cerebral embolism is the most serious type of stroke and is frequently fatal due to extensive bleeding into the brain tissue.

Notes

Chapter Outline

The chapter outline provides you with an organizational guide to the topics and ideas presented in this chapter of the text.

Structure and Function of the Skeletal System
  Bone Formation
  Bone Growth
Congenital Malformations
  Abnormal Bone Formation
  Malformation of Fingers and Toes
  Congenital Clubfoot (Talipes)
  Congenital Dislocation of the Hip
Arthritis
  Rheumatoid Arthritis
  Osteoarthritis
  Gout
Fracture
Osteomyelitis
  Hematogenous Osteomyelitis
  Osteomyelitis as a Result of Direct Implantation of Bacteria
  Clinical Manifestations and Treatment
Tumors of Bone
Osteoporosis
Avascular Necrosis
Structure and Function of the Spine
Scoliosis
Intervertebral Disk Disease
Structure and Function of Skeletal Muscle
  Contraction of Skeletal Muscle
  Factors Affecting Muscular Structure and Function
Inflammation of Muscle (Myositis)
  Localized Myositis
  Generalized Myositis
Muscular Atrophy and Muscular Dystrophy
Myasthenia Gravis

Study Questions

The following questions are provided as a test for comprehension and as a study guide for use with the text chapters. Additional study material is located at http://health.jbpub.com/humandisease/8e, which contains useful tools such as an A&P review, animated flashcards, an interactive online glossary, crossword puzzles, and web links.

Key Terms

Define the following terms:

1. Endochondral bone formation _____

2. Fracture _____

3. Intervertebral disks _____

4. Rheumatoid arthritis _____

Fill-in-the-Blank

1. In a long bone, the thick tubular part is called the _____, and the end is called the _____.

2. The active bone-forming cells are called _____. The mature cells that become incorporated in the bone as it forms are called _____, and the large multinucleated cells that are concerned with bone resorption are called _____.

3. In a movable joint, the ends of the bones forming the joint are covered by _____, and the interior of the joint is lined by _____, which secretes _____ to lubricate the joint.

4. The two types of bone formation are called _____ bone formation and _____ bone formation.

5. The hereditary condition characterized by disturbed endochondral bone formation that leads to a type of dwarfism in which the limbs are disproportionately short in relation to the trunk is called _____.

6. The congenital abnormality characterized by very thin, delicate bones that are easily broken under very minimal stress is called _____.

7. The name of the congenital condition in which the foot is turned inward on the ankle is called _____.

8. The inflammatory change in rheumatoid arthritis involves _____ initially, followed by spread of the inflammatory process over the surface of the joint.

9. A fracture in which the bone is broken into several fragments is called a _____ fracture.

10. A fracture in which the overlying skin is disrupted is called a _____ fracture.

11. The parts of the intervertebral disks are the _____ and the _____.

12. The condition characterized by a lateral curvature of the spine is called _____.

13. A systemic (collagen) disease characterized by inflammation of muscles and overlying skin is called _____ _____.

14. A disease characterized by atrophy of muscles resulting from degeneration of the nerve cells supplying the muscles is called _____.

15. A disease characterized by atrophy and degeneration of muscles caused by abnormalities in the muscle fibers is called _____.

16. The autoimmune disease characterized by muscle weakness that is caused by progressive autoantibody-mediated damage to acetylcholine receptors at the myoneural junction of the muscle fiber is called _____.

17. The two forms of muscular dystrophy are type _____ and type _____. The method of inheritance is _____. Sometimes the muscles of affected patients appear large because the muscle fibers have been replaced by _____.

True/False

Tell whether each statement is true or false. If false, explain why the statement is incorrect.

1. The blood and synovial tissues of rheumatoid arthritis (RA) patients contain an autoantibody directed against the patients' own gamma globulin. _____

_____

2. Immune complexes composed of gamma globulin and autoantibody are deposited in joints of RA patients. _____

_____

3. Antigen–antibody complexes activate complement and generate an inflammation within the joints in RA patients. _____

_____

4. Lymphocytes and macrophages attracted to the joints by the RA inflammatory process secrete cytokines (tumor necrosis factor) that damages joints. _____

_____

5. Drugs that block the effects of tumor necrosis factor have not been useful or effective in treating RA patients. _____

_____

Identify

1. Construct a table comparing the three main types of arthritis. (*Hint:* see Table 27-1.)

Characteristics	Rheumatoid Arthritis	Osteoarthritis	Gout

Matching

Match the types of arthritis on the right with each disease characteristic on the left.

1. ____ Affects primarily small bones of hands and feet   A. Osteoarthritis

2. ____ Autoantibodies formed   B. Rheumatoid arthritis

3. ____ Disturbed purine metabolism   C. Gout

4. ____ Major weight-bearing joints involved

5. ____ Fragmentation and degeneration of articular cartilage

6. ____ Destructive cytokines produced by inflammatory cells

7. ____ Uric acid deposit in and around joints

8. ____ May lead to kidney damage

Discussion Questions

1. What is a "slipped disk"? Why does it occur? Why does it sometimes produce pain radiating down the leg? How is it treated? _____

_____

_____

_____

2. Explain whether each of the following descriptors applies to rheumatoid arthritis.

   a. Primarily a degenerative change involving major weight-bearing joints _____

   _____

   b. Deformities result from joint instability caused by destruction of articular surfaces or joints _____

   _____

   c. Associated with autoantibodies _____

   _____

   d. Involves the synovial linings _____

   _____

   e. Responds to antibiotic therapy _____

   _____

3. List the features that characterize gout. _____

_____

_____

_____

4. What neoplastic processes may involve bone? _____

_____

_____

_____

5. What disease or condition affecting the skeletal system is due primarily to endocrine gland dysfunction?

_____

_____

_____

6. What is a herniated intervertebral disk? How does it occur? How is it detected? _____

_____

_____

_____

7. What is osteoporosis? What is the cause? How can it be prevented? _____

_____

_____

_____

Notes

Chapter 27

The Musculoskeletal System

Learning Objectives (1 of 2)

- Name common congenital abnormalities of the skeletal system
- Describe three major types of arthritis, pathogenesis, clinical manifestations, and treatment
- Describe causes and effects of osteoporosis, and methods of treatment
- Describe structure and functions of intervertebral disks; clinical manifestations of herniated disk

Learning Objectives (2 of 2)

- Describe pathogenesis, manifestations, and treatment of **myasthenia gravis**
- Describe manifestations, complications, and treatment of **scoliosis**
- Compare pathogenesis, common types, and clinical manifestations of muscular atrophy and dystrophy

Skeletal System (1 of 2)

- Skeleton: rigid supporting structure of the body
  - All bones have same basic structure
    - Cortex: outer layer of compact bone, the cortex
    - Trabeculae: inner spongy layer arranged in a loose meshed lattice of thin strands
    - Bone marrow: spaces between trabeculae consist of fat and blood-forming tissue
- Bone: specialized type of connective tissue
  - Composed of a dense connective tissue framework impregnated with calcium phosphate salts
  - Continually broken down and reformed

Skeletal System (2 of 2)

- Types of cells in bone
  - Osteoblasts
  - Osteocytes
  - Osteoclasts
- Strength and thickness of bones depend on activity
- Bones of skeleton are connected by joints
- Types of joints
  - Fibrous joint
  - Cartilaginous joint
  - Synovial joint

Bone Formation

- Intramembranous
  - Mesoderm transformed into osteoblasts that are converted into bone
- Endochondral
  - Cartilage model converted into bone

Congenital Malformations (1 of 2)

- Achondroplasia
  - Faulty endochondral bone formation
  - Impaired growth of extremities and formation of skull bones
  - Causes dwarfism with disproportionately short limbs
- Osteogenesis imperfecta
  - Thin and delicate bones easily broken
  - May be born with multiple fractures
  - Malformation of fingers and toes
  - Extra digits or polydactyly
  - Easily removed
  - Fused digits more difficult to correct

Congenital Malformations (2 of 2)

- Congenital clubfoot (talipes)
  - Multifactorial inheritance
  - Most common type: talipes equinavarus
  - Treatment: manipulation and casts
- Congenital dislocation of the hip
  - Multifactorial inheritance
  - More common in females
  - Shallow acetabulum causes femoral head to be displaced out of socket
  - Breech position favors development
  - Treatment: manipulation and casts

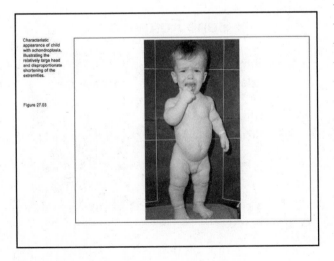

Characteristic appearance of child with achondroplasia, illustrating the relatively large head and disproportionate shortening of the extremities.

Figure 27.03

Notes

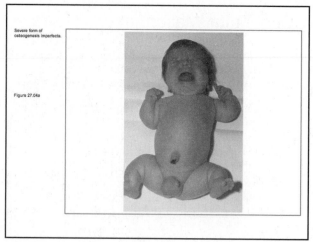

Severe form of osteogenesis imperfecta.

Figure 27.04a

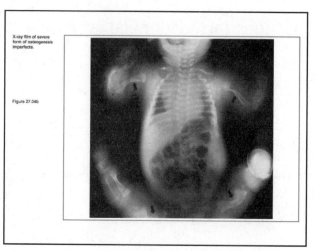

X-ray film of severe form of osteogenesis imperfecta.

Figure 27.04b

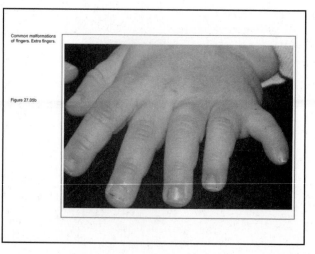

Common malformations of fingers. Extra fingers.

Figure 27.05b

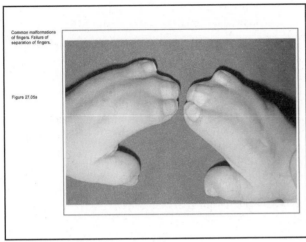

Common malformations of fingers. Failure of separation of fingers.

Figure 27.05a

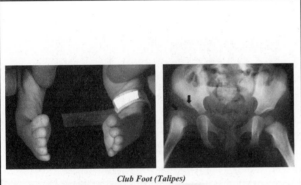

Club Foot (Talipes)

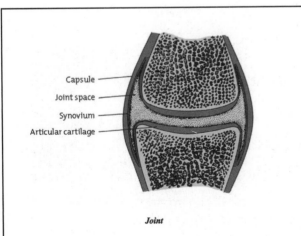

Capsule
Joint space
Synovium
Articular cartilage

Joint

Rheumatoid Arthritis (RA)

- Systemic disease affecting connective tissues throughout the body, specially the joints
- Produces chronic inflammation and thickening of synovial membrane
- Classified as an autoimmune disease
- Rheumatoid factor: autoantibody in blood and synovial tissues; produced by B lymphocytes directed against individual's own gamma globulin
- Encountered most frequently in young men and middle-aged women
- Usually affects small joints of hands and feet
- Dislocation from joint instability

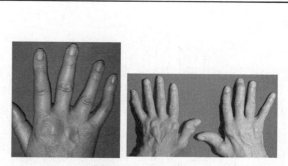

Rheumatoid Arthritis (RA)

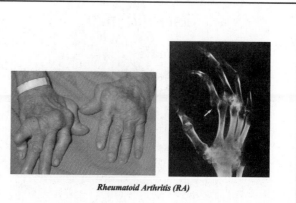

Rheumatoid Arthritis (RA)

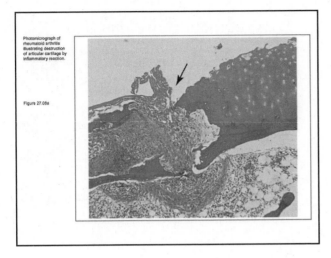

Photomicrograph of rheumatoid arthritis illustrating destruction of articular cartilage by inflammatory reaction.

Figure 27.08a

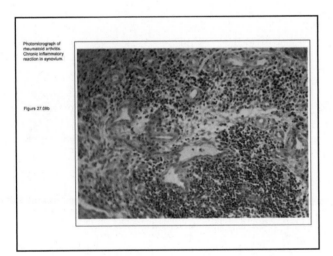

Photomicrograph of rheumatoid arthritis. Chronic inflammatory reaction in synovium.

Figure 27.08b

Osteoarthritis

- Not a systemic disease
- "Wear and tear" degeneration of one or more weight-bearing joints
- Causes degeneration of articular cartilage
- Seen in older adults, considered a manifestation of normal aging process
- Treatment: drugs; joint replacement if severe

Notes

Knee joint, illustrating smooth articular surface of femoral condyles.

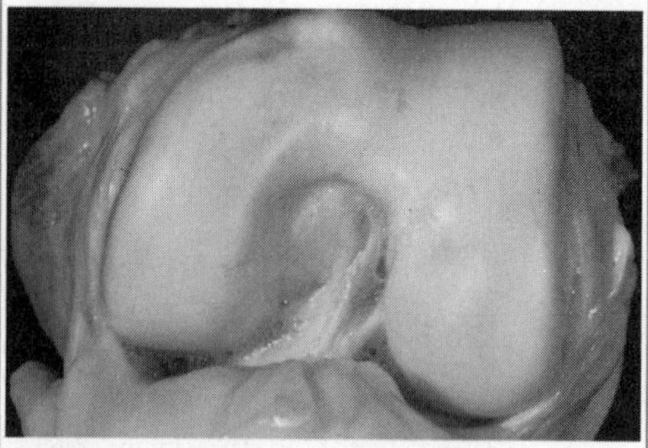

Figure 27.11a

Advanced osteoarthritis.

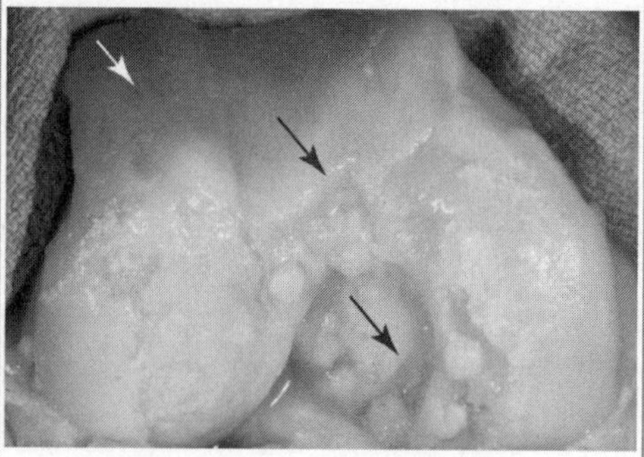

Figure 27.11c

Osteoarthritis.

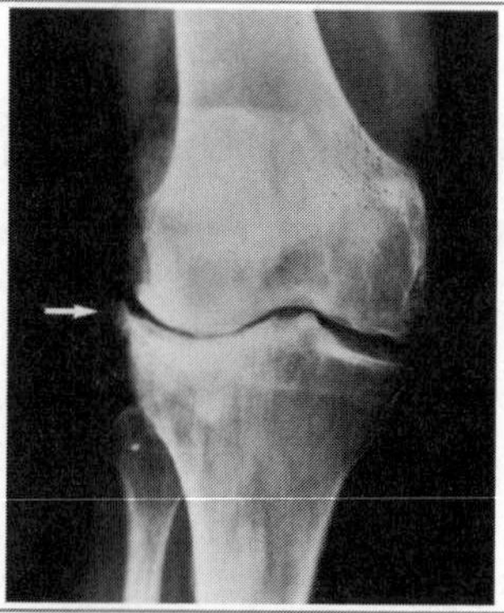

Figure 27.12

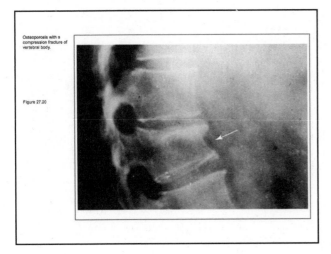

Osteoporosis with a compression fracture of vertebral body.

Figure 27.20

Gout

- Disorder of purine metabolism
  - Uric acid: an insoluble end-product of purine metabolism
  - Acute episodes caused by precipitation of uric acid crystals in joint fluid
  - Uric acid stones also may form within kidney and lower urinary tract
- Urate nephropathy: urate deposits plug tubules and damage kidneys
  - Treatment: diet and drugs that lower uric acid

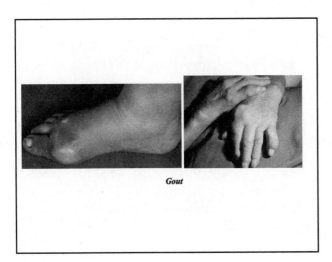

Gout

Notes

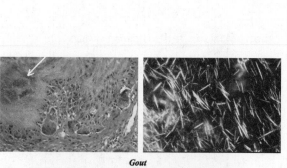

Gout
A. Mass of urate crystals with macrophages and fibrous tissue
B. Needle-like sodium urate crystals under polarized light

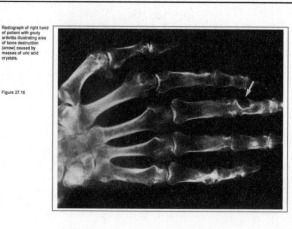

Radiograph of right hand of patient with gouty arthritis illustrating area of bone destruction (arrow) caused by masses of uric acid crystals.

Figure 27.16

Fractures

- Simple fracture: bone broken in only two pieces
- Comminuted fracture: bone shattered into many pieces
- Compound fracture: overlying skin is broken with potential for infection
- Pathologic fracture: fracture through a diseased area in the bone
- Treatment
  - Closed reduction: plaster cast
  - Open reduction: internal fixation

Osteomyelitis (1 of 2)

- Infection of bone and adjacent marrow cavity as a result of bacteria
- Organisms gain access to bone via
- Hematogenous
  - Bacteria carried to bone from an infection in body; occurs at ends of bones
  - Spread of infection may strip periosteum from cortex and devitalize bone
  - Mostly in children
  - In adults: infection may spread into joints
  - Infection in drug abusers tend to localize in vertebral bodies

Osteomyelitis (2 of 2)

- Organisms gain access to bone via direct implantation of bacteria
  - From conditions that expose bone to direct infection
  - Following trauma or surgery
- Manifestation
  - Fever, local pain and tenderness
- Diagnosis and treatment
  - X-ray reveals changes in bone
  - Antibiotics, possible surgery

Tumors of the Bone

- Usually metastatic tumors from prostate, breasts, other organs
- Multiple myeloma: plasma cell neoplasm
- Benign cysts and tumors: encountered occasionally
- Primary malignant bone tumors: unusual
  - Chondrosarcoma: malignant tumor of cartilage
  - Osteosarcoma: malignant tumor of bone-forming cells

Notes

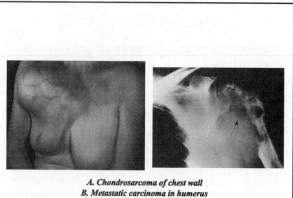

A. Chondrosarcoma of chest wall
B. Metastatic carcinoma in humerus

Osteoporosis

- Generalized thinning and demineralization of entire skeletal system
  - "Porous bones"
  - Most common in postmenopausal women
  - Loss of estrogen accelerates rate of bone resorption
  - Also develops in elderly men
- Treatment: high-calcium diet, estrogen

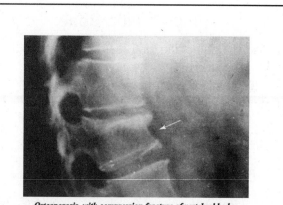

Osteoporosis, with compression fracture of vertebral body

Avascular Necrosis

- Interference in blood supply to the epiphysis of bones
- Results in necrosis and degeneration at ends of bone
- Disturbance in blood supply probably from injury
- Local pain and disability
- Common sites
  - Femoral head, tibial tubercle, articular surface of femoral condyle

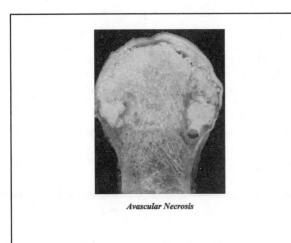

Avascular Necrosis

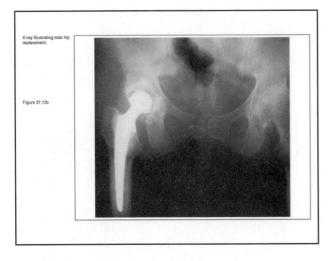

X-ray illustrating total hip replacement.

Figure 27.13b

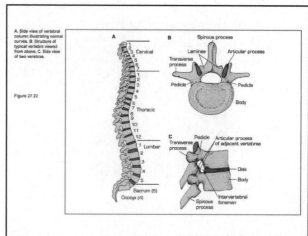

Spine

- Vertebral column forms the central axis of the body
  - Series of vertebrae joined by intervertebral disks and fibrous ligaments
  - Disks: fibrocartilaginous cushions interposed between adjacent vertebral bodies; function as shock absorbers
- 4 curves of vertebral column
  - Cervical and lumbar curves arch forward
  - Thoracic and sacral curves bend in opposite direction

A. Side view of vertebral column illustrating normal curves. B. Structure of typical vertebra viewed from above. C. Side view of two vertebrae.

Figure 27.22

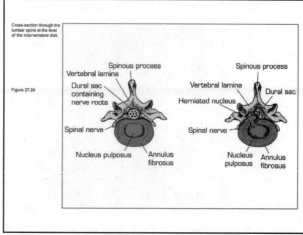

Cross-section through the lumbar spine at the level of the intervertebral disk.

Figure 27.24

Intervertebral Disk Disease

- Intervertebral disks undergo progressive wear-and-tear degeneration of both nucleus and annulus
- Nucleus pulposus may be extruded through tear in annulus fibrosus
- Manifestation
  - Sudden onset of back pain radiating down the leg
- Diagnosis: CT scan or myelogram
- Treatment: surgery

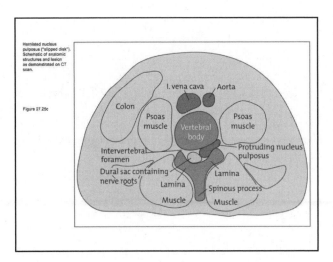

Herniated nucleus pulposus ("slipped disk"). Schematic of anatomic structures and lesion as demonstrated on CT scan.

Figure 27.25c

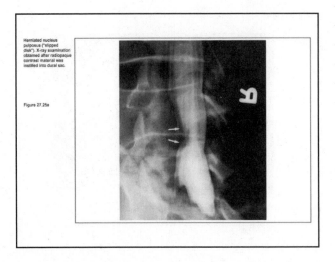

Herniated nucleus pulposus ("slipped disk"). X-ray examination obtained after radiopaque contrast material was instilled into dural sac.

Figure 27.25a

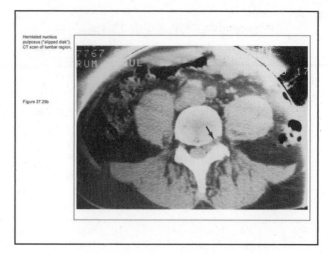

Herniated nucleus
pulposus ("slipped disk").
CT scan of lumbar region.

Figure 27.25b

Scoliosis

- Abnormal lateral curvature of spine
- Occurs in 4% of the population
- Most cases are idiopathic, occurs in adolescence
- Can lead to asymmetry of trunk and ↓ size of thoracic cavity
- One shoulder is higher than the other; pelvis is tilted
- Large curvatures cause pronounced disabilities
- Treatment: depends on extent of curvature

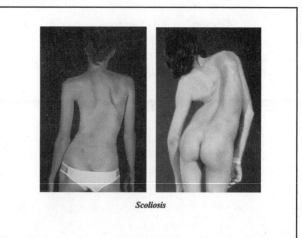

Scoliosis

Skeletal Muscle (1 of 3)

- Muscle contraction
  - Myofilaments slide together
  - Myoneural junction: communication between nerve and muscle
  - Nerve stimulation releases acetylcholine that interacts with receptors on surface of muscle fibers and initiates contraction
- Normal structural and functional integrity depends on
  - Intact nerve supply
  - Normal transmission of impulses across myoneural junction
  - Normal metabolic processes within muscle cell

Skeletal Muscle (2 of 3)

- Myositis: muscle inflammation
  - Localized
    - From injury or overexertion
  - Generalized
    - Systemic disease
    - Widespread degeneration and inflammation of skeletal muscle or polymyositis
- Dermatomyositis: type of polymyositis associated with swelling and inflammation of skin

Skeletal Muscle (3 of 3)

- Group of relatively rare diseases characterized by progressive atrophy or degeneration of skeletal muscle
- Categories
  - Progressive muscular atrophy
    - Secondary to motor nerve cell degeneration with secondary muscle atrophy
  - Muscular dystrophy
    - Primary muscle degeneration

Notes

Myasthenia Gravis

- Chronic disease characterized by abnormal fatigability of voluntary muscles due to abnormality at the myoneural junction
- Autoimmune disease; autoantibodies against acetylcholine receptors at myoneural junction
- Treatment: drugs that prolong action of acetylcholine

Discussion

- Arthritis pain that begins in one joint is usually characteristic of:
  - A. Rheumatoid arthritis
  - B. Osteoarthritis
- Joint pain accompanied by redness, swelling, warmth, and tenderness is usually characteristic of:
  - A. Rheumatoid arthritis
  - B. Osteoarthritis
- Type of arthritis that affects only joints and not internal organs.
  - A. Rheumatoid arthritis
  - B. Osteoarthritis